Health Promotion for People with Intellectual and Developmental Disabilities

Health Promotion for People with Intellectual and Developmental Disabilities

Edited by

Laurence Taggart and Wendy Cousins

Mc
Graw
Hill
Education Open University Press

Open University Press
McGraw-Hill Education
McGraw-Hill House
Shoppenhangers Road
Maidenhead
Berkshire
England
SL6 2QL

email: enquiries@openup.co.uk
world wide web: www.openup.co.uk

and Two Penn Plaza, New York, NY 10121-2289, USA

First published 2014

A catalogue record of this book is available from the British Library

ISBN-13: 978-0-335-24694-6
ISBN-10: 0-335-24694-X
eISBN: 978-0-335-24695-3

Library of Congress Cataloging-in-Publication Data
CIP data applied for

Typeset by Aptara, Inc.

Praise for this book

"This timely and important book synthesises current knowledge about health promotion interventions for people with intellectual disabilities. Written by leading researchers and practitioners, it should be on the bookshelves of everyone concerned with addressing the stark inequalities in health experienced by people with intellectual disabilities around the world."

Eric Emerson, Professor of Disability Population Health,
Centre for Disability Research and Policy, University of Sydney, Sydney, Australia
and Emeritus Professor of Disability and Health Research,
Centre for Disability Research, Lancaster University, UK.

"The editors and authors have done practitioners a great favour in bringing together in one volume a comprehensive account of how children and adults with intellectual disabilities can be supported to lead healthier lives. The increased risks they face across many health conditions are precisely defined as are the evidence-based strategies that can be used from an early age to promote better and longer lives. No more can it be said: "we didn't know what to do!"

Roy McConkey, Professor of Developmental Disabilities,
University of Ulster, N. Ireland, UK.

"I highly recommend this book to anyone working directly with people with an intellectual disability as well as professionals, academics and students who strive to promote issues and improve the lives of people with intellectual disabilities and their families. The book pulls together national and international expertise and translates knowledge gained from research into practical advice including useful, accessible tools. Using these simple, common sense resources should significantly contribute to improved health and well-being and tackle the unacceptable inequalities which current exist in terms of access to positive healthcare for these individuals."

Agnes Lunny OBE, Chief Executive of Positive Futures, N. Ireland, UK.

Contents

List of contributors

Editors:

Laurence Taggart
Laurence Taggart is a registered nurse for people with intellectual disabilities and a nursing lecturer. He is leader of the Research Centre for Intellectual and Developmental Disabilities at the University of Ulster, Northern Ireland. His main research interests focus on the physical and mental health of people with intellectual disabilities, health promotion, the needs of carers and innovative service developments. He is the 2013–2014 Chair of the International Association for the Scientific Study of Intellectual and Developmental Disabilities (IASSIDD) special interest group on health.

Wendy Cousins
Wendy Cousins is a chartered psychologist and an associate fellow of the British Psychological Society. Her research and publication activity is chiefly concerned with the health and social care of vulnerable populations. She is a member of the Research Centre for Intellectual and Developmental Disabilities at the University of Ulster, Northern Ireland where she is course director for degree programmes in health and wellbeing.

Contributors:

Jim Blair
Jim Blair is consultant nurse in intellectual disabilities at Great Ormond Street Hospital London, England and Honorary Principal Lecturer / Associate Professor in intellectual disabilities at Kingston University and St. George's University of London, England.

Penny Blake
Penny Blake is an intellectual disability psychiatrist working in Swansea, Wales. She has a particular interest in teaching and educating students and health professionals about intellectual disabilities.

Malin Broberg
Malin Broberg is a clinical psychologist and her research is focused on the wellbeing of children with intellectual disabilities and their families. She works as an associate professor with teaching and research roles at the Department of Psychology at the University of Gothenburg, Sweden.

Michael Brown
Michael Brown is reader in health and social care research at the Faculty of Health, Social and Life Sciences at Edinburgh Napier University, Scotland and nurse consultant with specialist intellectual disability health services with NHS Lothian. He has an interest in research and education relating to access to health, health inequalities, and health improvement.

Eddie Chaplin
Eddie Chaplin is the research and strategy lead for the Behavioural and Developmental Psychiatry Clinical Academic Group at the South London and Maudsley NHS Foundation Trust, England.

He currently leads the intellectual disability research programme at the Estia Centre and is co-chair of the Trust's Nursing and OT Research Council. He is also visiting researcher at the Department of Forensic and Neurodevelopmental Sciences, Institute of Psychiatry, King's College London, England.

Bob Davis

Bob Davis is the director of the Centre for Developmental Disability Health Victoria, Monash University, Australia. He works as a clinician, teacher, and researcher. His interests include the management of medical issues for people with intellectual disability and in particular those issues which impact on challenging behaviours. He is chair of the IASSIDD Health Special Interest Research Group. Bob is the foundation president of the Australian Association of Developmental Disability Medicine.

Gillian Eastgate

Gillian Eastgate is a general practitioner at the Queensland Centre for Intellectual and Developmental Disability, The University of Queensland, Brisbane, Australia. She has a particular interest in both clinical work and qualitative research in the field of sexual and reproductive health in people with intellectual disabilities.

Dora Fisher

Dora Fisher is a research specialist at the University of Illinois at Chicago, Disability and Human Development (UIC DHD), USA. Before her work at UIC DHD, she worked in gerontological health promotion programming and research. Her research interests include health promotion, the intersectionality of healthy ageing and disability, as well as critical approaches in gerontology and disability.

Paul Fleming

Paul Fleming is pro vice-chancellor for science and professor of health promotion and population health at the University of Canterbury, Christchurch, New Zealand. He has taught, researched, and published on a range of issues, including intellectual disability, workplace health, cancer education, and men's health.

Linda Goddard

Linda Goddard is senior lecturer in the School of Nursing, Midwifery and Indigenous Health at Charles Sturt University, Australia and senior clinician with Aspire Support Services, working to support families of children with disabilities. Her areas of expertise include intellectual disabilities, physical and mental health, chronic illness and families.

Tamar Heller

Tamar Heller is professor and head of the Department of Disability and Human Development, University of Illinois at Chicago (UIC), USA and director of its University Center of Excellence in Developmental Disabilities for the State of Illinois. She also directs the Rehabilitation Research and Training Center on Aging with Developmental Disabilities: Lifespan Health and Function.

John Heng

John Heng teaches philosophy and thanatology at King's University College of Western University in London, Canada. He previously worked at Surrey Place Centre, a University of Toronto affiliated centre that supports people with intellectual and developmental disabilities. He is a member of the Developmental Disabilities Primary Care Initiative of Ontario.

Thanos Karatzias
Thanos Karatzias is a clinical and health psychologist. He is a professor of mental health at the Faculty of Health, Life and Social Sciences at Edinburgh Napier University and consultant psychologist at Adult Mental Health Psychology Services in NHS Lothian, Scotland.

Mike Kerr
Mike Kerr is professor of intellectual disability psychiatry and honorary consultant in neuropsychiatry at Cardiff University, Wales. He initially trained as a general practitioner before deciding to train in psychiatry. His clinical practice is in the types of epilepsy associated with intellectual disability, and in the assessment and treatment of epilepsy and psychiatric disorders. He chairs the Epilepsy Action Wales Advisory Board.

Nick Lennox
Nick Lennox is a professor and director of the University of Queensland's Centre for Intellectual and Developmental Disability and president of the Australian Association of Developmental Disability Medicine. He is a researcher, educator, advocate, and medical clinician. He developed the Comprehensive Health Assessment Program (CHAP).

Tadhg Macintyre
Tadhg Macintyre is a chartered psychologist registered with the Health and Care Professions Council. He lectures in sport and exercise psychology at the University of Limerick, Ireland and is an accredited member of the Irish Institute of Sport.

Beth Marks
Beth Marks is a research associate professor in the Department of Disability and Human Development, and an associate director for research in the Rehabilitation Research and Training Centre on Aging with Developmental Disabilities, University of Illinois at Chicago, USA, and President of the National Organization of Nurses with Disabilities. Beth directs research programmes and has published articles and books on the empowerment and advancement of people with disabilities.

Jane McCarthy
Jane McCarthy is clinical director and consultant psychiatrist, St. Andrew's Healthcare Nottinghamshire, England, leading the development of the assessment and treatment models for autism spectrum disorders and intellectual disability secure pathways. She is also visiting senior lecturer in the Department of Forensic and Neurodevelopmental Sciences, the Institute of Psychiatry, King's College London, where she leads research and teaching on the health needs of adults with intellectual disability and autism spectrum disorders.

Judi Moyle
Judi Moyle is an experienced social worker who has worked extensively with children, adolescents, and adults with intellectual disabilities experiencing challenges in how they relate to people in their families, friendship networks, and other environments. In particular, for a number of years Judi has provided human relations consultancy and counselling as a clinician in the Centre for Developmental Disability Health Victoria, in the Faculty of Medicine, Nursing and Health Sciences of Monash University, Melbourne, Australia. She is now a lecturer in Social Work and Disability at Deakin University, Australia.

Karen Nankervis
Karen Nankervis is a professor and the director of the Centre of Excellence for Behaviour Support at the University of Queensland, Australia, utilizing research and practice leadership to improve

the lives of people with intellectual or cognitive disability and challenging behaviour. She has a clinical, educational, and research background with expertise including challenging behaviour, positive behaviour supports, evidence-based practice in service delivery for people with disabilities, forensic disability, parent training, staff satisfaction and stress, and relinquishment of family members with disabilities.

Ruth Northway
Ruth Northway is professor of intellectual disability nursing at the University of Glamorgan, Wales. Her areas of expertise include nursing, safeguarding, ethical issues, and participatory research.

Renée Proulx
Renée Proulx is the research and knowledge transfer director at the Centre de réadaptation en déficience intellectuelle et troubles envahissants du développement (CRDITED) de Montréal and adjunct professor, Department of Social and Public Communication, Université du Québec à Montréal, Canada.

Janet Robertson
Janet Robertson is a lecturer in health research at the Division of Health Research, Lancaster University, England. Janet has been involved in research within the field of intellectual disabilities since completing her PhD in 1993.

Cathy Ross
Cathy Ross has worked for over nine years producing information in multiple formats for the general public and medical professionals about cardiovascular disease and its prevention, including inherited heart conditions. In particular, she produced a DVD, booklet, and online information for individuals with intellectual disabilities, working closely with organizations with expertise in this area.

Jasmina Sisirak
Jasmina Sisirak is an associate project director in the Rehabilitation Research and Training Center on Aging with Developmental Disabilities (RRTCADD) in the Department of Disability and Human Development at the University of Illinois at Chicago (UIC), USA. Her research interests consist of nutrition, health literacy, and health promotion for persons with intellectual and developmental disabilities. She coordinates health promotion projects in the RRTCADD, and has written publications and presented papers in the areas of disability, health, and nutrition.

Eamonn Slevin
Eamonn Slevin is a reader in nursing at the University of Ulster, Northern Ireland. Having qualified as a registered intellectual disability and general nurse in the 1980s, Eamonn graduated with a diploma in nursing in 1990, PGDip in Education in 1992, a BSc (Hons) in 1993, and a PGDip in Advanced Nursing in 1995 from Ulster. In 1998, Eamonn was awarded a doctor of nursing science (DNSc) by the University of Ulster, for his thesis on the role of community nurses caring for people with challenging behaviours.

David Stewart
David Stewart OBE DL has worked with pupils with learning disabilities for over 40 years, the last 33 at Oak Field School (formerly Shepherd School) in Nottingham where he has been head teacher for 21 years. He has been a lead in the field of sex and relationship education, working closely with the late Anne Craft. He is the lead editor of *Living Your Life* (third edition) published in 2011 by Brook. With colleagues he has worked over many years with parents, arranging training and support and developing resources. David is an honorary doctor of the University of Nottingham and a Deputy Lieutenant of Nottinghamshire

William F. Sullivan
William F. Sullivan is associate professor in the Department of Family and Community Medicine, University of Toronto, and engages in service, teaching, and research at St. Michael's Hospital and at Surrey Place Centre, a University of Toronto affiliated centre that supports people with intellectual and developmental disabilities. He is the director of the Developmental Disabilities Primary Care Initiative of Ontario. He also has a PhD in philosophy and is the chair of the Ethics Committee of the College of Family Physicians of Canada.

Beverley Temple
Beverley Temple is an associate professor with the Faculty of Nursing and a researcher with the St. Amant Research Centre, Canada. Her research emphasis is on supporting families of children with intellectual disabilities and supporting the health of this population. This involves research about tobacco use, health promotion, and knowledge translation.

Hana Válková
Hana Válková is a professor at the Department of Adapted Physical Activity, Palacký University in the Czech Republic where she carries out research and teaching in sport psychology and adapted physical activity. She is a consortium member of the Erasmus-Mundus APA programme and recent president of the Czech Special Olympics Association.

Henny van Schrojenstein Lantman-de Valk
Henny van Schrojenstein Lantman-de Valk is professor of health care for people with intellectual disabilities at the Radboud University Medical Centre in Nijmegen, the Netherlands. The mission of her research is to support adequate healthcare provision for people with intellectual disabilities living in the community.

Foreword

Laurence Taggart and Wendy Cousins have brought together experts on the health of persons with intellectual and developmental disabilities from around the world in this thorough over-view, and in doing so have captured key areas of health of concern to this group of citizens such as vision, dental, nutrition, cancer, and health promotion. The authors of this text have pre-sented their research in a positive and informative manner, looking at health as a 'foundation for achieving human potential'.

Given that persons with disabilities are altogether too often researched and viewed from a defi-cit model, the approach the researchers have taken in this book is refreshing. The book presents many facts, research, and current trends in the field, tackling areas that are critical in today's world such as mental health, sexuality, and parenting.

Regardless of what area of health is being discussed, it is critical that persons with intellectual and developmental disabilities are educated and involved in discussions about health issues. The authors emphasize the need for individuals with intellectual and developmental disabilities to be involved in their health-related decisions; this philosophy is found throughout this book – an approach for which the authors are to be commended.

The book's thorough overview of health issues also has a practical element. The authors have not only focused on being informative, but have also brought in numerous recommendations and prac-tical approaches to issues. The chapters have summaries and vignettes, a format that is ideal for teach-ing students and even working with caregivers. The chapters also contain lists and facts that are easy to follow, and the authors have worked at ensuring the chapters are readable and comprehensive.

So often, we focus on traditional medical approaches to health and disability. This book goes beyond such a traditional approach, however, by emphasizing the environment and risk factors that affect the lives of persons with intellectual and developmental disabilities. The chapters on ageing and families take an interconnected view of the world for individuals with disabilities. The authors clearly demonstrate that the larger social systems in which we live often result in services and attitudes that limit the potential of persons with intellectual and developmental disabilities. The chapters highlight the importance of health at different stages of life, always with an eye to health promotion and education. This lifespan approach to health is a major strength of the book.

As President and Secretary of the International Association for the Scientific Study of Intellectual and Developmental Disabilities, we are aware of the importance of health matters to practitioners, caregivers, families, and individuals with disabilities. This excellent book provides an overview of health issues for persons with intellectual and developmental disabilities. It presents research in an accessible way, inspired by a philosophy of an inclusive and holistic approach to health. We highly recommend this book to healthcare educators, families, and service providers alike.

Vianne Timmons
President and Vice-Chancellor, University of Regina, Canada
President of IASSIDD, 2012–2016

Hélène Ouellette-Kuntz
Associate Professor at Queen's University, Canada
Secretary of IASSIDD 2008–2016

Introduction

Laurence Taggart and Wendy Cousins

The World Health Organization (WHO) has described health as:

> The extent to which an individual or group is able, on the one hand, to realize aspirations and satisfy needs, and on the other hand, to change or cope with the environment. Health is, therefore, seen as a resource for everyday life, not the object of living. It is a positive concept, emphasising social and personal resources as well as physical capabilities.
>
> (WHO 1984)

The significance of this definition comes with its recognition that health includes more than physical aspects and is more than just the absence of disease or underlying chronic health conditions. While terms like 'health education' and 'health promotion' are not commonly associated with people with intellectual disabilities, this conception of health as a multi-dimensional phenomenon, with multiple determinants and primarily defined by its positive rather than negative aspects, has relevance to the lives of this often overlooked section of society. Negative imagery, stereotypes, and stigma persist and disability is generally equated with incapacity. Globally there is a lack of appreciation of the range of capabilities of individuals with intellectual disabilities and low expectations of what they can achieve (Siperstein et al. 2003).

The concept of health as a foundation for achieving human potential, enabling and empowering people to become all that they are capable of becoming, has important implications for all those concerned with the care and wellbeing of people with intellectual disabilities. People with intellectual disabilities suffer from significantly more health problems than the general population and are much more likely than other citizens to have significant health risks and major health problems. Nevertheless, there is considerable evidence that people with intellectual disabilities are not receiving the same level of health education, health promotion opportunities, and health screening as other members of society.

As is the case for the non-disabled population, health promotion has the capacity to improve the lives of people with intellectual disabilities. Health promotion has been defined as the 'process of enabling people to increase control over, and to improve their health. It moves beyond a focus on individual behaviour towards a wide range of social and environmental interventions' (WHO 1998).

Health as a human right was first enunciated in the WHO's Constitution, which states that: 'Every human being is entitled to the enjoyment of the highest attainable standard of health conducive to living a life in dignity' (United Nations 1976). More recently, the United Nations (UN) Convention on the Rights of Persons with Disabilities (2007) has recognized that persons with disabilities have the right to the enjoyment of the highest attainable standard of health without discrimination on the basis of disability.

People with intellectual disabilities have similar physical, mental, and social health needs to the general population. However, they also have additional health needs posed by specific health risks associated with their intellectual disabilities. Cognitive, linguistic, and social impairments imposed by living with an intellectual disability may result in individuals being denied the opportunity to utilize health promotional literacy information, engage in health promotion initiatives, and to access and use health screening programmes on an equal footing with those who have the cognitive ability to read and understand such messages. There is considerable evidence that people with intellectual disabilities are not receiving the same level of health care as other members of society. A UK based Confidential Inquiry into premature deaths of people with intellectual disabilities (Heslop et al. 2013) estimated that 37% of deaths were potentially avoidable. Medical or health checks are given less often to people with intellectual disabilities than to the non-disabled population.

There is a strong need to challenge this inequality as an important human rights issue. Yet part of the reason why the health outcomes of this population are poor is because people with intellectual disabilities are too often reliant on both family carers and professional staff to promote healthy lifestyles and to make healthy choices on their behalf. However, many family carers and professionals may not be fully cognisant of the particular physical and mental needs of this population, or fully aware of the importance of health promotion and its related activities. Globally, a clear opportunity exists for health promotion efforts to improve the health prospects of people with intellectual disabilities and also improve the quality of life of this population. In addition, with greater gains in health, and improvements in the quality of life of people with intellectual disabilities, there will be reductions in healthcare costs.

Health is a multi-dimensional concept. Over the course of a person's lifespan, their health will change and develop – sometimes it will be good and at other times rather worse. A person with an intellectual disability will experience fluctuations in health across the course of their life in the same way as anyone else. However, as people with intellectual disabilities often start at the lower end of the health continuum and face additional challenges to their wellbeing, it could be argued that this is a particularly good reason for an enhanced focus on health promotion for this population. For people with intellectual disabilities, additional challenges in the form of even minor illnesses can have a significant impact on their capacities and potentially lead to an earlier decline in health and a greater dependency on other individuals for care (Rimmer 1999).

Just as health is a multi-factorial issue, health promotion is itself a multi-dimensional endeavour. Fleming (1999: 234) defines it as:

> Not a single activity, but an approach that encompasses a number of activities which produce health gain but which are derived from an overall aim to promote the health status of individuals and people groups. The increase of control implies the empowerment of individuals through a range of enabling measures, which may have policy, education and service provision implications.

The cardinal principle of health promotion is empowerment; it is fundamentally concerned with ensuring that individuals and communities make full use of their capabilities and potential. The empowerment model is one of mutual respect derived from the valuing of every human life. Empowerment may be a social, cultural, psychological or political process through which individuals and social groups are able to express their needs, present their concerns, devise strategies for involvement in decision making, and achieve political, social, and cultural action to meet those needs (WHO 1998). A distinction is made between individual and community empowerment: individual empowerment refers primarily to the individual's ability to make decisions and have control over their personal life, while community empowerment involves individuals acting collectively to gain greater influence and control over the quality of life in their community. For individuals with intellectual disabilities, the empowerment of their 'community of carers' – both families and professionals – is of key importance.

This volume is aimed at increasing family, professional, and public awareness of the importance of health education, health promotion initiatives, and health screening for people with intellectual and developmental disabilities across the lifespan. In highlighting the importance of health promotion for this population, the book aims to provide family carers and health and social care professionals with knowledge about key aspects of health for people with intellectual disabilities, and strategies to address these issues. We hope to enable and empower those who care for this population to act as mediators, or to act as catalysts for change, so they can empower people with intellectual disabilities to change their behaviours and enjoy healthier lives.

The book contains 20 chapters of empirically based reviews highlighting the holistic health needs of people with intellectual disabilities across the lifespan and in a variety of social contexts. It examines how psychological, physiological, environmental, and cultural factors are involved in promoting the health and wellbeing of people with intellectual disabilities. All of the contributing authors have adopted a knowledge transfer approach to outline clear, evidence-based strategies for putting research evidence into practice for each of the topic areas covered.

Structure of the book

There are three sections of the book. Each chapter provides readers with a short review of the current evidence base, and concludes with a summary of key points for ease of reference, and a list of internet-based resources and web resources to provide additional information. In the first section of the book, Chapter 1 offers readers a succinct current evidence base for what we know about the health of people with intellectual disabilities. Chapter 2 explores the difficulties of applying health promotion activities for people with intellectual disabilities and the importance of developing comprehensive health promotion programmes for this population.

The second section of the book examines the current evidence base of specific health conditions and mediating factors that affect people's health, offering readers practical strategies and solutions to the many challenges that families and professionals face in promoting the health of people with intellectual disabilities. The focus of this section is about the translation of research/knowledge to practice. Chapter 3 identifies the sensory problems (for example, vision, hearing, and oral health) experienced by this population. Chapter 4 explores how people with intellectual disabilities make decisions about the foods that they choose. Chapter 5 examines the growing topic of obesity and presents suggestions on how people with intellectual disabilities might be helped to achieve a normal healthy weight via health promotion activities. Chapter 6 identifies the risk factors for developing Type 2 diabetes and also illustrates how this condition can be prevented and provides readers with strategies for self-management. In Chapter 7, epilepsy and health promotion are examined. Chapter 8 explores cardiovascular disease: the risk factors and how to make appropriate lifestyle changes. Chapter 9 highlights the risk factors for developing gastrointestinal (i.e. stomach and gall-bladder), breast and cervical, and testicular cancers. Chapter 10 outlines the challenges, practice issues, and potential solutions for promoting the sexual health of people with intellectual disabilities. Chapter 11 examines the principles of promoting good mental health for people with intellectual disabilities. Chapter 12 identifies the risk factors for smoking, abusing alcohol, and using illicit drugs and examines the health promotion strategies that can be used to prevent such substances from being used. Chapter 13 draws from the innovative techniques in translational research as it relates to health promotion for older adults that may be applicable to adults with intellectual disabilities.

The third section examines different contexts in which health promotion can take place. Chapter 14 explores the value of embedding health promotion within the family. Chapter 15 illustrates how health promotion is integral to the overall learning of children and young people with intellectual disabilities in both mainstream and special school settings. Chapter 16 examines the importance of promoting exercise and sport for all people with intellectual disabilities. Chapter 17 considers the role that healthcare professionals can make in promoting the health of this population. Chapter 18 considers the importance of ensuring that health checks are conducted, as they clearly improve the health of people with intellectual disabilities. Chapter 19 identifies some of the ethical issues that can be encountered when empowering and supporting people with intellectual disabilities to make healthier lifestyle choices. Chapter 20 concludes the book and explores the key elements of evaluation planning and implementation in health promotion programmes, particularly as they affect people with intellectual disabilities.

We hope that this book will play an important part in identifying the health needs of this population and, more importantly, in identifying a range of practical strategies based upon evidence that will assist readers in their efforts to promote the health of people with intellectual disabilities.

References

Fleming, P. (1999) Health promotion for individuals, families and communities, in A. Long (ed.) *Interaction for Practice in Community Nursing*. Basingstoke: Macmillan.

Heslop, P., Blair, P.S., Fleming, P.J., Hoghton, M.A., Marriott, A.M. and Russ, L.S. (2013) *Confidential Inquiry into premature deaths of people with learning disabilities (CIPOLD)*: Final report. Bristol: Norah Fry Research Centre. Available at: http://www.bris.ac.uk/cipold/fullfinalreport.pdf [accessed 24 June 2013].

Rimmer, J.H. (1999) Health promotion for people with disabilities: the emerging paradigm shift from disability prevention to prevention of secondary conditions. *Physical Therapy*, 79: 495–502.

Siperstein, G.N., Norins, J., Corbin, S. and Shriver, T. (2003) *Multinational Study of Attitudes Towards Individuals with Intellectual Disabilities*. Washington, DC: Special Olympics, Inc.

United Nations (1976) *International Covenant on Economic, Social and Cultural Rights*. New York: United Nations.

United Nations General Assembly (2007) *Convention on the Rights of Persons with Disabilities: resolution adopted by the General Assembly*, 24 January 2007, A/RES/61/106. Available at: http://www.unhcr.org/refworld/docid/45f973632.html [accessed 11 December 2012].

World Health Organization (WHO) (1984) *Health Promotion: A Discussion Document on the Concept and Principles*. Copenhagen: WHO Regional Office for Europe.

World Health Organization (WHO) (1998) *Second International Conference on Health Promotion*, Adelaide, South Australia, 5–9 April.

Part I

The health and health promotion needs of people with intellectual disabilities

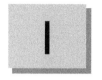

Health issues for people with intellectual disabilities: the evidence base

Robert Davis, Renée Proulx, and
Henny van Schrojenstein Lantman-de Valk

Introduction

People with intellectual disability experience significantly more health problems than the general population. Furthermore, there is considerable evidence that people with intellectual disability do not receive the same level of health care as other members of society. For example, health screening medical checks are given less often to people with intellectual disability than to the non-disabled population (Evenhuis et al. 2001), yet it has been shown consistently that health checks lead to detection of unmet health needs and lead to targeted actions to address health needs (Lennox et al. 2006; Robertson et al. 2007) (see Chapter 18). Jurisdictions across the world are signatories to the UN Convention on the Rights of Persons with Disabilities (2006), which states: 'parties recognize that persons with disabilities have the right to the enjoyment of the highest attainable standard of health without discrimination on the basis of disability'.

The UN Convention (2006) further states that parties shall 'provide persons with disabilities with the same range, quality and standard of free or affordable health care and programmes as provided to other persons, including . . . population-based public health programmes'. Another core point the UN made was that service providers should offer 'health services needed by persons with disabilities specifically because of their disabilities, including early identification and intervention as appropriate, and services designed to minimize and prevent further disabilities, including among children and older persons'. Access to health promotion and illness prevention services would be included within this remit.

While the gap is narrowing in some countries, on average people with intellectual disability have more significant health problems and die younger than their non-disabled peers, particularly those in the severe to profound range (Ouellette-Kuntz et al. 2005; Krahn et al. 2006). People with moderate to severe intellectual disabilities are three times as likely to die early than the non-disabled population (Turner 2011). This is due in part to the underlying cause of their disability and in part to predisposing and interrelated factors such as poverty, illiteracy and other social determinants. Improved health is likely to lead to improved quality of life for both the individuals with intellectual disability and their families. In this chapter, we review the evidence base for the major health problems of this population and provide readers with a synopsis of the up-to-date evidence of the health status of people with intellectual disability. We identify individual health targets and implications for health promotion, and examine the importance of the role of empirical evidence and how this needs to be clearly translated into practice.

Definitions

Intellectual disability

Intellectual disability is 'a disability characterised by significant limitations in intellectual functioning and in adaptive behaviour, which covers many everyday social and practical skills. This disability originates before the age of 18 years' (AAIDD 2012). One criterion for determining the presence of intellectual disability is a standardized measure of intellectual functioning or IQ test. Significant impairment measured through this rating is said to be two standard deviations below average, which translates to an IQ that is below 70. There are also standardized measures for adaptive behaviour that include conceptual, social and practical skills.

The term intellectual disability is synonymous with previous terms such as mental retardation and mental handicap, and with terms used in other jurisdictions such as learning disability. People with intellectual disability have a broad range of abilities and these abilities will significantly influence the way they interact with the community, the types of choices they have in their lives, and the degree to which others support them.

According to the World Health Organization intellectual disability can be categorized as follows:

- Mild (IQ of 50–70) – the ability to communicate effectively and live relatively independently with minimal support within the community.
- Moderate (IQ of 35–49) – individuals who, with lifelong support, will have significant relationships, can communicate, handle money, travel on public transport, make choices for themselves, and understand daily schedules.
- Severe or Profound (IQ <34) – individuals who are almost totally dependent on those around them and will require lifelong help with personal care tasks, communication, and accessing and participating in community facilities, services and activities.

There is a wide range of aetiologies for intellectual disability, including chromosomal, single gene deficits, a range of environmental factors that include intra-uterine infections (for example, maternal rubella), peri-natal trauma, nutritional deficits (for example, iodine deficiency), maternal alcohol abuse, and childhood neglect and deprivation. In approximately half of cases no cause has yet been identified. The variation in social, political, economic and environmental factors influence the prevalence of particular causes of intellectual disability in each country, as they do the health and nutritional status of the non-disabled population.

Developmental disability

Developmental disabilities are those that relate to 'differences in neurologically based functions that have their onset before birth or during childhood, and are associated with significant long-term difficulties' (Graves 2003). As such, developmental disability is an umbrella term that includes intellectual disability but also includes other disabilities that are acknowledged during early childhood. Some developmental disabilities are derived largely from physical impairments, such as cerebral palsy and epilepsy. Some individuals may have a condition that includes a physical and intellectual disability, such as Down syndrome or foetal alcohol syndrome. Other developmental disabilities, such as cerebral palsy or autism spectrum disorders (autism or pervasive developmental disorder [PDD]) are often associated with intellectual disability, further adding to the complexity of their physical and mental health needs.

Health problems of people with intellectual disability

People with intellectual disability have a range of health vulnerabilities when considered as a population; however, specific aetiologies of intellectual disability carry with them more defined risk profiles. Most of the large prevalence studies of health problems in this population are based on indirect assessments of the knowledge of staff of their clients' health status. The real prevalence tends to be underestimated because of the reduced ability of the individual with intellectual disability to present with symptoms, the difficulty for staff to recognize symptoms and signs, and limitations in the skills and available time of physicians to make their assessments (Haveman 2004). The prevalence of these problems has been found to be much higher in studies where direct assessment measures were undertaken by skilled clinicians.

People with intellectual disability are one of the most marginalized groups in our society, as they have extremely limited access to education, employment, and financial resources. They are subject to the very powerful social determinants of health, poverty, and social class. Epidemiological studies of the health of people with intellectual disability have looked at both their health in general as well as specific health problems (Van Schrojenstein Lantman-de Valk and Walsh 2008). These have shown that this group is particularly vulnerable to a range of chronic health problems that include:

- sensory problems (including vision, hearing and dental)
- poor nutrition
- constipation
- thyroid problems
- gastro-oesophageal reflux disease (GERD) and *Helicobacter pylori*
- obesity
- osteoporosis
- epilepsy
- cardiovascular disease
- Type 1 and Type 2 diabetes
- some types of cancers (particularly stomach and gall-bladder)
- mental health problems
- addictions
- ageing problems.

Furthermore, there is general agreement that people with intellectual disability do not use and engage fully in:

- health education/information
- health promotion programmes, such as those for healthy eating, weight reduction, physical activity, and exercise classes
- health screening programmes, including health checks, *Helicobacter pylori* screening, sexual health (for example, contraception), women's health (for example, breast and cervical cancer screening), men's health (for example, testicular cancer screening), and dementia screening.

The Health Special Interest Research Group of the International Association for the Scientific Study of Intellectual Disability (IASSID) met in 1999 under the auspices of the WHO to develop a consensus on health targets and recommendations for people with intellectual disability (see Web Resources).

Key determinants of health inequalities

According to Emerson (2011), there are five key determinants of health inequalities affecting people with intellectual disabilities:

1. Greater risk of exposure to social determinants of poorer health such as poverty, poor housing, unemployment and social disconnectedness.
2. Increased risk of health problems associated with specific genetic, biological, and environmental causes of intellectual disabilities.

3. Communication difficulties and reduced health literacy.
4. Personal health risks and behaviours such as poor diet and lack of exercise.
5. Deficiencies relating to access to healthcare provision.

Specific health issues in people with intellectual disability

Sensory problems (including vision, hearing, and oral health)

Research shows clearly that problems with vision are strongly associated with intellectual disability, and that the prevalence of these problems increases with age (Janicki and Dalton 1998). The condition is under-recognized; it has been shown that the assessment and management of poor vision in this population requires specialized skills (Evenhuis et al. 2001). Having deficiencies in vision when other faculties are already compromised has implications for mobility, learning, and behaviour. Monitoring sight and providing timely intervention is an important aspect of health care in this population (Evenhuis et al. 2009). Intervention not only involves improving the person's visual capabilities but also ensuring that health professionals are aware of the issues, so that the effect of the visual deficit is minimized by appropriate adjustments to the physical and interpersonal environment (see Chapter 3).

Hearing impairments in adults with intellectual disability who are aged 50 years and over range from 8 per cent to as many as 28 per cent in those with Down syndrome (van Schrojenstein Lantman-de Valk et al. 1994). There is a wide range of causes, some of which are similar to those in the non-disabled population while others are associated with the underlying aetiology (for example, Down syndrome, congenital rubella). The diagnosis is dependent on the awareness of people with intellectual disability to recognize their hearing impairments, as well as the awareness of those who support them: given the high prevalence there is need for regular hearing checks. As with visual impairments, advice on adjustment to the environment can make a major difference to people with hearing impairments (Meuwese-Jongejeugd et al. 2006) (see Chapter 3).

A higher proportion of people with intellectual disability have tooth extractions and filled teeth compared with the general population (Cumella et al. 2000). Access to regular dental review from an early age and throughout adult life is fundamental to good dental health. Proper dental hygiene in people with intellectual disability is as an important preventative health measure as it is in the wider population (see Chapter 3).

Nutrition

Many people with intellectual disability have less nutritional diets compared with the non-disabled population, and those with more severe and profound disability have higher rates of under-nutrition (Gravestock 2000) (see Chapter 4). The reason for this may be swallowing difficulties or concurrent problems with their gastrointestinal tract. Chronic malnutrition makes an individual vulnerable to infection; it can also compromise skeletal integrity and the resultant muscle weakness will often limit mobility. This is one of the major causes of morbidity and premature death in this population. Services need to monitor the diets and weights of this population and take appropriate action when problems are identified.

Obesity

The underlying problems of poor nutritional diet and inadequate activity and exercise that cause obesity in the non-disabled population, also impact on people with intellectual disability, who have higher rates of obesity (see Chapter 5). Obesity leads to many health problems and also brings with it an increased risk of cardiovascular disease and diabetes. People with intellectual disability have, to a large extent, not received the preventative health messages and programmes that have been directed to the rest of the community, and are thus less informed to make appropriate food choices. Their relative poverty makes cheaper and accessible sources of calories particularly attractive. People living independently make food choices for themselves, while those in supported settings are often reliant on support staff to make those choices for them. There is evidence that people in supported environments have healthier diets. The challenge for services supporting more independent options is to ensure that the message on diet and exercise gets through to this population.

Diabetes

People with intellectual disabilities are estimated to be three to four times more likely to have diabetes than the non-disabled population (see Chapter 6). Anwar et al. (2004) found that Type 1 diabetes was more prevalent in individuals with Down syndrome than those with other genetic causes of intellectual disability. Young people and adults with intellectual disabilities are more likely to develop Type 2 diabetes as a result of leading a more sedentary lifestyle, undertaking low levels of exercise and consuming high-fat diets, all of which can contribute towards obesity. Like the non-disabled population, people with intellectual disabilities are living longer, thereby making them more susceptible to developing Type 2 diabetes. There is a dearth of studies that have examined the extent to which their diabetes is managed or whether the quality indicators for diabetes care are met (Taggart et al. 2012).

Epilepsy

The prevalence of epilepsy in people with intellectual disability in the literature ranges from 14 to 44 per cent. This variation is associated with the degree of disability, the population, underlying aetiology, research methodology, and accommodation setting (Bowley and Kerr 2000) (see Chapter 7). Management not only includes the use and monitoring of appropriate medication but also the provision of a safe living environment, adjustments in lifestyle, setting appropriate safety standards, skills in the monitoring and reporting of seizures, and established protocols for responding to seizures.

Cardiovascular disease

Coronary heart disease (CHD) is the second largest cause of premature death for people with intellectual disabilities. They are more likely than the general population to have high blood pressure, be overweight or obese, and be inactive, all of which are risk factors for CHD (de Winter et al. 2012) (see Chapter 8).

Respiratory disease

A 25-year follow up of 2369 people with intellectual disability reported that those under 40 years were more than twice as likely to die as a result of a respiratory disease (87 per cent as a result of pneumonia) than the general population (Patja et al. 2000). Higher rates of aspiration pneumonia and inhalation of foreign bodies were also observed in this population. The risk of respiratory disease was found to increase with the degree of disability, gastro-oesophageal disease, dysmorphias in the oral cavity and a range of immunological deficits.

Cancer

Globally, it is estimated that over 12 million people are diagnosed with cancer every year. The global cancer burden doubled in the final 30 years of the twentieth century, and it is estimated that this will double again by 2020 and nearly triple by 2030. Overall, the incidence of cancer among people with intellectual disabilities has been reported to be lower than that of the general population (see Chapter 9). Research has shown that nearly half of all cancers in people with intellectual disabilities are gastrointestinal and oesophageal cancers; this may result from a higher incidence of *Helicobacter pylori* infection. The next main group of cancers is the urogenital cancers (for example, breast and cervical cancers for women, and testicular and prostate cancers for men) (Patja et al. 2001).

Sexual health

People with intellectual disabilities commonly experience opposition to sexual activity and face difficulties in expressing their sexuality in a safe and healthy way. Those supporting them face complex challenges (see Chapter 10). Lack of acceptance of the sexuality of people with intellectual disabilities has implications for their access to sexuality related health promotion, screening, and health care (Van Schrojenstein Lantman-de Valk et al. 2002). The key areas in sexual health promotion for this population include: relationship formation; sexual abuse and relationship violence; appropriate sexual behaviour; contraception, sterilization and menstrual management; pregnancy and parenting; and screening in sexual and reproductive health.

Mental health

The prevalence of mental health problems in people with intellectual disability varies depending on the diagnostic criteria and the research methodology. The overwhelming volume of research shows a much higher prevalence of mental health disorders compared with the non-disabled population (see Chapter 11). Cooper et al. (2007) found double the rate of all mental health problems using the DC-LD (Diagnostic Criteria for Psychiatric Disorders for Use with People with Adults with Learning Disabilities/Mental Retardation; Royal College of Psychiatrists 2001). This study indicated a prevalence of psychotic illness of 4.6 per cent compared with 0.4 per cent in the general population. Cooper and colleagues also showed that 6.6 per cent of people with intellectual disability suffered from affective disorders, and 3.6 per cent from anxiety disorders. Social and environmental factors can contribute to the development of mental health disorders in this population. Communication difficulties, social isolation, lack of employment opportunities, loss and grief when carers move on, and limitations in their choice of with whom and where they live are all significant stressors that need to be considered in the prevention and management of mental health problems.

Addictions

In the non-disabled population, cessation of smoking is one of the most significant preventative health programmes impacting on respiratory disease, cardiovascular health, cancer, and diabetes. Emerson (2005) reported that smoking was more prevalent in people with intellectual disability living in the community than those living in supported accommodation. This situation will evolve as public health policies in reference to smoke free environments are being implemented in different countries. A study of 1097 people with intellectual disability found that 17.3 per cent smoked tobacco and that asthma rates in those who smoked was double that of those who did not (Gale et al. 2009) (see Chapter 12).

In a review of 67 substance users with intellectual disability in Northern Ireland, Taggart et al. (2007) showed that alcohol was the main substance misused; in 20 per cent of cases this was in combination with illicit drugs and/or prescribed medication. There was an increased risk of substance abuse among males who were young with borderline/mild intellectual disability, living independently, and who had mental health problems. Problematic behaviours related to the addiction were also seen as an issue of concern (Taggart et al. 2006). Research has suggested a need for earlier identification to limit long-established patterns of use and associated behaviours (see Chapter 12).

Ageing

The authors of a critical review of the international literature from 1999 to 2009 that focused on age-related health risks, age-related oral health and lifestyle health risks in older people with intellectual disabilities, reported that cardiovascular disease is as prevalent and as common a cause of death among older people with intellectual disabilities as in the general population (Haveman et al. 2011). There are, however, variations in prevalence, which are culturally dependent: lifestyle health risks included poor nutrition, a lack of exercise, and poor mobility leading to higher obesity levels (Hilgenkamp et al. 2012) (see Chapter 13). As in the non-disabled population, healthier lifestyles, improved nutrition and increased exercise, as well as regular health checks to improve surveillance of health risks, are reported as key to improving the health status of older adults with intellectual disabilities (Evenhuis et al. 2012).

Medication

The efficacy and side-effects of medications used in this population are less reliant on patient reports and more reliant on the observations of others. People with intellectual disability are some of the highest consumers of psychotropic and anti-epileptic medications with high rates of potentially serious side-effects and the potential for significant interactions (McGillicuddy 2006; de Kuijper et al. 2010). If we are to prevent or minimize iatrogenic disease from medications, people with intellectual disabilities and their carers need to be active participants in both the reporting of outcomes and the observation of side-effects. As some side-effects, such as weight gain associated with certain medications, can be anticipated, active health promotion strategies around diet and exercise need to be put in place from the outset.

Systemic issues

Regular health checks, including physical examinations that include a record of blood pressure, weight, review of dentition, breast or testicular examination, and assessment of vision and hearing, should be part of a person's health management programme (see Chapter 18). Research has shown that when this is done regularly, health problems are identified earlier (Lennox et al. 2006). While this is becoming a requirement of support services in some jurisdictions, people with intellectual disability who live independently or with their families also need to be aware of the need for regular health checks that focus on their health vulnerabilities.

People with intellectual disabilities and the need for health promotion

Major progress in improving the health of the wider community has come about through public health measures targeting social disparities and through specific health education, health promotion programmes and health screening initiatives (see Chapter 2). This has proven to be a cost-effective way of tackling the major health problems in the community, especially when targeting chronic diseases.

People with intellectual disability have the same right to access these interventions as the non-disabled population (UN 2006). While people with intellectual disability are subject to the same range of major health problems as the general population, research has shown that they have particular vulnerabilities. The health promotional activities commonly used in the non-disabled population may need to be adapted for people with intellectual disability and their carers. Where greater health vulnerabilities have been identified health education, health promotion programmes, and health screening initiatives need to be better targeted.

Summary

The social determinants of health are extremely important for this population and lessons learnt from approaches used in other marginalized groups should be considered. Research and evaluation is critical to ensure that interventions achieve the expected outcomes in the most cost-effective manner (see Chapter 20). The challenge in establishing equitable health promotion programmes for people with intellectual disability is an issue in many countries. The need to measure health outcomes and to build new or extend existing partnerships with key stakeholders to improve access to health promotion activities is now widely recognized. Developing and promoting a good evidence base for health promotion activities in this population would help support services achieve better outcomes. Not only do priorities need to be established, it is also important to target interventions appropriately: times of transition, such as leaving school, the start of living independently, moving from the family home, or retirement, provide opportunities for targeted interventions. Better health is a key foundation for better lives in people with intellectual disability.

Useful resources

- *Health Inequalities and People with Learning Disabilities in the UK: 2012* (Emerson et al. 2012) summarizes the latest evidence about the extent, nature, and determinants of health inequalities experienced by people with learning disabilities in the UK. Available at: http://www.improvinghealthandlives.org.uk/publications/1165/Health_Inequalities_&_People_with_Learning_Disabilities_in_the_UK:_2012

Web resources

- Health Guidelines for Adults with an Intellectual Disability, IASSID: www.iassid.org/pdf/healthguidelines-2002.pdf

- The Improving Health and Lives Learning Disabilities Observatory are here to keep a watch on the health of people with learning disabilities and the health care they receive: www.improvinghealthandlives.org.uk/

- The following site offers fact sheets on common health problems for people with intellectual disabilities: www.nswcid.org.au/health/se-health-pages/standard-fact-sheets.html

References

American Association on Intellectual and Developmental Disabilities (AAIDD) (2012) *Definition of intellectual disability*. Washington, DC: AAIDD. Available at: www.aaidd.org/content_100.cfm?navID=21 [accessed September 2012].

Anwar, A., Walker, D. and Frier, B. (2004) Type 1 diabetes mellitus and Down syndrome: prevalence, management and diabetes complications. *Diabetic Medicine*, 15: 160–63.

Bowley, C. and Kerr, M. (2000) Epilepsy and intellectual disability. *Journal of Intellectual Disability Research*, 44(5): 529–43.

Cooper, S.A., Smiley, E., Morrison, J., Williamson, A. and Allan, L. (2007) Mental ill-health in adults with intellectual disabilities: prevalence and associated factors. *British Journal of Psychiatry*, 190(1): 27–35.

Cumella, S., Ransford, N., Lyons, J. and Burnham, H. (2000) Needs for oral care among people with intellectual disability not in contact with Community Dental Services. *Journal of Intellectual Disability Research*, 44(1): 45–52.

de Kuijper, G., Hoekstra, P., Visser, F., Scholte, F.A., Penning, C. and Evenhuis, H. (2010) Use of antipsychotic drugs in individuals with intellectual disability in the Netherlands: prevalence and reasons for prescription. *Journal of Intellectual Disability Research*, 54(7): 659–67.

de Winter, C.F., Bastiaanse, L.P., Hilgenkamp, T.I.M., Evenhuis, H.M. and Echteld, M.A. (2012) Cardiovascular risk factors (diabetes, hypertension, hypercholesterolemia and metabolic syndrome) in older people with intellectual disability: results of the HA-ID study. *Research in Developmental Disabilities*, 33(6): 1722–31.

Emerson, E. (2005) Health status and health risks of the 'hidden majority' of adults with intellectual disability. *Intellectual and Developmental Disabilities*, 49(3): 155–65.

Emerson, E. (2011) Health status and health risks of the 'hidden majority' of adults with intellectual disability. *Intellectual and Developmental Disabilities*, 49(3): 155–65.

Emerson, E., Baines, S., Allerton, L. and Welch, V. (2012) *Health Inequalities and People with Learning Disabilities in the UK: 2012*. Improving Health and Lives: Learning Disability Observatory. London: Public Health England.

Evenhuis, H., Theunissen, M., Denkers, I., Verschuure, H. and Kemme, H. (2001) Prevalence of visual and hearing impairment in a Dutch institutionalized population with intellectual disability. *Journal of Intellectual Disability Research*, 45(5): 457–64.

Evenhuis, H., Sjoukes, L., Koot, H. and Kooijman, A. (2009) Does visual impairment lead to additional disability in adults with intellectual disabilities? *Journal of Intellectual Disability Research*, 53(1): 19–28.

Evenhuis, H.M., Hermans, H., Hilgenkamp, T.I.M., Bastiaanse, L.P. and Echteld, M.A. (2012) Frailty and disability in older adults with intellectual disabilities: results from the Healthy Ageing and Intellectual Disability Study. *Journal of the American Geriatrics Society*, 60(5): 934–8.

Gale, L., Naqvi, H. and Russ, L. (2009) Asthma, smoking and BMI in adults with intellectual disabilities: a community-based survey. *Journal of Intellectual Disability Research*, 53(9): 787–96.

Graves, P. (2003) The child with a developmental disability, in M. Robinson and D. Roberton (eds.) *Practical Paediatrics*, 5th edn. Edinburgh: Churchill Livingstone.

Gravestock, S. (2000) Eating disorders in adults with intellectual disability. *Journal of Intellectual Disability Research*, 44(6): 625–37.

Haveman, M.J. (2004) Disease epidemiology and aging people with intellectual disabilities. *Journal of Policy and Practice in Intellectual Disabilities*, 1(1): 16–23.

Haveman, M., Perry, J., Salvador-Carulla, L., Walsh, P., Kerr, M., Van Schrojenstein Lantman-de Valk, H. et al. (2011) Ageing and health status in adults with intellectual disabilities: results of the European Pomona II study. *Journal of Intellectual and Developmental Disability*, 36(1): 49–60.

Hilgenkamp, T.I.M., Reis, D., van Wijck, R. and Evenhuis, H.M. (2012) Physical activity levels in older adults with intellectual disabilities are extremely low. *Research in Developmental Disabilities*, 33(2): 477–83.

Janicki, M. and Dalton, A. (1998) Sensory impairments among older adults with intellectual disability. *Journal of Intellectual and Developmental Disability*, 23(1): 3–11.

Krahn, G., Hammond, L. and Turner, A. (2006) A cascade of disparities: health and health care access for people with intellectual disabilities. *Mental Retardation and Developmental Disabilities Research Reviews*, 12(1): 70–82.

Lennox, N., Rey-Conde, T. and Cooling, N. (2006) Comprehensive health assessments during de-institutionalization: an observational study. *Journal of Intellectual Disability Research*, 50(10): 719–24.

McGillicuddy, N.B. (2006) A review of substance use research among those with mental retardation. *Mental Retardation and Developmental Disabilities Research Reviews*, 12: 41–7.

Meuwese-Jongejeugd, A., Vink, M., van-Zanten, B., Verschuure, H., Eichhorn, E., Koopman, D. et al. (2006) Prevalence of hearing loss in 1598 adults with an intellectual disability: cross-sectional population based study. *International Journal of Audiology*, 45(11): 660–9.

Ouellette-Kuntz, H., Garcin, N., Lewis, M.E., Minnes, P., Martin, C. and Holden, J.J. (2005) Addressing health disparities through promoting equity for individuals with intellectual disability. *Canadian Journal of Public Health*, 96(suppl. 2): S8–S22.

Patja, K., Livanainen, M., Vesala, H., Oksanen, H. and Ruoppila, I. (2000) Life expectancy of people with intellectual disability: a 35-year follow-up study. *Journal of Intellectual Disability Research*, 44(5): 591–9.

Patja, K., Eero, P. and Livanainen, M. (2001) Cancer incidence among people with intellectual disability. *Journal of Intellectual Disability Research*, 45: 300–7.

Robertson, J., Roberts, H., Emerson, E., Turner, S. and Gregg, R. (2007) The impact of health checks for people with intellectual disabilities: a systematic review of evidence. *Journal of Intellectual Disability Research*, 55(11): 1009–19.

Royal College of Psychiatrists (2001) *Diagnostic Criteria for Psychiatric Disorders for Use with People with Adults with Learning Disabilities/Mental Retardation*. Occasional Paper OP 48. London: Gaskell/Royal College of Psychiatrists.

Taggart, L., McLaughlin, D., Quinn, B. and Milligan, V. (2006) An exploration of substance misuse in people with intellectual disabilities. *Journal of Intellectual Disability Research*, 50(8): 588–97.

Taggart, L., McLaughlin, D., Quinn, B. and McFarlane, C. (2007) Listening to people with intellectual disabilities who misuse alcohol and drugs. *Health and Social Care in the Community*, 15(4): 360–8.

Taggart, L., Truesdale-Kennedy, M. and Coates, V. (2012) Management and quality indicators of diabetes mellitus in people with intellectual disabilities. *Journal of Intellectual Disability Research* (DOI: 10.1111/j.1365-2788.2012.01633.x).

Turner, S. (2011) *Health Inequalities and People with Learning Disabilities in the UK: Implications and Actions for Commissioners and Providers of Social Care*. Evidence into Practice Report #4, November. Improving Health and Lives: Learning Disabilities Observatory. London: Public Health England.

United Nations (2006) *United Nations Convention on the Rights of Persons with Disabilities*. Available at: http://www.un.org/disabilities/ [accessed 12 December 2012].

Van Schrojenstein Lantman-de Valk, H. and Walsh, P.N. (2008) Managing health problems in persons with intellectual disabilities. *British Medical Journal*, 337: a2507.

Van Schrojenstein Lantman-de Valk, H.M., Haveman, M.J., Maaskant, M.A., Kessels, A.G., Urlings, H.F. and Sturmans, F. (1994) The need for assessment of sensory functioning in ageing people with mental handicap. *Journal of Intellectual Disability Research*, 38(3): 289–98.

Van Schrojenstein Lantman-de Valk, H.M.J., Schupf, N. and Patja, K. (2002) Reproductive and physical health in women with intellectual disability, in P.N. Walsh and T. Heller (eds.) *Health of Women with Intellectual Disability*. Oxford: Blackwell.

2 Health promotion and people with intellectual disabilities

Beth Marks and Jasmina Sisirak

Introduction

The UN Convention on the Rights of Persons with Disabilities (2006) supports the global impetus for health promotion for people with intellectual disabilities with its 50 articles, which address the human rights and fundamental freedoms that must be guaranteed for all persons with disabilities to enjoy the highest attainable standard of health without discrimination. Unfortunately, people with intellectual disabilities continue to be excluded from many community-based health promotion programmes, despite the extensively documented benefits of health promotion and education to maintain health and control risk factors. Because personal health practices are just one of the determinants of health, programmes must address the socio-environmental, cultural, and access constraints that impact individuals with intellectual disabilities and their support persons as they experience widening inequities in healthcare services and poorer health outcomes compared with their non-disabled peers. Integrating health promotion strategies within existing community-based structures such as schools, churches, worksite settings, day programmes, and residential programmes for people with intellectual disabilities can provide the structure for continuous access to information, ongoing financial support, and participation in health promoting behaviours.

This chapter addresses the situation in the USA; it gives an overview of factors contributing to health and wellness for individuals with intellectual disabilities and discusses the importance of developing comprehensive health promotion programmes that include health education, nutrition, and physical activity to improve the lives, self-determination, and community engagement of people with intellectual disabilities. In addition, factors related to physical activity, fitness, nutrition, and diets for individuals with intellectual disability are presented. The challenges in developing and implementing health promotion programmes are also discussed, together with strategies that can be used by community-based service providers to implement programmes.

Health promotion and people with intellectual disabilities

When health officials noted increases in chronic disease in the USA in the 1920s, fundamental changes in research, practices, and policies were required (Fox 1989). Community-based health promotion programmes were seen as a viable public health approach to the promotion of health and prevention of disease. Over the past 40 years, community-based health promotion programmes have flourished with a variety of goals and approaches reaching many communities around the world (Baker and Brownson 1998). However, community-based programmes continue to routinely exclude people with intellectual disabilities despite the extensively documented benefits of health promotion and education to maintain health and control risk factors. People with intellectual disabilities can be healthy across the lifespan; health promotion similar to that for the general population is a key element in bridging equity gaps and advocating for policies to achieve optimal health and wellness (Pan American Health Organization 2001).

While health is a basic component of human development, health promotion involves a broader scope of action than that customarily handled by healthcare services and is essential in addressing individual and community health concerns (Pan American Health Organization/ Pan American Sanitary Bureau 1999). Specifically, health promotion is the process of enabling people to take control over, and to improve, their health (WHO 2002).

Determining health: what matters

Health outcomes can vary among groups of people based on age and socio-economic status. In general, essential requirements for health include food, housing, education, income, sustainable resources, social justice, equity, and peace (WHO 2001). Major determinants of preventable illness and death are often the result of inadequate and poor health literacy skills, limited social support, poverty, and unemployment. People with disabilities may age differently based on the nature and severity of their disability, co-existing health conditions, and chronic health conditions. How well people with intellectual disabilities age depends on their health behaviours throughout their lifetime (see Chapter 13).

Many of the problems associated with ageing across the lifespan are attributed to a 'high-risk lifestyle'. Hence, health promotion and disease prevention activities are seen as a way to age well by lowering the risk for disease and illness later in life by having control over determinants of health. Determinants of health status can be categorized into four broad areas:

1. Biological factors are the only immutable factors (e.g. syndrome- and gender-related conditions).
2. Socioeconomic and environmental factors.
3. Access to health care (for example, physical, communication, and programmatic aspects).
4. Behavioural factors (for example, lifestyle choices, health promotion/disease prevention practices) (Tarlov 1999).

To improve health or to modify conditions for people with intellectual disabilities, consideration of these four areas must be addressed.

Biological factors (syndromes and gender)

Individuals with intellectual disabilities who have syndrome-related conditions are predisposed to a myriad of health conditions based on their type of disability, making health promotion and disease prevention activities imperative. For example, people with intellectual disabilities may have syndrome-related conditions that result in difficulty eating or swallowing, dental problems, reduced mobility, bone demineralization, gastro-oesophageal reflux, arthritis, decreased muscle tone, and progressive cervical spine degeneration (White-Scott 2007). In addition, people with intellectual disabilities who are frequently prescribed psychotropic and anti-seizure medications on a long-term basis have a higher risk of developing osteoporosis (brittle bone disease), which is compounded by a lack of physical activity and diets deficient in calcium and vitamin D. Individuals also experience different conditions based on gender: while men are diagnosed with breast cancer, the prevalence rate is much lower compared with women, and women are more likely to suffer from osteoporosis and depression (Walsh and Heller 2002).

Socio-economic and environmental issues

Socio-economic and environmental factors affect health status. Where people live, work, and play matters, as does the amount of income people have. For people with intellectual disabilities, living in specific residential settings and participating in day programmes (for example, schools, worksites, day activity programmes) can affect health status. For example, in the USA research data show that adults living in the least restrictive community settings have the highest rates of obesity and a lower intake of fruits and vegetables (Rimmer et al. 1995; Sisirak et al. 2007). Limited social support, along with disruption of personal ties, loneliness, violence directed at individuals with disabilities, and conflicted interactions with peers and caregivers can be major sources of stress for people with intellectual disabilities. Inadequate social support is associated with an increase in mortality, morbidity, and psychological distress and a decrease in overall general health. Supportive social connections and intimate relations are vital sources of emotional strength and have a positive effect on health status.

Access to health care and health promotion

Access to health care, health promotion, and disease prevention is vital in being able to achieve and sustain community engagement. Like other underserved populations, health promotion activities can enable people to take control over and to improve their health (Pan American Health Organization 2001). People with intellectual disabilities often struggle to obtain accessible (affordable, available) and acceptable (culturally relevant, satisfactory) health care due to different developmental trajectories and limitations in communication and cognitive skills; healthcare delivery to people with intellectual disabilities is often ineffective or absent (Beange et al. 1995). Access barriers (for example, programmatic, physical, attitudinal, communication barriers, and limited health literacy skills) and inadequate professional education regarding disability issues frequently are not addressed in healthcare services. For people with intellectual disabilities, readily available sources of health information may not be tailored to their needs.

Programmatic and physical barriers

Many people with intellectual disabilities face obstacles to obtaining basic health care and health promotion and disease prevention services, and are thus especially vulnerable to the programmatic inadequacies of the healthcare system. Such barriers may include inflexible appointments that fail to accommodate transportation difficulties and the time needed to communicate with people who have complex needs; underinsured or no health insurance coverage; geographic unavailability of health services; lack of personal assistance, inaccessible washrooms, lack of accessible signage regarding entrances; physically inaccessible equipment; and a lack of transportation to community-based fitness and nutrition programmes.

Attitudinal and communication barriers

Many licensed and certified healthcare providers have not had adequate training or experience to provide healthcare services for people with intellectual disabilities (Phillips et al. 2004). People with disabilities report that healthcare professionals lack knowledge and sensitivities about their health needs, and focus more on their disabilities rather than their immediate health problems (Gill 1996). Professionals often inadvertently objectify people with disabilities as a 'diagnosis' or 'disease' that needs to be cured (or fixed): a perspective that sees people with intellectual disabilities as unhealthy and unable to benefit from health promotion. The vast majority of health educational materials are not in accessible formats or inclusive of people with a variety of learning styles and in need of different types of accommodations to receive information in an understandable format. For example, there is a lack of sign interpreters for people who are deaf, large print formats for people with low vision, and materials written at an appropriate level of intellectual functioning (Marks et al. 2010a). In community settings, people may not feel welcomed at fitness centres and may worry that no-one will assist them or that people may ridicule them.

Health literacy

Individuals with low health literacy are less likely to be able to manage their health and prevent disease, which can lead to higher utilization of treatment services, increased hospitalization and emergency services, and lower utilization of preventive services, resulting in higher healthcare costs (National Center for Education Statistics 2003; Baur 2007). Healthcare providers, support people, and individuals with intellectual disabilities themselves need to increasingly share responsibility for health-related decisions. People with intellectual disabilities and their care providers need specific skills to obtain, process, and understand basic health information and services to make appropriate health decisions and navigate the healthcare system. Moreover, families, community service providers, and health services providers need to improve health communication using multimodal strategies to ensure accessibility (Selden et al. 2000). People with limited or inaccurate knowledge about the body and the causes of disease may not understand the relationship between lifestyle factors (for example, diet, exercise) and health outcomes or recognize when they need to seek care.

Health behaviours

Health behaviours can directly influence the health status of people with intellectual disabilities and may be indirectly affected by environmental factors. Behavioural factors of health include getting adequate exercise, practising good nutritional habits, refraining from smoking, and understanding options and choices regarding decision making (Marks and Heller 2003). Removing or modifying behavioural risk factors associated with the acceleration of the disease process can postpone the development of common chronic diseases. In general, health behaviours maintain or enhance health status, control or remove harmful risk factors, and prevent the onset of chronic conditions. Dietary intake and physical activity patterns are major determinants of being overweight and being obese (WHO 2003). For the general population and for adults with intellectual disabilities, the combination of sedentary lifestyles, high fat diets, and low fruit and vegetable diets is a major contributor to increased risk for acquiring chronic health conditions.

Defining health and community: health promotion matters

Of the determinants of health, the biological factors are generally the only immutable factors, whereas the other three determinants of health – socio-environmental support, access issues, and behavioural factors – can be impacted by targeted health promotion activities in various community settings. While individual behaviours do impact upon health, many of the behaviours are influenced by broader socio-environmental and economic factors. In developing sustainable health promotion programmes, examination of definitions of health, health behaviours, and the determinants of health behaviours provides a foundation for identifying factors related to active participation in health promotion programmes.

'Point of view' for health

Understanding how people define their own health is critical, as it can result in conflicting expectations about approach modalities, priorities, and outcomes of healthcare services including health promotion activities (Hornsten et al. 2004). For example, if individuals do not perceive the importance or the relationship of different dimensions of health and health status, they may not embrace lifestyle behaviours that enhance health status. What we think about health comes from our own point of view with our minds and bodies working together to keep us healthy. While health and social service professionals often define health for people with intellectual disabilities using a one-dimensional domain – the absence of disease or impairment based on aetiology, diagnosis, physical changes, and treatment – people with intellectual disabilities do have multi-dimensional views of health (Marks 1996; Marks et al. 2008), similar to their non-disabled peers whose definitions include influences from daily life (Hornsten et al. 2004).

Health promotion: 'it's our health'

The WHO (2005) Bangkok Charter for Health Promotion in a Globalized World defined health promotion as 'the process of enabling people to increase control over their health and its determinants, and thereby improve their health' (p. 1). Conference participants noted that health promotion occurs by developing public policy that addresses the correlates of health such as income, housing, food security, employment, and quality working conditions. For people with intellectual disabilities, health promotion across the lifespan has lagged decades behind the health promotion initiatives for their peers without disabilities. In December 2002, the US Surgeon General held a conference on health disparities and intellectual disabilities to address growing concerns about the health status of individuals with intellectual disabilities. The report from this conference identified two essential goals related to health promotion:

1. Integrate health promotion into community environments of people with intellectual disabilities and
2. Increase knowledge and understanding of health through practical and useful information (US Public Health Service 2002).

By broadening the definition of health promotion, practitioners and researchers can expand the focus of health promotion programmes beyond health education and social marketing aimed solely at behavioural risk factors, to an integrative, whole system, and strategic approach (Bunton and Macdonald 2002).

Community settings for health promotion programmes

Investing in health promotion activities for people with intellectual disabilities can have a substantial impact on improving health and reducing the personal and financial costs associated with poor health. Physically inactive people are almost twice as likely to develop heart disease as active people (US Department of Health and Human Services, Office of Disease Prevention and Health Promotion 2002). This makes inactivity as strong a risk factor for heart disease as smoking, high blood pressure, and high cholesterol. Chronic health conditions are at least one underlying cause of increased health problems among people with disabilities. In developing community health promotion programmes for people with intellectual disabilities, defining and understanding the associated factors from their perspective is important. Being clear on how community-based health promotion programmes differ from health promotion classes offered in community settings is important (Baker and Brownson 1998).

Taking charge: matters of support

Consideration of 'the combination of educational and environmental supports for actions and conditions of living conducive to health' (Green and Kreuter 1993) is imperative in developing health promotion programmes. Over time, the term 'health education' has become more inclusive and begun to focus on possible harmful effects of certain behaviours, and their legal status (for example, laws mandating safety-related provisions, such as the use of car air bags or bicycle helmets) (Breckon et al. 1994). In addition, educational processes extend cognitive approaches (presenting the facts) to include affective models (changing attitudes), peer support models, decision-making models, and more recently, behavioural models.

Multi-pronged approach

Individual motivation combined with socio-environmental and organizational support is an effective approach to changing behaviour and promoting health. By recognizing the importance of environments for supporting healthy lifestyles, individuals will be better able not only to change their health behaviours but also to maintain their newly adopted health habits. In developing a strategic plan for community-based health promotion, having a multi-pronged approach to explain the multitude of factors that impact human behaviour is essential. Behavioural models/theories that can explain human behaviour, in relation to health education, can be classified on three levels: (1) individual (intrapersonal), (2) interpersonal, and (3) community.

Individuals with intellectual disabilities (intrapersonal level)

Developing effective and sustainable health promotion programmes requires consideration of processes related to modifying or changing individual health behaviours. Intrapersonal health behaviour models include the Transtheoretical Model of Behaviour Change (Prochaska and DiClemente 1992) and Social Cognitive Theory (Bandura 1977, 1986), which includes the construct of self-efficacy (Bandura 1994) – that is, the self-confidence in one's ability to successfully perform a specific type of action.

The Transtheoretical Model (TTM) of Behaviour Change and Bandura's Social Cognitive Theory (SCT) are useful in developing strategies aimed at behaviour change for people with intellectual disabilities, support persons, and organizational culture. Within TTM, motivating people to change their behaviour can be viewed as a continuum related to a person's readiness to change by using the five stages of TTM: *Precontemplation, Contemplation, Preparation, Action*, and *Maintenance*. People often go through these five stages at different rates in a cyclical pattern, moving back and forth between stages a number of times before they maintain their behaviour change goal. With support, people become increasingly motivated and ready to modify or change a particular behaviour, and specific processes (or activities) can be targeted based on an individual's particular stage. In using SCT along with TTM, strategies are tailored for movement towards behaviour change depending on a person's (1) perception of the pros and cons of change, (2) confidence in the ability to change, and (3) perceived level of social support to adopt a new behaviour. For people with intellectual disabilities, building individual health advocacy skills is of particular importance as a way of developing an individual's confidence in changing behaviour.

Social support (interpersonal level)

Most health educators today recognize the critical importance of the social environment; they thus advocate changes in the social ecology that support individual change leading to better health and a higher quality of life. The lives of people with intellectual disabilities incorporate a culture of interdependency in that many people live their entire lives relying on their family members and multiple professionals for support (Carnaby 1998). For people with intellectual disabilities, the tyranny of no to low expectations and a lack of personal control over situations and practices dramatically influence their definitions of health and their health status.

Caregiver support The need to build collective efficacy in the community among proxy agents such as healthcare professionals and direct care professionals is imperative to advocate for health (Hanna et al. 2011). Building collective efficacy to support self-direction among people with intellectual disabilities requires an understanding of the following (for more information about collective efficacy):

- historical factors that impact attitudes, beliefs, and treatment of people with intellectual disabilities
- determinants of health issues and health promotion and disease prevention during all developmental stages
- concepts related to achieving physical, communication, and programmatic access (for example, universal design and strategies); and
- information about culturally relevant care incorporating a social model of disability versus an illness/medical model.

Developing collective self-efficacy for health advocacy can strengthen a common voice, improve health advocacy and increase group and self-directedness to promote social change in health care for people with intellectual disabilities (Bandura 2000).

The provision of caregiver support can provide accountability for both people with intellectual disabilities and their supports. Health promotion programmes should ensure all programme partners are willing and eager to participate. Scheduling preliminary meetings with people with disabilities, service providers, family members, and community partners provides an opportunity to present the proposed programme, address concerns, and respond to questions related to programme implementation. Lastly, having a strong working relationship with community partners is paramount to achieving a wide spectrum of successful health promotion that will ensure active, ongoing participation from everyone and ensure long-term positive health benefits.

Peer support For people with intellectual disabilities, peer support has the potential to increase awareness and engagement for changing behaviour. People with intellectual disabilities can contribute to their own wellbeing by becoming knowledgeable about their health and health resources, and by becoming active participants in health promotion activities. The Peer to Peer: Health Messages Program (Marks et al. 2012) provides an evidence-based programme for people with intellectual disabilities to become Healthy Lifestyle Coaches (HLCs) and deliver health messages to their peers. Healthy Lifestyle Coaches are leaders who can give their peers new health information and can show them how to take better care of their bodies over a period of time. Through weekly health messages booklets and health messages wristbands, peers are encouraged to 'take charge' and 'pass on' the weekly health message. This programme provides tools for people with intellectual disabilities to increase confidence, knowledge, and health advocacy by becoming peer HLCs.

Supportive environments (community level)

Developing supportive environments on a community level can be structured around four types of models/theories. The first is *community organization*, which has been identified as a method whereby individuals, groups, and organizations engage in planned action to influence a mutually identified social problem through consensus-building activities. Second, *Diffusion of Innovations Theory* is used to convey the processes of how new ideas, products, and social practices diffuse or spread within a society or from one society to another. A third approach, *organizational change theories*, directs health education strategies at several layers at once as a way of achieving both desired and sustainable results. Finally, health education incorporating an *ecological model* focuses attention on the individual and the social environmental factors as the targets. By directing attention away from terms such as 'lifestyle' and 'health behaviour', the focus shifts from changing individuals to a focus on changing the social and physical environment that may create unhealthy behaviours. With an ecological approach, practitioners and researchers seek

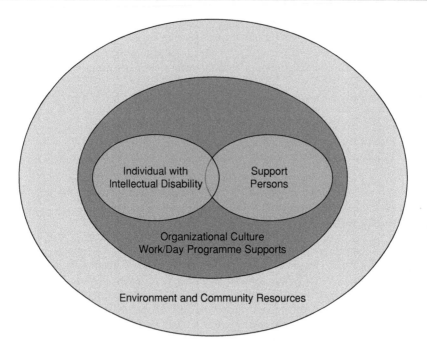

Figure 2.1 Ecological model for changing the social and physical environment

understanding between the individual and the environment. Figure 2.1 depicts an ecological approach to these factors (McLeroy et al. 1988).

Community-based organizations supporting people with intellectual disabilities in their family homes, and residential and day programmes are now beginning to consider the impact of environmental factors on healthy lifestyles both for people receiving services and their employees. Constraints regarding group living, service structures, unclear policy guidelines, and resource limitations may predetermine and limit the availability of health promotion programming, leisure time that fosters physical activities, and the availability of healthy food options (Messent et al. 1999; Harris et al. 2003). Sustainable, comprehensive health promotion programmes for people with intellectual disabilities require a supportive environment and supportive attitudes within community-based organizations.

A supportive environment refers to the policies and procedures relating to health and safety and the provision of support for engaging in healthy behaviours. Supportive attitudes are also necessary to promote healthy lifestyles for both staff and individuals with intellectual disabilities. Important steps to starting a health promotion programme include getting support from key stakeholders and leaders, creating selling points, and recruiting others to join a health promotion programme.

Champions to coordinate successful programmes

When initiating conversations about health promotion programmes, creating a core group of early adopters is a good starting point. Identifying key stakeholders at all levels who express interest in a new health promotion initiative (for example, people with intellectual disabilities, administrators, board members, parents, support staff) is important in supporting a successful launch of the programme; such people may become the programme *champions*. Many organizations will have some early adopters who are interested in promoting health and who want to learn more about it and try out new ideas with the people with whom they support.

Getting a small group of interested co-workers who are *early adopters* excited about creating an environment of health and wellness can serve as a core group who are able to sustain interest and enthusiasm. Early adopters are more likely to work through the inevitable glitches and setbacks that occur in the early stages of a new programme.

Gaining an understanding of the expectations and motivations among your core group of champions within an organization is also important in securing ongoing support. Within your core group, having individuals who can model positive health behaviours and have a collaborative relationship with individuals with intellectual disabilities and their support persons can influence decision-making processes.

Additional support can come from volunteers in a variety of settings, such as a volunteer pool, board members, and service learning projects. Strategic service learning projects can be a 'win–win' situation for students enrolled in health professions' training (for example, adapted physical education, nursing, social work, psychology, nutrition, health education, exercise physiology, physical therapy, occupational therapy, and recreational therapy) and for the community organization: the student can fulfil coursework requirements and the organization can receive a variety of services at no cost.

Once key stakeholders are identified, the primary goal should be to increase awareness of the need for health promotion initiatives, so that everyone has a consistent message as to the key issues supporting the need for a health promotion programme. A secondary goal should be to propose a health promotion programme plan addressing all the issues. Proposed plans should note that health promotion programmes do not have to be expensive! Many organizations are often hesitant to spend money on health promotion programmes, especially when there are other, competing priorities.

Finally, the benefits of the programme should be presented to people with intellectual disabilities. People with intellectual disabilities and their support persons can benefit from health promotion programmes in a number of ways, including health benefits, economic benefits such as being able to maintain employment and lower health insurance premiums, fewer visits to accident and emergency departments, fewer acute-care office visits, and fewer/shorter hospital stays. Controlling healthcare costs through the health promotion programme is one of the least expensive and potentially most beneficial economic strategies.

Strategic action plans for health promotion programmes

Once stakeholders in community organizations make a commitment to health promotion, developing a strategic action plan based on a comprehensive organizational assessment can support a viable health promotion programme. Evaluating organizational needs and capacity for developing a health promotion action plan includes an assessment of programmes/services, environmental supports, resources, culture, and employee knowledge and skills to undertake health-promoting activities. By benchmarking organizational capacity to promote health among clients and employees, targeted strategic action plans for health promotion programming can be developed (Marks and Sisirak 2009).

Assessing organizational culture (such as commitment and policies), employees' self-efficacy, health promotion knowledge, and available resources is important in creating a strategic action plan. Based on the results of your organizational assessment, sample targeted objectives may include the following:

- review and revision of the organization's vision, mission, policies, and job descriptions related to health promotion activities
- implementation of training workshops to increase employee knowledge and skills; and
- provision of resources for food preparation and physical activity.

Sustaining health promotion programmes: health matters!

Health promotion must be based on the needs and lifestyle preferences of individuals. In addition, health promotion programmes for people with intellectual disabilities that incorporate the concepts of choice, self-determination, self-efficacy, self-advocacy, rights, and responsibility have the potential to achieve maximum involvement of people with intellectual disabilities. The support of direct caregivers and organizational support in the provision of health promotion, rather than curative activities, can encourage people with intellectual disabilities in developing and achieving their health promotion goals, achieving full and sustained community engagement, and improving health outcomes.

Evidence-based programmes

Few evidence-based health promotion curricula developed and tested with people with intellectual disabilities exist: Steps to Your Health, part of the South Carolina Disabilities and Health Project (Ewing 1999), and the Health Matters programme from the University of Illinois at Chicago's Rehabilitation, Research, and Training Center on Aging with Developmental Disabilities (Marks and Sisirak 2008) are two notable exceptions. The first step is identifying training materials based on theories and theoretical frameworks and then determining if the materials have been documented to show successful outcomes (for example, increased support for healthy behaviours, enhanced self-efficacy, improved health status, reduced healthcare costs, and better quality of care). Appropriate evaluation is a key factor in evidence-based practice. Evidence-based, community-based programmes may include the following defining characteristics:

- the use of an ecological framework addressing individual needs, interpersonal supports, community social and economic factors, organizational issues, and governmental factors
- they are tailored to meet individual and community needs; and
- they provide an opportunity for people with intellectual disabilities to participate in (and influence) programme development, implementation, and evaluation.

The Health Matters Train-the-Trainer: Certified Instructor Workshop (Marks and Sisirak 2008) is an example of an evidence-based, interactive capacity-building programme for support persons in the community. Participants are provided with organizational and individual resources to implement a tailored 12-week physical activity and health education programme that can be personalized to meet the needs of people with intellectual disabilities. This programme uses the evidence-based curriculum entitled Health Matters: The Exercise and Nutrition Health Education Curriculum for People with Developmental Disabilities (Heller et al. 2004; Marks et al. 2010b).

Community academic partnerships for evidence-based practice

Caregivers in community disability services can play a role in meeting the many training needs related to improving health among people with intellectual disabilities and their families/support people. Community providers may also collaborate with academic institutions to meet the educational needs of professional caregivers and healthcare providers. Community academic partnerships have the unique power of working together to find practical solutions by using evidence-based curricula and training to improve health. HealthMatters™ CAP is a collaboration between two community-based organizations and an academic institution that aims to enhance health status and optimize full community participation of people with developmental disabilities across the lifespan (www.HealthMattersProgram.org). HealthMatters™ CAP is the only known community academic partnership building an infrastructure to facilitate and sustain healthy choices and behaviours among people with intellectual disabilities to improve health status through the following: (1) workforce capacity development for health promotion in community sectors; (2) health advocacy capacity building for people with intellectual disabilities; and (3) active participation among people with intellectual disabilities in health promotion.

Health promotion culture

Successful health promotion programmes include comprehensive targeted activities that recognize that both individual and organizational factors are related to behaviour change. Many models continue to focus only on motivating individuals to change their behaviours. Unfortunately, many people will return to unhealthy behaviours because their environment does not recognize the influence and importance of supportive attitudes, organizational policies, and 'corporate cultures' on individual behaviour change. In developing a health promotion programme for people with intellectual disabilities, it is important not only to consider the individual with a disability, but the interconnectedness of their families, caregivers and support professionals, the organizational culture of a service-related programme (including work/day programme and residential supports), and the environmental issues, community resources, and policy-related factors at local, state, and national level.

Summary

- Including people with intellectual disabilities in community-based health promotion programmes is essential for increasing access to health care and reducing health disparities.
- Broadening the definition of health promotion can expand the focus of health promotion programmes beyond health education and social marketing aimed solely at behavioural risk factors, to an integrative, whole system, and strategic approach.
- Evaluating organizational needs and capacity for developing a health promotion action plan includes an assessment of programmes/services, environmental supports, resources, culture, and employee knowledge and skills to implement health-promoting activities.
- Targeting comprehensive activities that recognize both individual and organizational factors related to behaviour change can lead to sustainable community-based health promotion programmes.

Acknowledgement

This document was produced under grant number H133B080009 awarded by the US Department of Education's National Institute on Disability and Rehabilitation Research to the Rehabilitation Research and Training Center on Aging with Developmental Disabilities-Lifespan Health and Function at the University of Illinois at Chicago. The contents of this chapter do not necessarily represent the policy of the US Department of Education, and should not be assumed as being endorsed by the US Federal Government.

Web resources
- Easyhealth provides excellent accessible health information with over 250 free-to-download materials: www.easyhealth.org.uk

References

Baker, E.A. and Brownson, C.A. (1998) Defining characteristics of community based health promotion. *Journal of Public Health Management and Practice*, 4(2): 1–9.

Bandura, A. (1977) *Social Learning Theory*. Englewood Cliffs, NJ: Prentice-Hall.

Bandura, A. (1986) *Social Foundations of Thought and Action: A Social Cognitive Theory*. Englewood Cliffs, NJ: Prentice-Hall.

Bandura, A. (1994) Self-efficacy, in V.S. Ramachaudran (ed.) *Encyclopedia of Human Behavior*. New York: Academic Press.

Bandura, A. (2000) Exercise of human agency through collective efficacy. *Current Directions in Psychological Science*, 9(3): 75–8.

Baur, C. (2007) Health literacy and adults with intellectual and developmental disabilities: achieving accessible health information and services. Paper presented at the *State of Science in Aging with Developmental Disabilities Symposium*, Atlanta, GA.

Beange, H., McElduff, A. and Baker, W. (1995) Medical disorders of adults with mental retardation: a population study. *American Journal on Mental Retardation*, 99: 595–604.

Breckon, D.J., Harvey, J.R. and Lancaster, B. (1994) *Community Health Education: Setting Roles and Skills for the Twenty-First Century*, 3rd edn. Gaithersburg, MD: Aspen.

Bunton, R. and Macdonald, G. (2002) *Health Promotion: Disciplines, Diversity, and Developments*, 2nd edn. London: Routledge.

Carnaby, S. (1998) Reflections on social integration for people with intellectual disability: does interdependence have a role? *Journal of Intellectual and Developmental Disability*, 23(3): 219–28.

Ewing, G. (1999) *Steps to Your Health (STYH)*, South Carolina Disabilities and Health Project, Available at: http://www.sciodh.com/materials/#Training-Manuals [accessed 11 January 2013].

Fox, D. (1989) Health policy and changing epidemiology in the United States: chronic disease in the twentieth century, in R.C. Maulitz (ed.) *Unnatural Causes: The Three Leading Killer Diseases in America*. New Brunswick, NJ: Rutgers University Press.

Gill, C.J. (1996) Becoming visible: personal health experiences of women with disabilities, in D.M. Krotoski, M.A. Nosek and M.A. Turk (eds.) *Women with Physical Disabilities: Achieving and Maintaining Health and Well-Being*. Baltimore, MD: Paul H. Brookes.

Green, L. and Kreuter, M. (1993) *Health Promotion Planning: An Educational and Environmental Approach*. Mountain View, CA: Mayfield.

Hanna, L.M., Taggart, L. and Cousins, W. (2011) Cancer prevention and health promotion for people with intellectual disabilities: an exploratory study of staff knowledge. *Journal of Intellectual Disability Research*, 55(3): 281–91.

Harris, N., Rosenberg, A., Jangda, S., O'Brien, K. and Gallagher, M. (2003) Prevalence of obesity in International Special Olympic athletes as determined by body mass index. *Journal of the American Dietetic Association*, 103(2): 235–7.

Heller, T., Hsieh, K. and Rimmer, J. (2004) Attitudinal and psychological outcomes of a fitness and health education program on adults with Down syndrome. *American Journal on Mental Retardation*, 109(2): 175–85.

Hornsten, A., Sandstrom, H. and Lundman, B. (2004) Personal understandings of illness among people with Type 2 diabetes. *Journal of Advanced Nursing*, 47(2): 174–82.

Marks, B. (1996) *Conceptualizations of Health among Adults with Intellectual Impairments*. Unpublished doctoral dissertation, University of Illinois at Chicago.

Marks, B.A. and Heller, T. (2003) Bridging the equity gap: health promotion for adults with developmental disabilities. *Nursing Clinics of North America*, 38(2): 205–28.

Marks, B. and Sisirak, J. (2008) *HealthMatters Train-theTrainer: Certified Instructor Workshop*. Chicago, IL: Rehabilitation Research and Training Center on Aging with Developmental Disabilities (www.RRTCADD.org).

Marks, B. and Sisirak, J. (2009) *HealthMatters Assessments*. Chicago, IL: Rehabilitation Research and Training Center on Aging with Developmental Disabilities (www.HealthMattersProgram.org).

Marks, B., Sisirak, J. and Cutler, A. (2008) *Building Capacity to Promote Health Advocacy among People with Developmental Disabilities*. Chicago, IL: Rehabilitation Research and Training Center on Aging with Developmental Disabilities (www.RRTCADD.org).

Marks, B., Sisirak, J. and Heller, T. (2010a) *Health Matters: Establishing Sustainable Exercise and Nutrition Health Promotion Programs for Adults with Developmental Disabilities.* Philadelphia, PA: Brookes Publishing.

Marks, B., Sisirak, J. and Heller, T. (2010b) *Health Matters: Exercise and Nutrition Health Education Curriculum for Adults with Developmental Disabilities.* Philadelphia, PA: Brookes Publishing.

Marks, B., Sisirak, J., Medlen, J. and Magallanes, E. (2012) *Peer to Peer HealthMessages Program: Becoming a Healthy Lifestyle Coach.* Chicago, IL: Rehabilitation Research and Training Center on Aging with Developmental Disabilities (www.RRTCADD.org).

McLeroy, K.R., Bibeau, D., Steckler, A. and Glanz, K. (1988) An ecological perspective on health promotion programs. *Health Education and Behavior,* 15(4): 351–77.

Messent, P.R., Cooke, C.B. and Long, J. (1999) What choice? A consideration of the level of opportunity for people with mild and moderate learning disabilities to lead a physically active healthy lifestyle. *British Journal of Learning Disabilities,* 27: 73–7.

National Center for Education Statistics (2003) *NAAL 2003: Overview.* Available at: http://nces.ed.gov/naal.

Pan American Health Organization (2001) *Promoting Health in the Americas.* Annual Report of the Director 2001. Washington, DC: PAHO.

Pan American Health Organization/Pan American Sanitary Bureau (1999) *Strategic and Programmatic Orientations, 1999–2002.* Document #291. Washington, DC: PAHO.

Phillips, A., Morrison, J. and Davis, R.W. (2004) General practitioners' educational needs in intellectual disability health. *Journal of Intellectual Disability Research,* 48(2): 142–9.

Prochaska, J.O. and DiClemente, C.C. (1992) Stages of change in the modification of problem behaviors, in M. Hersen, R.M. Eisler and P.M. Miller (eds.) *Progress in Behavior Modification.* Sycamore, IL: Sycamore Press.

Rimmer, J.H., Braddock, D. and Marks, B.A. (1995) Health characteristics and behaviors of adults with mental retardation residing in three living arrangements. *Research in Developmental Disabilities,* 16: 489–99.

Selden, C.R., Zorn, M., Ratzan, S. and Parker, R.M. (2000) *Health Literacy, January 1990 through October 1999.* Bethesda, MD: National Library of Medicine.

Sisirak, J., Marks, B., Heller, T. and Riley, B. (2007) Dietary habits of adults with intellectual and developmental disabilities residing in community-based settings. Paper presented at the *135th Annual Meeting and Exposition of the American Public Health Association,* Washington, DC, 6 November.

Tarlov, A.R. (1999) Public policy frameworks for improving population health. *Annals of the New York Academy of Sciences,* 896: 281–93.

United Nations (2006) *United Nations Convention on the Rights of Persons with Disabilities.* Available at: http://www.un.org/disabilities [accessed 20 June 2013].

US Department of Health and Human Services, Office of Disease Prevention and Health Promotion (2002) Physical activity and fitness – improving health, fitness, and quality of life through daily physical activity. *Prevention Report,* 16(4): 1–15.

US Public Health Service (2002) *Closing the Gap: A National Blueprint for Improving the Health of Individuals with Mental Retardation.* Report of the Surgeon-General's Conference on Health Disparities and Mental Retardation, Washington, DC.

Walsh, P.N. and Heller, T. (2002) *Health of Women with Intellectual Disabilities.* London: Blackwell Science.

White-Scott, S. (2007) Health care and health promotion for aging individuals with intellectual disabilities. Paper presented at the *State of Science in Aging with Developmental Disabilities Symposium,* Atlanta, GA.

World Health Organization (WHO) (2001) *Health Promotion.* Report by the Secretariat. Fifty-fourth World Health Assembly A54/8, 2001. Geneva: WHO.

World Health Organization (WHO) (2002) *Active Aging: A Policy Framework. A Contribution of the World Health Organization to the Second United Nations World Assembly on Ageing,* Madrid, Spain, April 2002. Geneva: WHO.

World Health Organization (WHO) (2003) *Diet, Nutrition and the Prevention of Chronic Diseases.* Geneva: WHO.

World Health Organization (WHO) (2005) *The Bangkok Charter for Health Promotion in a Globalized World.* Sixth Global Conference on Health Promotion. Geneva: WHO.

Part 2 — Health promotion evidence applied to practice

3 | Vision, hearing, and oral health

Michael Brown and Linda Goddard

Introduction

Meeting the sensory and oral health needs of people with intellectual disabilities is the focus of this chapter. We provide an overview of the issues relating to the care and management of sensory and oral health needs, and the application of clinical guidelines as a means to ensure equity and standard of care. The specific needs relating to the sensory and oral care treatment of people with intellectual disabilities will be presented and supported by a case example from practice.

Vision

Visual impairment is a severe reduction in vision that cannot be corrected with standard glasses or contact lenses and reduces the ability to function and perform tasks. The WHO estimates that some 314 million people across the world experience a visual impairment and that 39 million suffer from blindness (WHO 2010a). The International Classification of Diseases-10 (ICD-10; WHO 1992) sets out four categories of vision:

- Normal vision
- Moderate visual impairment
- Severe visual impairment
- Blindness.

The most common visual impairments (43 per cent) are due to uncorrected refractive errors such as myopia, hyperopia and astigmatism, with another 33 per cent due to cataracts, which are the leading cause of blindness; glaucoma accounts for 10 per cent of visual loss (WHO 2010b) (see Table 3.1). Correctable refractive errors are common in children and young people and conditions such as cataracts and glaucoma become more common with increasing age.

With assessment and treatment, much visual impairment is correctable and preventable. There has been a decrease in visual impairment over the past 20 years due to national prevention programmes and improvements in the availability of screening. Central to the detection, prevention and treatment of visual impairments is a structured assessment (WHO 2010b). The essential elements of a visual assessment are set out in Table 3.2.

Vision and people with intellectual disabilities

People with intellectual disabilities experience a wide range of visual impairments that, when coupled with those associated with hearing, result in what can be significant sensory

Table 3.1 Definitions of common visual impairments

Impairment	Definition
Amblyopia	When the vision in one eye does not develop fully during early childhood
Astigmatism	A condition in which blurred vision due to an irregular curving of the cornea results in light rays not focusing correctly on the retina
Cataract	A clouding of the lens in the eye that affects vision
Cortical visual impairment	Disturbed or reduced vision due to brain abnormalities
Glaucoma	A group of eye diseases that result in abnormally high intraocular fluid pressure that damages the optic disc and results in partial to complete loss of vision
Hyperopia	A visual defect in which close objects appear blurred because the image is focused behind the retina rather than on it; also called far-sightedness
Myopia	A visual defect in which distant objects appear blurred because the image is focused in front of the retina rather than on it; also called short-sightedness
Refractive error	The inability of the lens of the eye to focus an image accurately, as occurs in near-sightedness and far-sightedness.

impairments. Some 40 per cent of people with intellectual disabilities experience visual impairments that increase with the severity of the disability (Warburg 2001), and can lead to further disability (Evenhuis et al. 2009). Refractive errors were found to be common during the screening of over 3500 Special Olympic athletes with intellectual disabilities: 25 per cent of individuals experienced problems with distance while 10 per cent were unable to see up close (Special Olympics 2005). There can be differences in each eye; 26.4 per cent of athletes required glasses while others required a new prescription (Woodhouse et al. 2003).

Visual impairment is associated with specific genetic conditions, such as Down syndrome and Williams syndrome (Carvill 2001). The incidences of cataracts, nystagmus and optic nerve anomalies are much higher in this population (Woodhouse 2010). The person's specific visual need must be assessed and corrected. Assessing vision can be challenging; it is important that people with intellectual disabilities and their carers are provided with support to enable full assessments to be undertaken, as there is evidence that they do not always occur (Starling et al. 2006). This is necessary to determine the form and level of visual impairment present and ensure that refractive errors are corrected and treatment provided (Cregg et al. 2001).

Providing information about visual impairments and the options available is important, as well as enabling access to optometry, primary care and ophthalmology services to detect visual impairments and provide treatments and interventions as indicated (Starling 2006). When visual aids are required, such as spectacles, some people with intellectual disabilities may struggle to adapt and cope. Therefore, timely additional support may be required through appropriate written instruction and advice to families and carers that is built into their personal plans (Sjoukes et al. 2010). People with intellectual disabilities with visual impairments may need additional support from families and carers to help them compensate, as well as time to adjust to unfamiliar settings and situations. Health education for people with intellectual disabilities, their families and carers is necessary to ensure that regular reviews are undertaken on an annual basis, or as indicated, to monitor vision and ensure that remedial correction is taken; this is increasingly important with ageing (Evenhuis et al. 2001; Melville et al. 2009).

Table 3.2 Elements of a comprehensive visual assessment

Element	Description
Clinical presentation	Clinical history regarding onset, sudden or persistent symptoms, rapidity of symptoms, monocular or binocular visual disturbance, severity of pain, visual ocular examination, permanent or transient visual loss, facial trauma or injury, presence of 'flashers' and 'floaters'
Past medical history	Cardiovascular disease, diabetes, hypertension, past ocular incidents and outcome, recurrent ocular loss, neurological and vascular incidents
Ophthalmic history	Past ocular history is of importance and includes the wearing of spectacles and contact lens. The presence of corneal ulceration needs to be assessed along with recent red eye, infections and ocular surgery for conditions such as cataracts and glaucoma
Medication history	An accurate medication history is required to identify possible associations with vision loss
Physical examination	• Baseline assessment of blood pressure and oxygen saturation • Examination of the head and neck for trauma • Visual acuity readings • Peripheral vision testing • The assessment of pupillary defects to identify retinal or optic nerve dysfunction • Pupillary reaction • Extra-ocular motility assessment • Eyelid and ocular surface examination to identify intra-ocular inflammation, corneal irregularity and cataracts • Fundoscopy to review the optic discs, fundi and posterior poles of the eye
Blood tests	Consider deferring tests to ophthalmologists in most sub-acute and chronic cases. For sudden monocular vision loss, full blood counts, erythrocyte sedimentation rates and C-reactive protein levels may be indicated. Patients with transient vision loss may require lipid profiles and full blood counts
Radiological examination	Vision loss and abnormal ocular motility require urgent imaging. Neuroimaging may be indicated due to bilateral loss such as hemianopia or other bilateral symptoms, suggestive of an intracranial disorder. Computed tomography (CT) or magnetic resonance imaging (MRI) scanning may be indicated if intracranial haemorrhage is suspected. Where ischaemia is suspected as a result of transient visual changes, carotid Doppler may be required

Hearing impairment

Globally it is estimated that more than 275 million people have some form of moderate or profound hearing impairment, although population-based studies are limited (Stevens et al. 2013). Hearing impairment can occur in one or both ears and refers to complete or partial loss of the ability to hear. There are two types of hearing impairment, conductive and sensorineural. Conductive hearing impairment relates to issues in the outer or middle ear, such as chronic middle ear infections, which if untreated results in problems with the conduction of sound waves through the middle chamber of the ear. Sensorineural hearing impairment relates to issues within the inner ear and the cochlear nerve (Mathers et al. 2000).

There are a range of congenital causes of hearing loss that can lead to deafness at, or soon after, birth. Congenital causes can be inherited and passed on from a parent with a hearing loss. Hearing impairments can also result from issues during pregnancy and childbirth and include premature birth, foetal anoxia, rubella, and syphilis. The primary causes of hearing impairment include infectious diseases such as measles, mumps, meningitis, and ear infections, which, if untreated, become chronic, resulting in hearing loss as well as head and ear injury, foreign bodies and ear wax, and overexposure to excessive noise. Early detection and screening is therefore a central part of hearing loss (WHO 2010c). Hearing loss is also common in older age and is referred to as presbycusis. Half of all hearing loss is avoidable through primary prevention such as immunization, prenatal screening, good maternity care, and early diagnosis and treatment of ear infections, and the provision of protective devices to minimize exposure to noise (WHO 2010c). For hearing loss that does not receive early intervention, later treatment can be provided medically or surgically by way of hearing aids and cochlear implants.

Hearing and people with intellectual disabilities

Evidence highlights that hearing loss is 40–100 times higher in people with intellectual disability than among the non-disabled population (Carvill 2001). The screening of 3500 Special Olympic athletes for hearing impairments identified hearing deficits in 30 per cent of athletes, with the incidence increasing with age (Special Olympics 2005). More recently, Hild et al. (2008) identified deficits in 25 per cent of 552 Special Olympic athletes, 48 per cent of whom required referral to a hearing specialist, while 42 per cent required removal of wax. These assessments were carried out on people with mild to moderate intellectual disability; the potential for hearing deficits in people with more severe and profound disabilities may be much higher, which can impact on their interactions and subsequent behaviour. People with intellectual disabilities experience hearing loss a decade earlier compared with the general population and in those with Down syndrome it is apparent three decades sooner (Carvill 2001; Meuwese-Jongejeugd et al. 2006). In babies and young children with intellectual disabilities, early detection and treatment of hearing loss is important and has a significant impact on language development and progression in education and personal relationships. Hearing is essential for the development of spoken language, yet carers may fail to identify impairments experienced by their family member with an intellectual disability (Evenhuis et al. 2001; Starling et al. 2006). As a result, screening and hearing assessments are important to detect deficits and provide treatments and remedial supports such as hearing aids (Lennox et al. 2007). It is important to identify the person's level of understanding with regard to the use of hearing aids and to offer pictorial cues and careful instructions (Meuwese-Jongejeugd et al. 2007).

There may be signs of hearing loss that are indicated by the slow and poor development of speech with developmental milestones not being achieved. Full specialist hearing assessments are therefore necessary to ensure that possible treatments are provided at an early age, such as cochlear implants (Henderson et al. 2007). Early intervention programmes involving speech and language therapists may be indicated (see Chapter 17). Behavioural challenges such as head banging and poking and picking of the ears may also be evident in some people with intellectual disabilities, which can impact on and damage their hearing. Health education and information is required by people with intellectual disabilities, their families and carers to support effective communication (Melville et al. 2009).

Oral health

Oral health is defined as:

> A state of being free from chronic mouth and facial pain, oral and throat cancer, oral sores, birth defects such as cleft lip and palate, periodontal (gum) disease, tooth decay and tooth loss, and other diseases and disorders that affect the oral cavity.
>
> (WHO 2012: 1)

The WHO Global Oral Health Programme aimed to make links between policies and strategies relating to chronic disease prevention and health promotion, thereby seeking to prevent and reduce oral health problems (WHO 2006). Oral diseases are some of the most common of the chronic diseases and are important public health problems because of their prevalence and their impact on society and individuals due to the expense of treatment. The prevalence of oral disease varies globally by geographical region and is affected by the availability and accessibility of oral health services.

There are a range of risk factors associated with poor oral health, including cardiovascular diseases, HIV, cancer, respiratory diseases and diabetes, unhealthy diets with a high sugar intake, tobacco and alcohol use, facial injuries, and poor oral care and hygiene (Petersen et al. 2005). A range of strategic public health approaches need to be implemented so as to impact on whole populations, including people with intellectual disabilities (Department of Health 2005). Public health approaches, such as water fluoridation, oral health education programmes, and pre-school screening for children, seek to minimize oral disease, thereby avoiding dental decay and costly treatments and interventions, and to enhance the quality of life of the individual (Watt 2005).

A range of interrelated approaches to the delivery of oral public health policy and strategies and health promotion are necessary to minimize the burden of chronic oral diseases and are central to effective long-term oral health care (Petersen et al. 2005). The oral public health approaches include:

- Decreasing sugar intake and maintaining a well-balanced nutritional intake to prevent tooth decay and premature tooth loss.
- A diet comprising fruit and vegetables to protect against oral cancer.
- Eliminating tobacco use and decreasing alcohol consumption to reduce the risks of oral cancer, periodontal disease, and tooth loss.
- Ensuring adequate and proper oral hygiene.
- Ensuring the use of protective sports equipment to prevent facial injuries.
- The promotion of safe physical environments, thereby preventing facial injuries.

Oral health and people with intellectual disabilities

Public health approaches need to recognize and reflect the specific and distinct oral care needs of people with intellectual disabilities. Poor oral care can ultimately impact on an individual's quality of life when there is difficulty eating, pain, problems sleeping, and low self-esteem (Anders and Davis 2010). National and local policy needs to take account, and reflect the needs, of the population and ensure practitioners are prepared with the knowledge and skills to respond appropriately (Cumella et al. 2000; Nunn et al. 2004; Brookes and Master 2010). Central to the identification and management of the oral health needs of people with intellectual disabilities is the need for access to services and assessment to undertake regular oral reviews and check-ups that includes education and treatment within the context of person-centred care (Gallagher and Fiske 2007). Where possible self-care is enabled and families and carers provided with the support and information necessary to enable the effective prevention, detection, and management of the oral care needs of people with intellectual disabilities (Owens et al. 2006).

The approach to effective oral and dental care involves a systematic assessment and review of the needs of the individual with the aim of moving away from a reactive, restorative approach to care to one that is preventative. This involves long-term management and care that is built upon a person-centred assessment of need and risk, with the aim of enabling and supporting people to manage their own oral health wherever possible (NHS Education for Scotland 2011).

The core elements of comprehensive oral health care are:

- an oral health assessment and review
- a personal and oral health history

- the assessment of oral health status
- a diagnosis and risk assessment
- a personal care plan and
- a regular Focused Oral Health Review (FOHR).

People with intellectual disabilities experience significant health issues, and require care and treatment from all health services, from primary through to general hospital care and specialist intellectual disability health and social care services (Department of Health 2008; Brown et al. 2010). This is central to the assessment and identification of needs, as some people with intellectual disabilities experience co-morbid health issues such as physical disabilities including kyphosis, scoliosis, epilepsy, sensory impairments, autism, mental illness, and behavioural challenges that require services to take account of, and plan for, their additional needs (Krahn et al. 2006; Kwok and Cheung 2007; Emerson and Baines 2010).

Poor oral health impacts on the individual, both physically and psychologically, in relation to growth and development, language development, eating and drinking, socializing and participation in society (Department of Health 2005). People with intellectual disabilities have the right to access oral health care appropriate to their needs; however, historically it is an issue that has been neglected, despite the evidence of their poor oral health (Owens et al. 2011). Central to enabling an oral health assessment and review are equal access to services and the provision of adjustments to ensure that assessment and treatment care be provided and take account of the physical and psychological needs of the individual (British Society for Disability and Oral Health 2012). There are oral health issues that are common in people with intellectual disabilities (see Table 3.3).

Promoting good oral and dental care and the prevention of complications associated with poor care is necessary. Health promotion regarding the need to ensure that people with intellectual disabilities receive care and support appropriate to their needs is necessary, as poor care impacts on their health and quality of life. Education needs to be individualized to ensure that people with intellectual disabilities, their families and carers recognize the need for good oral care and regular dental review and treatment. Dental caries and gum disease, periodontal disease and root caries are common and result in poor nutritional intake, pain and discomfort and, as a consequence, higher numbers of extractions and the use of sedation and general anaesthetics. Responding to these issues is important, as some people with intellectual disabilities may experience gastric oesophageal reflux disorder (GORD), which if untreated results in pain and discomfort as well as contributing to dental disease. People with intellectual disabilities may experience issues in relation to their weight and diet (see Chapter 5); health promotion

Table 3.3 Oral health issues found within people with intellectual disabilities

Condition	Definition
Excessive salivation	Poor lip closure and head control, resulting in the build-up of saliva in the mouth and thus drooling
Bruxism	The grinding and clenching of the teeth that, if persistent and chronic, can result in degeneration of teeth, oral pain, and tooth loss
Tooth erosion	The chemical or mechanochemical destruction of tooth material
Dental caries	The destructive process causing decalcification of the tooth enamel that leads to continued destruction of enamel and dentin, and cavities of the tooth
Gingivitis	An inflammation of the gingiva
Periodontal disease	Periodontal disease is a group of diseases that affect the tissues that support and anchor the teeth

and education, therefore, needs to focus on healthy eating and nutrition and take account of food and drinks that can contribute to dental disease and decay.

Behavioural issues may be apparent; changes in behaviour and routine should not be ignored and need to be fully assessed to exclude oral and dental problems. Health promotion activities therefore should focus on early and regular oral and dental assessment where additional support may be required to access care and treatment. Chronic diseases such as obesity, diabetes and caries are increasing in developing countries, with the implication that quality of life related to oral health, as well as general quality of life, may deteriorate.

Case study

Daniel is 19 years old and lives at home with his parents. He has a 24-hour community support package with visiting support workers who supplement the care he receives from his parents. Daniel was born prematurely at 23 weeks gestation and suffered from foetal anoxia that resulted in profound and multiple intellectual disabilities and significant co-existing mental and physical disabilities. He has cerebral palsy, urinary incontinence, constipation, epilepsy, GORD, oral health problems associated with sugary medications, feeding difficulties, and aspiration. He has both a hearing impairment and a visual impairment. Daniel requires access to health services to assist with the assessment and management of his needs as well as a range of healthcare interventions to maintain his health. Daniel is only able to communicate his basic needs: his facial expression and body language indicate his pleasure or displeasure at activities; he has a communication board with a limited number of pictures at which he can point. (See Table 3.4 for an example care plan for Daniel).

Table 3.4 Health promotion care plan

Needs and priorities	Aims and objectives	Resources required
General health: Daniel has exhibited some behavioural changes, full health assessment required. This is in response to the 'felt need' of Daniel's parents based on the changes in his behaviour	To improve and maintain Daniel's overall health and participation in daily activities	Daniel's medical practitioner, his past health diary or healthcare plan Daniel's health assessment (if in place) completed prior to appointment by nurse/carer Medication information
Oral health: Daniel's family have found him reluctant to have his teeth cleaned and think he may be experiencing pain	To seek assessment and advice about Daniel's oral health To develop education programme related to cleaning Daniel's teeth	A suitable dentist with experience with people who have intellectual/physical disabilities Daniel's family and their knowledge of his needs Daniel, who communicates through noises, facial expressions and through his communication board
Vision: Daniel experiences near-sightedness and the distance is blurred, and strabismus (squint)	To seek assessment and advice about Daniel's visual health from an ophthalmologist	An ophthalmologist who has experience with a person with intellectual disabilities Information on Daniel's past experience with glasses His parents (as above)

(continued)

Table 3.4 Health promotion care plan (*Continued*)

Needs and priorities	Aims and objectives	Resources required
Hearing: Daniel regularly experiences ear infections. He had wax build-up in the past and is thought to have a hearing deficit but does not tolerate hearing aids	To seek assessment and advice from an audiologist To obtain pictorial information on use of hearing aids for Daniel and family/carers	An audiologist who has experience with a person with intellectual disabilities Information on Daniel's past experience and hearing aids if used His family (as above)

The Action Plan – interventions	Plan implementation	Evaluation
General health: Assist Daniel's parents to organize appointments with general practitioner (GP) attend if required	All appointments attended Health care needs identified Any actions listed in Daniel's healthcare plan Follow up appointment made Explanations/clarification with family as required	Increased awareness of Daniel's healthcare needs via feedback from parents Daniel will appear more comfortable, as demonstrated by his facial expression and body language, with increased participation in activities and feedback from family and carers
Oral health: Appointment made with dentist and oral hygienist Request regarding use of electric toothbrush Request pictorial directions for cleaning teeth	Daniel attended dental clinic Oral hygiene plan in place with pictures and instructions for using electric toothbrush for Daniel, his family and carers Observe for any signs of pain or discomfort and record in health diary	Daniel will be responsive to having his teeth cleaned Daniel will be free from pain, indicated by facial expression and body language Feedback from family will clarify Daniel's comfort or any issues
Vision: Appointment made with ophthalmologist Request advice regarding the use of glasses, times, etc.	Visual deficits identified Plan in place for the use of glasses with pictures and instructions for Daniel, his family and carers Responses recorded in health diary	Daniel will demonstrate increased responsiveness to his environment, as indicated by his facial expression, body language and feedback from family/carers
Hearing: Appointment made with audiologist Request pictorial and written instructions regarding the use of hearing aids	Hearing deficits identified Plan in place for the use of hearing aids for Daniel, his family and carers Record responses in health diary	Daniel able to tolerate wearing hearing aids and be more responsive to his environment Family/carers will offer feedback

Summary

- There is global recognition of the prevalence of visual, hearing and oral issues experienced by the general population that require assessment, treatment, and management.
- People with intellectual disabilities experience particular needs in relation to their visual, hearing, and oral health, which, when not addressed, impact significantly on their health, wellbeing, and quality of life.

- Clinical guidelines and evidence-based standards have been developed for the general population that provide the standards that people with intellectual disabilities can expect in relation to their visual, hearing, and oral health.
- Access to effective assessment and treatments is necessary to detect visual, hearing, and oral health conditions and disorders that can be effectively treated and managed.
- Health promotion plays an important part in enabling people with intellectual disabilities, their families and carers to ensure that visual, hearing, and oral health needs are addressed by adopting person-centred approaches.

Useful resources

- Easyhealth allows people to find 'accessible' health information. 'Accessible' information that uses easy words with pictures: http://www.easyhealth.org.uk/

- The Improving Health and Lives Learning Disabilities Observatory keeps watch on the health of people with learning disabilities and the health care they receive: http://www.improvinghealthandlives.org.uk/

- A DVD about eye care for people with intellectual disabilities, 'You and Eye': http://www.seeability.org/about_us/video_gallery/you_and_eye_main_page.aspx

---

Web resources

- Dental: http://www.easyhealth.org.uk/listing/teeth-(leaflets)
- Going to the dentist: http://www.easyhealth.org.uk/listing/going-to-the-dentist-(leaflets)
- Hearing: http://www.easyhealth.org.uk/listing/ear-problems-(leaflets)
- Vision: http://www.easyhealth.org.uk/listing/eye-problems-(leaflets)
- Going to the optician: http://www.easyhealth.org.uk/listing/going-to-the-opticians-(leaflets)

References

Anders, P.L. and Davis, E.L. (2010) Oral health of patients with intellectual disabilities: a systematic review. *Special Care Dentist*, 30: 110–17.

British Society for Disability and Oral Health (2012) *Clinical Guidelines and Integrated Care Pathways for Oral Health Care of People with Learning Disabilities*. London: Faculty of Dental Surgery.

Brookes, V. and Master, S. (2010) Developing a highly skilled workforce. *Journal of Disability and Oral Health*, 11(4): 183–6.

Brown, M., MacArthur, J., McKechanie, A., Hayes, M. and Fletcher, J. (2010) Equality and access to general healthcare for people with learning disabilities: reality or rhetoric? *Journal of Research in Nursing*, 15(4): 351–61.

Carvill, S. (2001) Review: Sensory impairments, intellectual disability and psychiatry. *Journal of Intellectual Disability Research*, 45: 467–83.

Cregg, M., Woodhouse, J.M., Pakeman, V.H., Saunders, K.J., Gunter, H.L., Parker, M. et al. (2001) Accommodation and refractive error in children with Down syndrome: cross-sectional and longitudinal studies. *Investigative Ophthalmology and Visual Science*, 42(1): 55–63.

Cumella, S., Ransford, N., Lyons, J. and Burnham, H. (2000) Needs for oral care among people with intellectual disability not in contact with Community Dental Services. *Journal of Intellectual Disability Research*, 44(1): 45–52.

Department of Health (2005) *Choosing Better Oral Health: An Oral Health Plan for England.* London: Department of Health.

Department of Health (2008) *Health Care for All: Independent Inquiry into Access to Health Care for People with Learning Disabilities.* London: HMSO.

Emerson, E. and Baines, S. (2010) *Health Inequalities and People with Learning Disabilities in the UK: 2010.* Improving Health and Lives: Learning Disability Observatory. London: Public Health England.

Evenhuis, H.M., Theunissen, M., Denkers, I., Verschuure, H. and Kemme, H. (2001) Prevalence of visual and hearing impairment in a Dutch institutionalized population with intellectual disability. *Journal of Intellectual Disability Research*, 45(5): 457–64.

Evenhuis, H.M., Sjoukes, L., Koot, H.M. and Kooijman, A.C. (2009) Does visual impairment lead to additional disability in adults with intellectual disability? *Journal of Intellectual Disability Research*, 53(1): 19–28.

Gallagher, J. and Fiske, J. (2007) Special care dentistry: a professional challenge. *British Dental Journal*, 202(10): 619–29.

Henderson, A., Lynch, S.A., Wilkinson, S. and Hunter, M. (2007) Adults with Down's syndrome: the prevalence of complications and health care in the community. *British Journal of General Practice*, 57: 50–5.

Hild, U., Hey, C., Baumann, U., Montgomery, J., Euler, H.A. and Neumann, K. (2008) High prevalence of hearing disorders at the Special Olympics indicate need to screen persons with intellectual disability. *Journal of Intellectual Disability Research*, 52(6): 520–8.

Krahn, G., Hammond, L. and Turner, A. (2006) A cascade of disparities: health and health care access for people with intellectual disabilities. *Mental Retardation and Developmental Disabilities Research Reviews*, 12: 70–82.

Kwok, H. and Cheung, P. (2007) Co-morbidity of psychiatric disorder and medical illness in people with intellectual disabilities. *Current Opinion in Psychiatry*, 20: 443–9.

Lennox, N., Ware, R., Bain, C., Taylor Gomez, M. and Cooper, S.-A. (2007) Effects of screening for adults with intellectual disabilities: a pooled analysis. *British Journal of General Practice*, 61: 193–6.

Mathers, C., Smith, A. and Concha, M. (2000) *Global Burden of Hearing Loss in the Year 2000.* Geneva: WHO.

Melville, C., Hamilton, S., Miller, S., Boyle, S., Robinson, N., Pert, C. et al. (2009) Carer knowledge and perceptions of healthy lifestyles for adults with intellectual disabilities. *Journal of Applied Research in Intellectual Disabilities*, 22: 298–306.

Meuwese-Jongejeugd, A., Vink, M., van Zanten, B., Verschuure, H., Eichhorn, E., Koopman, D. et al. (2006) Prevalence of hearing loss in 1598 adults with an intellectual disability: cross-sectional population based study. *International Journal of Audiology*, 45: 660–9.

Meuwese-Jongejeugd, A., Verschuure, H. and Evenhuis, H.M. (2007) Hearing aids: expectations and satisfaction of people with an intellectual disability. A descriptive pilot study. *Journal of Intellectual Disability Research*, 51(11): 913–22.

NHS Education for Scotland (2011) *Oral Health Assessment and Review: Guidance in Brief.* Edinburgh: NHS Education for Scotland.

Nunn, J., Boyle, C., Thompson, S. and Wilson, K. (2004) Developing an undergraduate curriculum in special care dentistry. *Journal of Disability and Oral Health*, 6: 3–15.

Owens, P., Kerker, B., Zigler, E. and Horwitz, S. (2006) Vision and oral health needs of individuals with intellectual disability. *Mental Retardation and Developmental Disabilities Research Reviews*, 12: 28–40.

Owens, J., Mistry, K. and Dyer, T. (2011) Access to dental services for people with learning disabilities: quality care? *Journal of Disability and Oral Health*, 12: 17–30.

Petersen, E., Bourgeois, D., Ogawa, H., Estupinan, S. and Ndiaye, C. (2005) The global burden of oral disease and risks to oral health. *Bulletin of the World Health Organisation*, 83: 661–9.

Sjoukes, L., Kooijman, A., Koot, H. and Evenhuis, H. (2010) Rehabilitation of low vision in adult with intellectual disabilities: the influence of staff. *Journal of Applied Research in Intellectual Disabilities*, 23: 186–91.

Special Olympics (2005) *Changing Attitudes, Changing the World: The Health and Health Care of People with Intellectual Disabilities.* Special Olympics, Inc. Available at: www.specialolympics.org [accessed 23 June 2013].

Starling, S., Willis, A., Dracup, M., Burton, M. and Pratt, C. (2006) 'Right to sight': accessing eye care for adults who are learning disabled. *Journal of Intellectual Disabilities*, 10(4): 37–55.

Stevens, G., Flaxman, S., Brunskill, E., Mascarenhas, M., Mathers, C.D. and Finucane, M. (2013) Global and regional hearing impairment prevalence: an analysis of 42 studies in 29 countries. *European Journal of Public Health*, 23(1): 146–52.

Warburg, M. (2001) Visual impairment in adult people with intellectual disability: literature review. *Journal of Intellectual Disability Research*, 45: 424–38.

Watt, R. (2005) Strategies and approaches in oral disease prevention and health promotion. *Bulletin of the World Health Organization*, 83: 711–18.

Woodhouse, J.M. (2010) Systems disorders: eye diseases and visual impairment, in J. O'Hara, J. McCarthy and N. Bouras (eds.) *Intellectual Disability and Ill Health: A Review of the Evidence*. Cambridge: Cambridge University Press.

Woodhouse, J.M., Adler, P.M. and Duignan. A. (2003) Ocular and visual defects amongst people with intellectual disabilities participating in Special Olympics. *Ophthalmic and Physiological Optics*, 23: 221–32.

World Health Organization (WHO) (1992) *The International Classification of Diseases-10 (ICD-10)*. Geneva: WHO.

World Health Organization (WHO) (2006) *Oral Health: Action Plan for Promotion and Integrated Disease Prevention*. Geneva: WHO.

World Health Organization (WHO) (2010a) *Global Data on Visual Impairment*. Geneva: WHO.

World Health Organization (WHO) (2010b) *Action Plan for the Prevention of Avoidable Blindness and Visual Impairment, 2009-2013*. Geneva: WHO.

World Health Organization (WHO) (2010c) *Newborn and Infant Hearing Screening: Current Issues and Guiding Principles for Action*. Geneva: WHO.

World Health Organization (WHO) (2012) *What is Oral Health?* Fact sheet #318. Geneva: WHO.

4 Framing food choices to improve health

Jasmina Sisirak and Beth Marks

Introduction

Food is an integral part of our life. What we eat is influenced by numerous external and internal factors. Over our lifetimes, eating habits can protect us from chronic health conditions and help us enjoy longer and healthier lives. Poor diet may also be a risk factor contributing to obesity and chronic health conditions, such as Type 2 diabetes. Many people with intellectual disabilities living in developed countries have insufficient nutrition knowledge, limited food preparation skills, diets that are high in fat and calories, low consumption of fruits and vegetables, and limited incomes, which lead to poor food choices and potential health issues.

This chapter discusses strategies to support healthy food choices among people with intellectual disabilities using the Ecological Framework of Food Choice (EFFC). The EFFC is a useful guide for understanding how people with intellectual disabilities make food choices and creating environmental and social changes that will allow people with intellectual disabilities to actively participate in food planning, purchasing, and preparation within their communities. This chapter presents issues related to the factors and determinants of food choice using a multi-level approach derived from ecological models of health behaviour, the principles of the Primary Health Care Model, Person-Centred Planning, and Social Cognitive Theory. Information on how people with intellectual disabilities make food choices is discussed to provide insight in developing appropriate, accessible, effective, and successful health promotion and education programmes while promoting community integration in this population.

Nutrition, obesity and choice

Nutrition and obesity

In the United States, the prevalence of overweight and obese adults with intellectual disabilities has been estimated to be either equal to or higher than the general population, ranging from 34 to 48 per cent (Harris et al. 2003; Jansen et al. 2004; Yamaki 2005; Rimmer and Yamaki 2006; Melville et al. 2007). Yamaki (2005), in the first US population-based study of adults with intellectual disabilities, reported combined prevalence of overweight and obesity at 64 per cent, and the prevalence of obesity alone at 35 per cent. (For more information about obesity and people with intellectual disabilities, see Chapter 5.)

For people with intellectual disabilities, the combination of a sedentary lifestyle, high fat diet, and low fruit and vegetable intake increases their susceptibility to health conditions, including obesity, cardiovascular disease (CVD), osteoporosis, hypertension, Type 2 diabetes, and depression (Beange et al. 1995; Fujiura et al. 1997; Draheim et al. 2002; Yamaki 2005; Rimmer and Yamaki 2006; Taggart et al. 2012). Cardiovascular disease is one of the most common causes of death among adults with intellectual disabilities (Hayden 1998; Janicki et al. 1999) and the onset of CVD is strongly associated with a lack of physical activity and poor nutrition (see Chapter 8). While poor nutrition is a risk factor for many health conditions, there is very limited research on how people with intellectual disabilities choose the food that they eat. It is believed that only 45 per cent of people with intellectual disabilities in community settings choose the food that they eat and the majority of them have little or no involvement in food shopping (66 per cent), meal planning (68 per cent) or meal preparation (59 per cent) (Sisirak et al. 2007). Furthermore, the existing literature contains no information as to the factors that affect food choice-making among adults with intellectual disabilities.

Defining and supporting food choice

To support people with intellectual disabilities in making food choices, having an understanding of the meaning of choice is critical. While the term 'choice' has multiple definitions, such as a 'performative' action given the specific situation (Rawlings et al. 1995) and a 'perceived range of available options' (Harris et al. 2003), for the purpose of making food choices, we use the definition 'a process through which an individual makes a decision regarding different options available' (Harris et al. 2003). Within this definition, choice is a multidimensional concept affected by cognitive activity and the interaction of the individual and the environmental setting and its social context.

Using the EFFC to create healthy food environments

The EFFC supports a systematic and comprehensive understanding of food choice-making among people with intellectual disability. The EFFC draws on several perspectives and disciplines, including the Primary Health Care (PHC) Model (McElmurry et al. 2002) and the philosophy of Person-Centred Planning (PCP) (O'Brien et al. 1997), in supporting choices related to food planning, purchasing, and preparation to be accessible (for example, affordable, available) and acceptable (for example, culturally relevant, satisfactory). The level of participation and cultural relevancy are important factors in bringing people 'to the table'. The person with intellectual disabilities needs to be involved and central to any decision-making process. Person-Centred Planning incorporates the individual's unique characteristics, including their disability, and the interaction of the individual and their disability.

The EFFC also incorporates Social Cognitive Theory (SCT) (Bandura 1977) and an ecological perspective to clarify the important factors related to food choice for people with intellectual disabilities. Social Cognitive Theory is widely used within health education and health promotion practice to explain, predict, and guide behaviour change related to choosing foods (Whitehead 2001). Within SCT, carers can examine the interaction between personal factors, behaviour, and environment, known as reciprocal determinism (Bandura 1977, 1986; Baranowski et al. 2002). Examining the interaction of personal characteristics, knowledge, attitudes, social supports, and environment from an ecological perspective helps carers to have a better appreciation of the food choices being made by adults with intellectual disabilities. By using the EFFC, we can determine how personal factors, behaviour, and environmental influences may be interrelated and impact upon food choices. This will guide the development of programmes that build capacity for self-efficacy (confidence) and empower people with intellectual disabilities, and enhance the social supports that exist for this population.

Lastly, the EFFC also provides the tools for creating dynamic multi-level ecological programmes to create healthy food environments through the work of Sorensen et al. (2003, 2007). By including the social context of health behaviours across different levels as illustrated in Figure 4.1, the EFFC for people with intellectual disabilities consists of three components: personal characteristics,

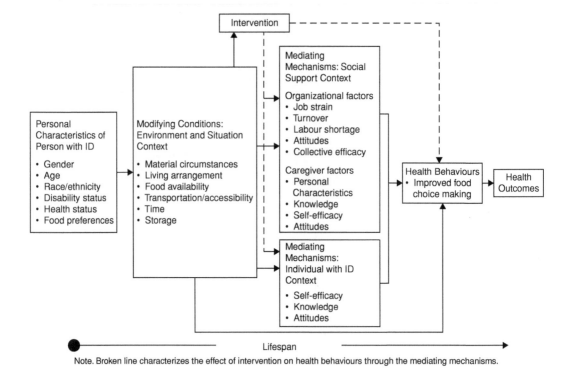

Figure 4.1 Ecological Framework of Food Choice (EFFC) (ID = intellectual disability)

Source: Adapted from Sorensen et al. (2003)

modifying conditions, and mediating mechanisms. Modifying conditions are the variables that have an impact on the health outcome but are not manipulated by an intervention, whereas mediating mechanisms are factors that are on the pathway between the intervention and health outcome. Mediating mechanisms are directly influenced by an intervention.

Practical ways to support food choices

Personal factors

In supporting people with intellectual disabilities to make healthy food choices, caregivers need to consider personal characteristics that affect such choices. Personal factors include the following: biological (for example, gender, age, disability status), physiological (for example, health status, hunger, ageing, post-ingestive/absorptive effects), and psychological (for example, personality, preferences, mood, familiarity with food) (Hamilton et al. 2000; Wetter et al. 2001; Conner and Armitage 2002). The interconnectedness of these factors can be seen as they relate to taste: evidence suggests that taste has a major influence on food selection and preferences in the general population; the concept of food taste is guided by the chemical senses of taste and smell and perceptions of texture (physiological), as well as the hedonic or pleasure-inducing effect of food (psychological) (Drewnowski 1997; Nestle et al. 1998; Hamilton et al. 2000; Conner and Armitage 2002).

Due to their higher rates of nutrition-related health issues (Stewart 2003) and living arrangements that may limit food selection, the influence of taste may be under-recognized among people with intellectual disabilities. Altered food taste from poor oral health, dysphagia, medication use, including polypharmacy, and ageing-related physiological changes affect food selection, alter food preferences, and potentially limit food choices (Cumella et al. 2000; Robertson et al. 2000; Stewart 2003; Samuels and Chadwick 2006). Over half of adults with intellectual disabilities have unmet oral health needs, including gingivitis, decay, missing teeth, heavy wear due to tooth grinding, and tooth enamel deficiency (Cumella et al. 2000; Pezzementi and Fisher 2005). Long-term use of anticonvulsants, psychotropic medications, antibiotics, anticonvulsants, antidepressants, antihypertensives, lipid-lowering agents, and laxative medications alter taste and smell (Bromley 2000). All of these factors require the use of a multi-level framework for developing tailored programmes that address the unique needs of people with intellectual disabilities to achieve sustainable behavioural changes within a supportive environment.

The physiological characteristics of an individual may affect that person's choices regardless of understanding of the choice (Conner and Armitage 2002). Food choice is affected by disability-related characteristics and by eating disorder conditions (Drewnowski 1997). For example, due to their disability, people with Prader-Willi syndrome lack satiety triggers. The constant feeling of hunger in some instances is so severe that the person can put their life in danger by extreme overeating. However, a person's distinctive characteristic should not be the sole focus of providing a plausible solution to support individuals with Prader-Willi in living a healthful lifestyle; instead, external supports and influences need to be considered in finding an acceptable solution.

Environment and situational supports

Where people live and the types of environment in which they reside can control (or modify) their food choices. These factors are not easily changed and people often have little control over them. Environment is a physically external factor that affects a person's behaviour (Baranowski et al. 2002); in relation to food this includes availability and accessibility, cost, cultural and religious practices, and media advertising (Conner and Armitage 2002). Situation is a real, distorted or imagined representation of one's cognitive perspective of environment. When we consider the interaction between personal factors, behaviour, and environment (Social Cognitive Theory) and person-centred planning, programme development can incorporate the dynamic characteristics of dietary intake throughout the life cycle given the natural rhythm of environmental and situational changes that will occur within a person's life (O'Brien et al. 1997; Bandura 1998; Baranowski et al. 2002).

Cost, shopping, the time that it takes to prepare foods, storage space limitations, and accessibility were identified as barriers to a healthy diet among the general population (Nestle et al. 1998; Shankar and Klassen 2001). Food availability in grocery stores, homes, and vending machines was also a determinant of food intake. Fruit and vegetable consumption increases when grocery stores carry more fresh produce, workplace cafeterias offer more choices at lower prices, and more healthy choices are available in vending machines (Nestle et al. 1998). Constraints regarding group living, service structures, unclear policy guidelines, and resource limitations may predetermine and limit the availability of foods for making fully informed choices (Messent et al. 1999; Harris et al. 2003).

The participants in a study of people with intellectual disabilities residing in group homes reported that they had no choice over what they were eating by having to accommodate their roommates and follow the requirements of state meal plans. In addition, they had limited or no involvement in grocery shopping while barriers to meal preparation included caregiver concerns about safety and breaking organizational rules that limited involvement with cooking (Rodgers 1998). Limited time for food preparation and menu planning leads to greater purchasing of processed and convenience foods, which are usually higher in fat and calories but easier to prepare (Nestle et al. 1998). Furthermore, limited community exposure and increased routines in the everyday lives of people with intellectual disabilities have decreased experience and exposure to different foods, making fully informed choice difficult (Rawlings et al. 1995).

Social supports

Social support from caregivers, friends, and family members plays an important role in the promotion of independence for people who live in community-based settings and ensuring that they make informed choices. Although over 60 per cent of people with intellectual disabilities in the USA live with members of their families (Fujiura 1998), 52 per cent receive day or employment support services where the work of professional staff is essential (Braddock et al. 2005). Front-line staff work with, support, and assist people with disabilities to lead self-fulfilling and directed lives in their communities. Research suggests that front-line staff often have a low level of health knowledge and poor health habits themselves (Rodgers 1998; Marks and Sisirak 2012). Results from one descriptive research study of health outcomes of staff showed that 60 per cent of the participants had a body mass index (BMI) greater than 25, and that 70 per cent of the participants were smokers (Marks et al. 2005). The few studies that have looked at health promotion interventions for front-line staff showed that staff benefit from educational seminars and personal exercise, and that this can increase the long-term stability of the workforce (White et al. 2006).

Front-line staff and family caregivers have a direct influence on a person's food choice by being role models and gatekeepers for food, and they can influence food choice by their own knowledge of menu planning and grocery shopping, food preparation, and attitudes and beliefs about food. Food preparation and menu planning are mostly staff responsibilities, even in residential settings (Rodgers 1998). High staff turnover in many countries have been found to range from 50 to 75 per cent annually, resulting in inadequate training, education, and staffing levels, which decreases the quality of social and emotional supports for people with intellectual disabilities (Hatton et al. 2001; Research and Training Center on Rural Rehabilitation Services 2002).

Support persons are vital in teaching and supporting people with intellectual disabilities to achieve more healthy food choice-making (Smyth and Bell 2006). The ability of caregivers not just to inform but to teach nutrition information increases the likelihood of a person with intellectual disabilities making a more informed choice. Providing staff with the necessary information, skills, and confidence to teach people with intellectual disabilities necessitates training that can occur only with strong organizational and management support. Community-based organizations are facing a challenge with high turnover rates, increased job strain, and labour shortages that may lead to poor attitudes and low collective efficacy to improve the health of people they support. Furthermore, support personnel may not perceive that teaching their clients is a part of their job and may view it as an unnecessary burden on their already busy schedule (Heller et al. 2000).

Attitudes

Attitudes are predecessors of determinants of behaviour. People anticipate what will happen as a result of their behaviour and given situation. These anticipations or outcome expectations have been learned from previous personal experiences and situations (doing), observing others in similar situations (seeing), and hearing about these situations from others (hearing) (Baranowski et al. 2002). There are three major types of outcome expectations (Bandura 1998). The first type of outcome expectations is the physical effect of the behaviour. This can be a pleasant sensory experience, such as taste that induces physical pleasure, or a negative physical reaction that induces discomfort. The second type of outcome is social expectation, more specifically outcomes related to an individual's social network such as family, community-based organizations, caregivers, and peers. The last outcome expectation is related to the self-evaluative response to one's behaviour. This response can be positive or negative (Bandura 1998; Baranowski et al. 2002). Self-evaluative response and social outcome expectation produce motivation to comply with a social norm (Bandura 1998).

Although food preferences are linked to exposure to food items, exposure is a function of cultural norms. People are exposed to foods that are in their culture and are accepted by their culture. Social psychological variables such as attitudes and beliefs may reveal more direct and modifiable factors of food choice (Conner and Armitage 2002).

Attitudes also depend on the value a person puts on a specific outcome. Bandura (1986) labels these incentives as outcome expectancies. Outcome expectations and outcome expectancies combined form attitudes towards behaviour. Expectancies have been used in research and shown to influence consumption of fruits and vegetables among children and adults (Domel et al. 1995; Reid et al. 2005).

Self-efficacy

Growing evidence suggests that self-efficacy (self-confidence) is one of the most influential determinants of health status and functioning (Bandura 1998; Anderson et al. 2001). Self-efficacy is one's personal confidence in the ability to perform and overcome barriers of specific activity (Bandura 1986, 1994; Baranowski et al. 2002). Four constructs influence a person's belief of self-efficacy.

First, performance accomplishment or mastery of experience has the strongest effect on increasing self-efficacy (Bandura 1994). People with intellectual disabilities who are introduced to different types of food and encouraged to try them will have a more robust opportunity and fullness of making choices, while boosting their self-efficacy through lived experience. Second, through vicarious or observational learning, behaviour is affected by the person's perceived resemblance to the model or person whose activity is being observed (Bandura 1994). Peer and caregiver modelling can play a major role and influence self-efficacy of food choice of individuals with disability. The third construct used to strengthen a person's self-efficacy is social or verbal persuasion; this involves encouragement and the giving of verbal cues so that people can master skills and become more likely to work harder than people who are not self-confident (Bandura 1994).

The last source of influence for self-efficacy is based on a person's emotional state. Self-efficacy affects emotions, goals, outcome expectations, motivation, and behaviour. Consequently, emotional states, such as depression, can affect self-efficacy, which in turn influences health functioning (Bandura 1994, 2000; Schnoll and Zimmerman 2001). Self-control, self-management, and goal setting are the targets of health education, so performing health behaviours will be under the individual's control (Schnoll and Zimmerman 2001; Baranowski et al. 2002). For example, individuals who are given a choice between several different food items can make a choice fully knowing the consequences of that choice.

Increased interdependence of human experience is based on collective agency and group belief; more power for change is built thorough collective action (Bandura 2000). Many people with intellectual disabilities live their entire lives relying on their family members, multiple professionals, and peers for support (Carnaby 1998). As such, in addition to focusing on building skills among individuals with intellectual disabilities, building collective efficacy among proxy agents (for example, staff, caregivers) is often a necessary component in efforts to build and obtain the necessary resources and expertise. While building individual efficacy increases the person's confidence (including staff) in changing behaviour as well as role-modelling to peers, encouraging collective efficacy builds collective voice, empowerment, and self-advocacy, increases group and self-directedness, and can promote social change (Bandura 1994, 2000).

Knowledge and sources of information

Limited educational opportunities, and inaccurate and inaccessible sources of information have resulted in scarce knowledge of healthy eating or health in general (Jobling 2001) and less ability to make informed decisions, including making healthy food choices. Television has been reported as a major, and probably the most widely used, source of health information second only to health professionals (O'Malley et al. 1999). Due to lower levels of employment and high barriers to alternative community-based leisure time activities, people with intellectual disabilities tend to watch more television than the general population (Frey et al. 2005; Bowe 2006). In addition, media messages have been found to confuse this population regarding information related to health and food choice (Rodgers 1998).

Changing health through food choices

By using the EFFC, caregivers can build collective efficacy to support people with intellectual disabilities in making food choices and living successful lives in community-based settings. Focusing on individual factors and building individual efficacy of the dyad of the person with the disability and caregiver increases collective efficacy (Bandura 1998). The challenge lies in organizational support, training, and establishing guidelines of what constitutes a true choice for a person with intellectual disabilities (Rawlings et al. 1995; Rodgers 1998; Harris et al. 2003; Smyth and Bell 2006).

The EFFC can guide understanding of how people with intellectual disabilities make food choices, reduce the risk of disease, manage existing health conditions, promote healthy ageing, increase wellbeing and self-efficacy, empower, and create opportunities for individuals to become active participants in making decisions regarding their health.

Furthermore, community-based organizations that provide support and services for people with intellectual disabilities can use a systematic process for planning, implementing, and evaluating interventions. They can gain a clearer understanding of targeted health behaviours on individual, organizational, and environmental levels taking into consideration ecological concepts of intrapersonal factors, interpersonal processes and primary groups, institutional factors, community factors, and public policy and still work within the principles of equity, accessibility, acceptability, and availability. Using the EFFC can promote a better understanding about the following questions: (1) How are people choosing the foods that they eat? (2) What are the issues that we need to know about before we develop and implement intervention programmes? (3) How can we focus our programmes to ensure success? And (4) how will we evaluate our programmes? Lastly, personal self-assessment will lead to greater independence, empowerment, community integration, taking charge of one's own body, and a decrease in the cost of training and service delivery.

Case study

Dottie is a 36-year-old female with Down syndrome. She is living in a community home with three other roommates with 24-hour staff supervision. Dottie has expressed a desire to learn how to prepare meals independently, including planning a meal and grocery shopping. Dottie also has Type 2 diabetes and a slight visual disability and she needs large print to be able to read. Using the EFFC, use the following questions to create a plan for Dottie to realize her goal to prepare her meals independently.

1   What are Dottie's personal characteristics (for example, gender, age, types of disabilities, and health status that may require accommodations, food preferences) that may influence her goal?
2   What are the modifying conditions (e.g. living arrangement, available foods, and transportation to fresh food markets or grocery stores, storage issues)?

3   What are mediating mechanisms (e.g. organizational capacity for food planning, purchasing, and preparation, labour shortage, employee turnover rates)?
4   Are there members of staff in the home who can teach Dottie how to plan a meal, purchase, and prepare food (caregiver knowledge, self-confidence, and attitudes towards food planning, purchasing, and preparation)?
5   What knowledge does Dottie have about meal planning, grocery shopping, and food preparation?
6   What knowledge does Dottie have about her health condition?
7   What knowledge do staff members have about Dottie's health condition?

Summary

- The EFFC can be used to understand how people with intellectual disabilities make food choices and can guide the development of appropriate, accessible, effective, and successful health promotion and education programmes while promoting community integration in this population.
- Material circumstances, living arrangement, food availability and accessibility affect a person's food choices.
- Influencing individual and collective factors such as attitudes, nutrition knowledge, efficacy, and organizational elements, including job strain, turnover rates, and labour shortages may have a direct effect on improving food choices and health behaviours.

Acknowledgements

This document was produced under grant number H133B080009 awarded by the US Department of Education's National Institute on Disability and Rehabilitation Research to the Rehabilitation Research and Training Center on Aging with Developmental Disabilities-Lifespan Health and Function at the University of Illinois at Chicago. The contents of this chapter do not necessarily represent the policy of the US Department of Education, and should not be assumed as being endorsed by the US Federal Government.

Useful resources

- Marks, B., Sisirak, J. and Heller, T. (2010) *Health Matters: The Exercise, Nutrition and Health Education Curriculum for People with Developmental Disabilities*. Baltimore, MD: Brookes Publishing.

- Marks, B., Sisirak, J. and Heller, T. (2010) *Health Matters for People with Developmental Disabilities: Creating a Sustainable Health Promotion Program*. Baltimore, MD: Brookes Publishing.

- Marks, B., Sisirak, J., Medlen, J. and Magallanes, E. (2012) *HealthMessages Program: Healthy Lifestyle Coaches Coaching Manual*. HealthMattersProgram.org.

- Medlen, J.E. (2006) *The Down Syndrome Nutrition Handbook: A Guide to Promoting Healthy Lifestyles*, 2nd edn. Portland, OR: Phronesis Publishing.

- Medlen, J.E. (2011) *Cooking by Color: Recipes for Independence*. Portland, OR: Phronesis Publishing.

Web resources

- Different types of food: http://www.easyhealth.org.uk/categories/different-types-of-food- (leaflets)

References

Anderson, E.S., Winett, R.A., Wojcik, J.R., Winett, S.G. and Bowden, T. (2001) A computerized social cognitive intervention for nutrition behavior: direct and mediated effects on fat, fiber, fruits, and vegetables, self-efficacy, and outcome expectations among food shoppers. *Annals of Behavioral Medicine*, 23: 88–100.

Bandura, A. (1977) *Social Learning Theory*. Englewood Cliffs, NJ: Prentice-Hall.

Bandura, A. (1986) *Social Foundations of Thought and Action: A Social Cognitive Theory*. Englewood Cliffs, NJ: Prentince-Hall.

Bandura, A. (1994) Self-efficacy, in V.S. Ramachaudran (ed.) *Encyclopedia of Human Behavior*. New York: Academic Press.

Bandura, A. (1998) Health promotion from the perspective of social cognitive theory. *Psychology and Health*, 13: 623–49.

Bandura, A. (2000) Exercise of human agency through collective efficacy. *Current Directions in Psychological Science*, 9: 75–8.

Baranowski, T., Perry, C.L. and Parcel, G.S. (2002) How individuals, environments, and health behavior interact: social cognitive theory, in K. Glanz, B.K. Rimer and F.M. Lewis (eds.) *Health Behavior and Health Education: Theory, Research, and Practice*, 3rd edn. San Francisco, CA: Jossey-Bass.

Beange, H., McElduff, A. and Baker, W. (1995) Medical disorders of adults with mental retardation: a population study. *American Journal on Mental Retardation*, 99: 595–604.

Bowe, F.G. (2006) *Video and People with Disabilities*. Hempstead, NY: Hofstra University.

Braddock, D., Hemp, R., Rizzolo, M.C., Coulter, D., Haffer, L. and Thompson, M. (2005) *The State of the States in Developmental Disabilities: 2005*. Washington, DC: American Association on Mental Retardation.

Bromley, S.M. (2000) Smell and taste disorders: a primary care approach. *American Family Physician*, 61: 427–36.

Carnaby, S. (1998) Reflections on social integration for people with intellectual disability: does interdependence have a role? *Journal of Intellectual and Developmental Disability*, 23: 219–28.

Conner, M. and Armitage, C.J. (2002) *The Social Psychology of Food*. Buckingham: Open University Press.

Cumella, S., Ransford, N., Lyons, J. and Burnham, H. (2000) Needs for oral care among people with intellectual disability not in contact with Community Dental Services. *Journal of Intellectual Disability Research*, 44: 45–52.

Domel, S.B., Baranowski, T., Davis, H.C., Thompson, W.O., Leonard, S.B. and Baranowski, J. (1995) A measure of outcome expectations for fruit and vegetable consumption among fourth and fifth grade children: reliability and validity. *Health Education Research*, 10: 65–72.

Draheim, C.C., Williams, D.P. and McCubbin, J.A. (2002) Physical activity, dietary intake, and the insulin resistance syndrome in nondiabetic adults with mental retardation. *American Journal of Mental Retardation*, 107: 361–75.

Drewnowski, A. (1997) Taste preferences and food intake. *Annual Review of Nutrition*, 17: 237–53.

Frey, G.C., Buchanan, A.M. and Sandt, D.D.R. (2005) 'I'd rather watch TV': an examination of physical activity in adults with mental retardation. *Mental Retardation*, 43: 241–54.

Fujiura, G.T. (1998) Demography of family households. *American Journal of Mental Retardation*, 103: 225–35.

Fujiura, G.T., Fitzsimons, N., Marks, B. and Chicoine, B. (1997) Predictors of BMI among adults with Down syndrome: the social context of health promotion. *Research in Developmental Disabilities*, 18: 261–74.

Hamilton, J., McIlveen, H. and Strugnell, C. (2000) Educating young consumers – a food choice model. *Journal of Consumer Studies and Home Economics*, 24: 113–23.

Harris, N., Rosemberg, A., Jangda, S., O'Brien, K. and Gallagher, M. (2003) Prevalence of obesity in International Special Olympic athletes as determined by body mass index. *Journal of the American Dietetic Association*, 103: 235–7.

Hatton, C., Emerson, E., Rivers, M., Mason, H., Swarbrick, R., Mason, L. et al. (2001) Factors associated with intended staff turnover and job search behaviour in services for people with intellectual disability. *Journal of Intellectual Disability Research*, 45: 258–70.

Hayden, M.F. (1998) Mortality among people with MR living in the United States: research review and policy application. *Mental Retardation*, 36: 345–59.

Heller, T., Miller, A., Hsieh, K. and Sterns, H.(2000) Later life planning: promoting knowledge of options and choice-making. *Mental Retardation*, 38: 395–406.

Janicki, M., Dalton, A., Henderson, C. and Davidson, P. (1999) Mortality and morbidity among older adults with intellectual disability: health service considerations. *Disability Rehabilitation*, 21: 284–94.

Jansen, D.E.M.C., Krol, B., Groothoff, J.W. and Post, D. (2004) People with intellectual disability and their health problems: a review of comparative studies. *Journal of Intellectual Disability Research*, 48: 93–102.

Jobling, A. (2001) Beyond sex and cooking: health education for individuals with intellectual disability. *Mental Retardation*, 39: 310–21.

Marks, B. and Sisirak, J. (2012) What about staff? Impact of HealthMatters Train-the-Trainer for direct support professionals. Presented at the *2012 IASSID World Congress*, Halifax, Nova Scotia, Canada.

Marks, B., Sisirak, J., Heller, T. and Hsieh, K. (2005) Health status, perceptions, and behavior of staff working with people with intellectual and developmental disabilities. Presented at the *133rd Annual Meeting and Exposition of the American Public Health Association*, Philadelphia, PA.

McElmurry, B. J., Marks, B. and Cianelli, R. (2002) *Primary Health Care in the Americas: Conceptual Framework, Experiences, Challenges and Perspectives*. Geneva: WHO.

Melville, C.A., Hamilton, S., Hankey, C.R., Miller, S. and Boyle, S. (2007) The prevalence and determinants of obesity in adults with intellectual disabilities. *Obesity Reviews*, 8(3): 223–30.

Messent, P.R., Cooke, C.B. and Long, J. (1999) What choice? A consideration of the level of opportunity for people with mild and moderate learning disabilities to lead a physically active healthy lifestyle. *British Journal of Learning Disabilities*, 27: 73–7.

Nestle, M., Wing, R., Birch, L., Disogra, L., Drewnowski A., Middleton, S. et al. (1998) Behavioral and social influences on food choice. *Nutrition Reviews*, 56: S50–S64.

O'Brien, C.L., O'Brien, J. and Mount, B. (1997) Person-Centered Planning has arrived . . . or has it? *Mental Retardation*, 35: 480–4.

O'Malley, A.S., Kerner, J.F. and Johnson, L. (1999) Are we getting the message out to all? Health information sources and ethnicity. *American Journal of Preventive Medicine*, 17: 198–202.

Pezzementi, M.L. and Fisher, M.A. (2005) Oral health status of people with intellectual disabilities in the southeastern United States. *Journal of the American Dental Association*, 136: 903–12.

Rawlings, M., Dowse, L. and Shaddock, A. (1995) Increasing the involvement of people with an intellectual disability in choice making situations: a practical approach. *International Journal of Disability, Development and Education*, 42: 137–53.

Reid, M., Bunting, J. and Hammersley, R. (2005) Relationships between the Food Expectancy Questionnaire (FEQ) and the Food Frequency Questionnaire (FFQ). *Appetite*, 45: 127–36.

Research and Training Center on Rural Rehabilitation Services (2002) Direct service staff turnover in supported living arrangements: preliminary results and observations. *Rural Disability and Rehabilitation Research Progress Report*. Missoula, MT: Research and Training Center on Rural Rehabilitation Services.

Rimmer, J.H. and Yamaki, K. (2006) Obesity and intellectual disability. *Mental Retardation and Developmental Disabilities Research Reviews*, 12: 22–7.

Robertson, J., Emerson, E., Gregory, N., Hatton, C., Kessissoglou, S. and Hallam, A. (2000) Receipt of psychotropic medication by people with intellectual disability in residential settings. *Journal of Intellectual Disability Research*, 44: 666–76.

Rodgers, J. (1998) 'Whatever's on her plate': food in the lives of people with learning disabilities. *British Journal of Learning Disabilities*, 26: 13–26.

Samuels, R. and Chadwick, D.D. (2006) Predictors of asphyxiation risk in adults with intellectual disabilities and dysphagia. *Journal of Intellectual Disability Research*, 50: 362–70.

Schnoll, R. and Zimmerman, B.J. (2001) Self-regulation training enhances dietary self-efficacy and dietary fiber consumption. *Journal of the American Dietetic Association*, 101: 1006–11.

Shankar, S. and Klassen, A. (2001) Influence on fruit and vegetable procurement and consumption among urban African-American public housing residents, and potential strategies for intervention. *Family Economics and Nutrition Review*, 13: 34–46.

Sisirak, J., Marks, B., Heller, T. and Riley, B. (2007) Dietary habits of adults with intellectual and developmental disabilities residing in community-based settings. Presented at the *135th Annual Meeting and Exposition of the American Public Health Association*, Washington, DC, 6 November.

Smyth, C.M. and Bell, D. (2006) From biscuits to boyfriends: the ramifications of choice for people with learning disabilities. *British Journal of Learning Disabilities*, 34: 227–36.

Sorensen, G., Emmons, K.M., Hunt, M.K., Barbeau, E.M., Goldman, R., Petersonb, K. et al. (2003) Model of incorporating social context in health behavior interventions: applications for cancer prevention for working-class, multiethnic populations. *Preventive Medicine*, 37: 188–97.

Sorensen, G., Stoddard, A.M., Dubowitz, T., Barbeau, E.M., Bigby, J., Emmons, K.M. et al. (2007) The influence of social context on changes in fruit and vegetable consumption: results of the healthy directions studies. *American Journal of Public Health*, 97: 1216–27.

Stewart, L. (2003) Development of the Nutrition and Swallowing Checklist, a screening tool for nutrition risk and swallowing risk in people with intellectual disability. *Journal of Intellectual and Developmental Disability*, 28: 171–87.

Taggart, L., Truesdale-Kennedy, M. and Coates, V. (2012) Management and quality indicators of diabetes mellitus in people with intellectual disabilities. *Journal of Intellectual Disability Research* (DOI: 10.1111/j.1365-2788.2012.01633.x)

Wetter, A.C., Goldberg, J.P., King, A.C., Sigman-Grant, M., Baer, R., Crayton, E. et al. (2001) How and why do individuals make food and physical activity choices? *Nutrition Reviews*, 59: S11–S20.

White, P., Edwards, N. and Townsend-White, C. (2006) Stress and burnout amongst professional carers of people with intellectual disability: another health inequity. *Current Opinion in Psychiatry*, 19: 502–7.

Whitehead, D. (2001) A social congitive model for health education/health promotion practice. *Journal of Advanced Nursing*, 36: 417–25.

Yamaki, K. (2005) Body weight status among adults with intellectual disability in the community. *Mental Retardation*, 43(1): 1–10.

5 Obesity

Eamonn Slevin and Ruth Northway

Introduction

Evidence suggests that people with an intellectual disability are more susceptible to being overweight/obese than others. This chapter presents information on how overweight/obesity can be measured, and provides an overview of the extent of overweight/obesity in people. This is followed by a discussion of the impacts that can result from being obese. Details on the main causative factors of overweight/obesity, including barriers to maintaining a healthy body weight, are presented. Within the chapter we present suggestions on how people with intellectual disabilities might be helped to achieve a normal healthy weight via health promotion activities. The overall emphasis of the chapter is that success in obtaining a normal healthy body weight requires commitment to making lifelong changes, and that health promotion for people with intellectual disabilities needs to take this into account.

Definitions and screening

Overweight/obesity can be defined as abnormally high body fat content that usually will impair health – if not at present, then in the future. A number of assessments can be used to classify if an individual is overweight or obese, and three main approaches are presented below.

Body mass index

Body mass index (BMI) is the most widely used measure for identifying overweight/obesity. An individual's BMI is calculated by dividing their weight in kilograms by the square of their height in metres (kg/m^2). The WHO (2011) states that for adults a BMI of 25 or over is overweight, while a BMI of 30 or over indicates obesity. Table 5.1 shows the various BMI weight classifications.

The BMI classification of children is not as straightforward and needs adjustment based on age and gender. In children, BMI cut-off points for age and gender are used and a number of these cut-off points have been developed. One of the most common is that developed from across

Table 5.1 Weight classifications according to BMI

BMI	Weight classification
Less than 18.5	Underweight
18.5 to 24.9	Healthy weight
25.0 to 29.9	Overweight
30 or higher	Obese

Table 5.2 An example of BMI cut-off classifications for children

Age (years)	BMI Male	BMI Female	BMI Male	BMI Female
	> = Overweight		> = Obese	
4	17.55	17.28	19.29	19.15
4.5	17.47	17.19	19.26	19.12
5	17.42	17.15	19.30	19.17
5.5	17.45	17.20	19.47	19.34

international countries by Cole et al. (2000) for the International Obesity Task Force (IOTF). This sets cut-off points for overweight and obesity for children aged 2–18 years of age differentiating by sex. Table 5.2 shows an example of this for some ages.

It is important to note that BMI alone is not meant to diagnose overweight/obesity but to function as a screening measure. This is because BMI correlates with the amount of body fat rather than directly measuring it. A good example of this limitation is a professional boxer who may have a BMI in the overweight classification but have little or no excess body fat. Body mass index is a useful population surveillance screening measure but other criteria may be required to identify overweight in individuals.

Waist circumference

Waist circumference is a useful measure of central body fat and a strong predictor of health problems if waist size is higher than recommended. The British Government and WHO (2008) state that men with a waist circumference of 37 inches (94 cm) or more, and women with a waist circumference of 31 inches (80 cm) or more are at greater risk of developing health problems. As waist circumference increases above these values, so too do the health risks.

As with BMI, different waist circumference measurements should be used for children based on their age and sex. There are not as many published cut-off points for waist circumference in children but some have been published (see, for example, McCarthy et al. 2003).

Bioelectrical measures of body fat

Bioelectrical impedance using a BodyStat Composition Analyser can be used to measure the fat content of the body. This is a small battery-operated device, which, with electrodes placed on the person's hand and foot to record their body fat, indicates if their fat content is high, medium or low for their age and gender.

The extent of overweight/obesity in intellectually disabled people

Research indicates that significantly higher percentages of people with an intellectual disability are overweight/obese compared with non-intellectually disabled individuals. This evidence is widely reported internationally for children. Stewart et al. (2009) reported the prevalence of overweight/obesity in Scottish children with intellectual disability to be 37 per cent for boys (versus 20 per cent for non-intellectually disabled boys) and 36 per cent girls (versus 15 per cent for non-intellectually disabled girls). In France, Salaun and Berthouze-Aranda (2011) reported that over 45 per cent of a sample of school pupils with intellectual disability had excessive body fat and over 30 per cent had high ratings of abdominal fat. These authors also reported that overweight/obesity according to BMI was 26 per cent for the sample of intellectually disabled pupils compared with 17.8 per cent for similarly aged children without intellectual disability. When some specific conditions related to intellectual disabilities have been researched, much higher rates of overweight/obesity have been identified. Rimmer et al. (2010: 792) reported that in young people with autism, Down syndrome, and spina bifida, overweight and obesity is 'two to four times higher than in non-disabled youths matched on age and gender'.

The tendency to be overweight in children persists into adulthood. Thomas and Kerr (2011) evaluated a health promotion intervention with 191 adults with an intellectual disability. At the beginning of the programme, 31 per cent of the participants were overweight, 31 per cent were obese, and 7 per cent were morbidly obese (BMI ≥40). After two years, approximately half of the participants who were deemed 'at risk' based on their BMI maintained a stable weight, and while 25 per cent showed an improvement in weight status, almost as many (22 per cent) got worse.

Gale et al. (2009) gathered data concerning 1097 adults with intellectual disabilities and found that BMI status was only available for 688 (62.8 per cent of the total sample). They suggest that this lack of data for a large percentage of the sample indicated that primary care services do not routinely record up-to-date measurements for many people with intellectual disabilities. When data were available, it was found that more than a quarter of the sample was overweight and one-third was obese. Significantly more women than men had a higher than desired BMI. Melville et al. (2008) conducted a cross-sectional study of 945 adults with intellectual disabilities aged from 16 to over 75. They also found that women were significantly more likely to be obese than men but that there was no correlation between BMI and age for either sex.

Impact of being overweight/obese

As stated above, people with intellectual disabilities are more likely to be overweight/obese than those without such disabilities. This is a major concern, as this population are often already disadvantaged because of their disability, and it could be argued that due to their susceptibility to being overweight they are doubly disadvantaged. This may lead to negative impacts in a number of areas.

Physical health impacts

Physical health impacts include:

- cardiac and circulatory problems including hypertension, heart disease, stroke, and increased risk for other circulatory problems (see Chapter 8). There is also evidence that the increased cholesterol associated with being overweight may hasten the onset of some dementias
- respiratory problems, such as shortness of breath, negative impacts on asthma symptoms, and sleep disorders such as sleep apnoea
- some cancers are increasingly being associated with obesity, including stomach and colon, breast, endometrial, and prostate cancers (see Chapter 9)
- musculoskeletal problems, such as joint pains, muscle cramps, arthritis, severe limitations to or loss of mobility
- gastric problems, including tooth decay due to a diet high in sugar, gallbladder problems, excessive gases and gastric bloating, liver problems, and potentially increases in a number of gastric cancers
- endocrine disorders, the most common being the very strong association between Type 2 diabetes and overweight/obesity.

Psychological and emotional

Research has found that from as early as 5 years of age, higher body weight is associated with lower self-concept, and that parental concern about a child's weight reinforces the child's negative self-evaluation (Davison and Birch 2001). Friedman et al. (2002) reported that the degree of obesity is correlated with body-image evaluation, and that this is related to both depression and self-esteem.

Social isolation

A child or adult with intellectual disability who has behavioural problems, such as being antisocial, anxious, dependent, depressed or withdrawn, has an increased likelihood of becoming obese. Obesity may lead to a child or adult being stigmatized and experiencing isolation and despondency, as they are viewed as being a 'fat person' rather than a 'person'. Social isolation may even be manifested in schools, as research has found teachers to show more positive attitudes to thinner pupils. Such attitudes have led to the identification of what has been called the 'obesity bias': this can result in isolation of pupils with disorders related to their body perception

Family impact

Health or psychological problems that affect people with intellectual disabilities due to overweight/obesity can add to the stress of family members and caregivers. If a young person with an intellectual disability is distressed and unhappy because of their weight, or they are being bullied in school (see Chapter 15), caregiving parents feel the emotional labour of this as personal distress. In addition, research on obese children has shown that the degree of obesity within the family is an important predictor of body weight in adulthood (Zeller et al. 2007). Various factors may impact negatively on parents; for example, they may feel guilty if they think their child is obese, frustrated at not being able to help their child lose weight, and angry if their child is subject to prejudice because they are fat.

Causative factors and barriers

It might seem that the causes of being overweight/obese are simple, namely that higher nutritional intake than required coupled with less energy expenditure leads to overweight. However, it is much more complex than this, as evidenced by the great difficulty most overweight people face in attempting to lose weight. Rimmer et al. (2007) suggest that the potential antecedents of obesity unique to adolescents and children with disabilities are lack of physical activity, nutrition, knowledge or awareness, and social participation. These in turn may be influenced by an array of genetic, psychological, social, cultural, and financial issues.

Genetic and physical factors

Some conditions and syndromes associated with intellectual disability predispose this population to be more overweight than others, such as Prader-Willi syndrome and Down syndrome. Co-morbid health problems such as cerebral palsy, spina bifida or other conditions that limit mobility may also lead to overweight (Rimmer et al. 2010). In addition, some people with autism may rigidly adhere to a diet that leads to overweight/obesity. It should be noted, however, that although these conditions may predispose the person to be overweight, it should not be considered inevitable that all people with such conditions will be overweight.

Psychological factors

Psychological influences can have a major impact on the body weight of people with intellectual disability. Food is a strong reinforcement of behaviour and some carers may inadvertently provide sugary or other high-calorie foods to pacify the person with an intellectual disability. If lacking stimuli in other areas of their life, people may turn to food as a comfort. Co-morbid mental health problems such as depression, emotional problems or fatigue can lead to the person both overeating and lacking in motivation to be physically active, which then leads to overweight. Mental health problems and behaviours that challenge can lead to the person being prescribed antipsychotic medications. There are also high numbers of people with intellectual disability on anti-epileptic drugs. Many of these or other psychotropic medications have the side-effect of weight gain (Singh et al. 2010) (see Chapter 7).

The cognitive understanding of the person with an intellectual disability can in itself influence body weight, as the individual may not have the necessary understanding to adhere to a healthy diet and adequate physical activity.

Social and cultural factors

There may be issues of overprotection leading to children and adults being prevented from going out independently and thus having reduced levels of physical activity. Or there may be negative social attitudes towards them using leisure facilities, joining in sports with others or forming friendships with non-disabled peers. This can lead to social exclusion of the person and limit their activity levels as well as impacting on their esteem.

Some caregivers may hold attitudes about nutritional intake for the person with an intellectual disability such as 'what else have they got?' or 'food keeps them happy' and they therefore do not see the need to encourage healthy nutritional habits. In addition, in some staffed residential settings there might be similar overprotective cultures and in various settings clients have little choice in their diet and activities undertaken.

Financial and other barriers

International research in the last decade or so indicates that obesity is associated with families of lower socio-economic status (Utter et al. 2010). These studies reported an association between increased obesity and lower socio-economic status in all populations. A comparison of families supporting a child with and without intellectual disability found that families with intellectual disability were '(1) more likely to be poor, (2) more likely to become poor, and (3) less likely to escape from being poor' (Emerson et al. 2010: 224). Research undertaken by one of the authors of this chapter found that school children with an intellectual disability who lived in areas of low socio-economic status had significantly higher levels of overweight and obesity than both intellectually disabled and non-disabled children who lived in areas of higher socio-economic status (Slevin et al. 2008). This study also identified various barriers to maintaining a healthy lifestyle for the intellectually disabled pupils and their families (see Figure 5.1).

There is evidence that adiposity laid down in childhood leads to overweight and obesity in adulthood. When children and adolescents reach adulthood, additional barriers might include overuse of alcohol to fit in with peers or lack of work, which can lead to dejection (see Chapter 12).

Rather than one causative factor of overweight/obesity for people with intellectual disabilities, the condition can be seen as a propelling cycle of events (as presented in Figure 5.2), which, if not broken or countered, may persist throughout life, ultimately shortening longevity for the obese person.

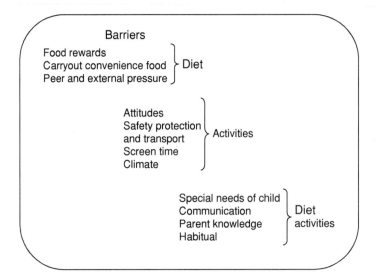

Figure 5.1 Barriers to maintaining a healthy weight

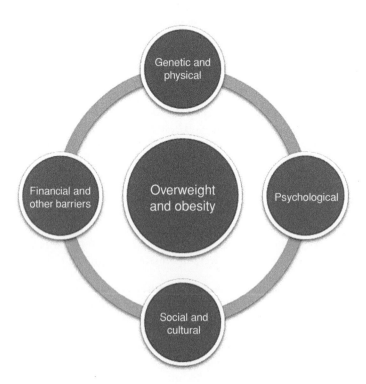

Figure 5.2 Factors that cause or influence overweight and obesity

Health promotion strategies

To help individuals with intellectual disabilities who are obese, input will be required in four areas: individual, family, services, and community/society (see Chapter 2). Aspects that can help people with intellectual disabilities maintain a healthy body weight are presented below; these draw on recognized recommendations from across international guidelines, including NICE (2006) guidelines in the UK, the WHO in Europe and further afield, and the US Department of Agriculture, and Department of Health and Human Services.

Individual

National Institute for Health and Care Excellence (NICE 2006: 10) stated that, 'Weight management programmes should include behaviour change strategies to increase people's physical activity . . . improve eating behaviour and . . . reduce energy intake'. They also stated that 'A person needs to be in "energy balance" to maintain a healthy weight: that is, their energy intake (from food) should not exceed the energy expended through everyday activities and exercise' (NICE 2006: 13). Individuals with an intellectual disability who are overweight will need to change their dietary and physical activity behaviours but they need help to do this.

Nutrition

Nutrition is addressed in the previous chapter, so it is not discussed in detail here other than to say that the person should be educated and supported to eat a balanced diet that is low in fat, sugar, and salt but contains the recommended five portions of fruit and vegetables a day. Portion sizes should be controlled, meals should not be missed, and snacking between meals should be reduced. In the UK, the Department of Health, in association with the Welsh Government, the Scottish Government, and the Food Standards Agency in Northern Ireland, recommends that foods should be taken in accordance with the portions outlined in the Eat Well Plate (see Figure 5.3).

For many years, the US Department of Agriculture, and Department of Health and Human Services recommended a food pyramid as a guide to healthy nutrition; this has now been replaced

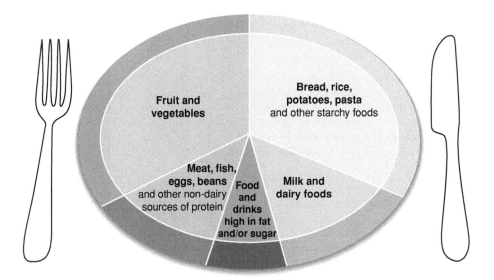

Figure 5.3 The food group quantities as recommended on the NHS 'Eat Well Plate'

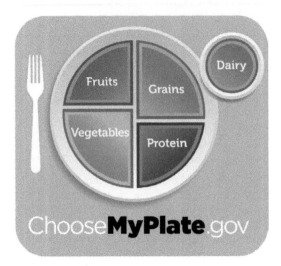

Figure 5.4 Myplate as used in the USA
Source: © US Department of Agriculture

with a much simpler symbol called Myplate (see Figure 5.4). This plate indicates that half of the diet should be made up of fruit and vegetables, followed by grains and then proteins. Dairy products are placed outside the plate and these should be eaten in fewer proportions in the diet. Myplate provides a simple guide to follow and it is adapted in accordance with need and age; for example, if someone does not want to eat dairy products, they can use alternatives such as soy.

Both the Eat Well and Myplate government sites offer additional guidance on meal portion sizes, replacing sugary drinks with water, and reducing fat and sugary foods.

Physical activity

Physical activity is necessary to help reduce body weight but the more obese the person is, the more unfit they are and the less motivation they have to exercise (see Chapter 16). This chain needs to be broken if successful weight loss is to occur. The following will help the person with an intellectual disability to lose weight:

- Set small and achievable goals – aim to lose 1–2 pounds (0.45–0.9 kg) per week.
- Select forms of physical activity that the person enjoys.
- Aim for at least 30 minutes of moderate activity on at least five days per week.
- Build activity into all normal day actions, including taking stairs rather than lifts, walking to school or work rather than using transport.
- Gradually reduce sedentary activities and replace with more activity.

Education

Individuals with intellectual disabilities should be taught in small steps the various health problems to which obesity can lead. For those with the most limited communication, pictures, videos, and computer packages are helpful. As well as educating individuals with intellectual disabilities about health problems, they need education and support to reduce weight if overweight/obese. Health promotion programmes should be based on the following:

- Person-centred and tailored to the individual.
- Empowering individuals to take control of their life.

- Behaviour change promoted by reinforcing a healthier lifestyle.
- Providing practical support for the individual to be active.
- Use of persuasion and motivation geared to the individual.
- Support the person to address barriers to their health with respect to weight.
- Health assessments and treatments of factors influencing body weight, including review of medications.
- Providing social support, as losing weight with others is helpful.

Family

The family of the person with an intellectual disability needs attention in two respects. First, they are important role models for the person with the intellectual disability. Second, they may need education on how to help the person with an intellectual disability achieve and maintain a healthy weight. George et al. (2011) reported significant associations between family health habits, parents' activity levels, and high BMI values in their children with intellectual disability. The factors above that are identified for an individual with an intellectual disability also need consideration in relation to the family.

Nutrition

Family members need encouragement to purchase healthy foods and reduce the consumption of convenience meals. The importance of eating together as a family should be emphasized, and people with an intellectual disability discouraged from eating alone or eating sitting watching TV. Children with intellectual disabilities should be provided with healthy lunch packs if they take lunches to school and similarly for adults who work.

Physical activity

Family members can do a number of things to help and support the individual with an intellectual disability with their weight, including:

- Taking part in physical activities such as walking, cycling, and going to leisure centres as a family.
- Discouraging their son/daughter from spending long periods of time on sedentary activities.
- Not driving the person with an intellectual disability everywhere, but walking as much as possible.
- A family dog is a good way of encouraging walking and the person with intellectual disability can be encouraged to help with its care.
- Some technologies can help, for example video exercise programmes and games such as the Wii for motion-controlled active sports or play can be used indoors. Use of step pedometers can also be a fun way for the person to record their walking progress. The various smartphones and tablets that are available now also have a vast array of 'apps' that can be used to record and help encourage physical activity; people of all ages are increasingly finding these easy to use.

Education

Education should not only be for the person with intellectual disability but include the family. The following aspects will help:

- Parents need to be discouraged from using unhealthy foods such as sweets as rewards.
- They may require financial advice, as sometimes there is a view that healthy foods are more expensive when in fact many fast foods are more expensive.

- If the family is experiencing poverty, they should be provided with support to make sure they are accessing all the benefits they are entitled to.
- Family attitudes are very important and views such as 'their food is all they have' about their son/daughter should be discouraged.
- Families should be educated to view health holistically and think of future problems that can result from obesity.
- Although families do have a protective role for the person with intellectual disabilities in relation to health vigilance, they should not overprotect the person to an extent that they disempower them.

Residential/supported living and day care services

People with intellectual disabilities who live in residential accommodation/supported living settings and attend day care may be dependent upon their support staff to ensure that they receive an appropriate diet. However, staff work different shifts and staff turnover within individual settings can sometimes make continuity of support difficult. Good communication therefore needs to be maintained to ensure that a balanced diet is offered. In addition, living in group settings can mean choice of diet might be determined by the preferences of other tenants or staff. Melville et al. (2009) suggest that paid carers may require training in relation to the promotion of healthy diets and exercise, and that it should be part of their induction programme. They add that adults with intellectual disabilities are a diverse group with widely differing needs: this diversity must be reflected in the training.

People with mild intellectual disabilities are less likely to receive the support of specific intellectual disabilities services, since they often live unsupported in community settings. They may also face challenges in accessing mainstream health services potentially impacting negatively on their health status, including their weight (Melville et al. 2008). Intellectual disability services need to work closely with primary care providers to ensure that the health promotion needs of this group are both recognized and appropriately addressed. For example, primary care providers need to be encouraged to include people with mild intellectual disabilities within their regular health promotion initiatives and health checks to maintain records of everyone's weight (see Chapter 18).

Community and society

It has been suggested that health promotion interventions aimed at the general population may not be effective for people with intellectual disabilities (Melville et al. 2008). However, inclusion within the wider community has been a key principle underpinning the provision of support for people with intellectual disabilities for many years. Thus, people with intellectual disabilities should be enabled to attend community health promotion activities such as weight loss classes should they wish to do so. This provides valuable peer support and a structured approach to weight loss. Support may be required both for the person with intellectual disabilities and for those leading such classes, to ensure that they are beneficial: professionals working with people with intellectual disabilities could have a key role here.

Ethical aspects

It is important to consider the ethics involved when intervening with a view to changing the weight of individuals with intellectual disabilities. Many ethical frameworks and principles regarding these issues are available but perhaps the most widely used is that proposed by Beauchamp and Childress (2009). They identify four ethical principles: autonomy, non-maleficence, beneficence, and justice.

Autonomy relates to the capacity of individuals to be self-determining and this is often an area of concern in relation to people with intellectual disabilities who may have problems with understanding information, and using this to make an informed decision. In recent years, health promotion materials that are easier to understand have been developed and so information should be more readily accessible both in terms of physical availability and ease of understanding. Linked to person-centred approaches to planning care this can promote outcomes that are acceptable to all involved. However, in a literature review of obesity interventions for people with intellectual disabilities, Jinks et al. (2010) note that few papers reviewed make specific reference to the tension that can arise between respecting client autonomy and a duty of care. They question whether professionals should accept that people with intellectual disabilities (like the general population) may make a conscious decision that they wish to remain overweight. There is a danger that the views of people with intellectual disabilities may be respected as long as they concur with those of other people, but they are deemed to lack capacity if they choose a different course of action.

A tension can arise between the different ethical principles: those supporting people with intellectual disabilities do not generally wish to cause harm (*non-maleficence*) and not enabling an individual to lose weight may cause them physical and psychological harm. Moreover, most people would wish to do good (*beneficence*) and to promote greater wellbeing through promoting weight loss. Both of these principles would be challenged if a person with intellectual disabilities expresses the wish to remain overweight and to continue with their current lifestyle, and those supporting them wish to respect their autonomy.

It is important to be clear as to whether the individual concerned does understand the consequences of their actions both in the short term and – which may be more challenging – in the long term. If they do not have the capacity to make an informed decision, it may be necessary to act in their best interests. It is essential, however, that individual rights are upheld (*justice*) and this may lead to ethical dilemmas for those supporting people with intellectual disabilities

Case study

Jim is in his mid-40s with an intellectual disability. Throughout most of his life he has maintained a healthy body weight with a BMI of 20–24. However, in the past ten years he has gradually put on weight and his BMI has increased to 35. He lives alone in a flat and is fairly independent but tends to eat a lot of junk food and he takes part in very little physical activity. Jim notices that he now becomes out of breath easily when he walks up the stairs to his flat and he also feels a little depressed because many of his clothes no longer fit him.

Jim's community nurse, Ann, has discussed the importance of maintaining a healthy body weight with him and she has educated him on this. She also notes that his blood pressure is high for his age. Together they work on a health living plan that Jim agrees to undertake. They begin by assessing Jim's eating pattern: how often he eats, types of food consumed, and portion sizes. Together they also explore Jim's level of physical activity. Ann provides Jim with a diary in which he records, over a one-week period, the food he eats and the amount of physical activity he undertakes.

Jim eats high-fat foods three to four nights per week and also a lot of sugary foods, such as cakes and biscuits. In addition, he drinks excessive amounts of sugary lemonade and cola drinks (one or two litres every day). His physical activity is very limited and the only time that he leaves his flat is to go to buy food.

Ann develops a written healthy living plan with Jim that is person-centred and includes health promotion interventions that Jim agrees to. He decides to reduce the high-fat takeaway foods from three to four times a week to once a fortnight. He also agrees to start taking a diet high in fruit and vegetables, eat high-fibre bread rather than the white bread he always buys, only eat cake once per week, and to reduce his sugary drinks to diet drinks only and to drink more water. Ann supports him by going food shopping with him when she can, until he has the knowledge of the types of food he should buy. She arranges for him to attend cookery classes, as Jim felt he was not competent in cooking healthy foods. Jim starts a walking programme, incrementally increasing until he takes a brisk walk on at least five days each week. Ann supports Jim to join a weight-watchers club. Jim sticks to the programme, even though he has some lapses but he gets through these with the help of Ann.

Summary

The incidence of overweight among individuals with intellectual disabilities is increasing. Overweight/obesity is a major concern with significant health impacts. Individuals should aim to achieve a better energy balance and a healthy weight as follows:

- Reduce energy intake of total fats and shift fat consumption away from saturated fats to unsaturated fats and towards the elimination of trans-fatty acids.
- Increase consumption of fruits and vegetables, and legumes, whole grains, and nuts.
- Limit the intake of sugary foods.
- Limit salt (sodium) consumption from all sources.
- Find a physical activity that is FUN.
- Gradually increase participation in physical activity as appropriate.
- Be active with family members – both in the home and outside.
- Reduce sedentary habits such as watching TV.

Useful resources

- Bolton, A., Dwyer, T. and Hardcastle, M. (1999) *Promoting Physical Well-being in Mental Health and Learning Disabilities*. Brighton: Pavilion Publishing. This training pack is for those who wish to set up and run a healthy living group that will be fun and interactive for individuals and groups, including adults with intellectual disabilities. Possible outcomes for service users include improved physical activity, weight management, healthy eating, improved self-esteem, increased confidence, and social inclusion.

- *The 3 Fives: Five Keys to Safer Food, Five Keys to a Healthy Diet, Five Keys to Appropriate Physical Activity.* WHO information leaflet: http://www.who.int/foodsafety/consumer/3x5_SA_en.pdf

- The following documents are from the Caroline Walker Trust – *Eating Well at Schools* is available at http://www.cwt.org.uk/pdfs/EatingWellatSchool.pdf, while *Nutrient-based Standards for School Food* is available at http://www.cwt.org.uk/pdfs/eatingwell.pdf

Web resources

- Food and exercise: http://www.easyhealth.org.uk/categories/food-and-exercise/
- Information from WHO about the health implications of obesity: http://www.who.int/topics/obesity/en/
- Eat Well Plate: http://www.nhs.uk/Livewell/Goodfood/Pages/eatwell-plate.aspx
- Myplate: http://www.choosemyplate.gov/food-groups/

References

Beauchamp, T.L. and Childress, J.F. (2009) *Principles of Biomedical Ethics*, 6th edn. Oxford: Oxford University Press

Cole, T.J., Bellizzi, M.C., Flegal, K.M. and Dietz, W.H. (2000) Establishing a standard definition for child overweight and obesity worldwide: international survey. *British Medical Journal*, 320(7244): 1240–5.

Davison, K.K. and Birch, L.L. (2001) Child and parent characteristics as predictors of change in girls' body mass index. *International Journal of Obesity*, 25(12): 1834–42.

Emerson, E., Shahtahmasebi, S., Lancaster, G. and Berridge, D. (2010) Poverty transitions among families supporting a child with intellectual disability. *Journal of Intellectual and Developmental Disability*, 35(4): 224–34

Friedman, K., Reichman, S., Costanzo, P. and Musante, G. (2002) Body image practically medicates the relationship between obesity and psychological distress. *Obesity Research*, 10(1): 33–41.

Gale, L., Naqvi, H. and Russ, L. (2009) Asthma, smoking and BMI in adults with intellectual disabilities: a community-based survey. *Journal of Intellectual Disability Research*, 53(9): 787–96.

George, V.A., Shacter, S.D. and Johnson, P.M. (2011) BMI and attitudes and beliefs about physical activity and nutrition of parents of adolescents with intellectual disabilities. *Journal of Intellectual Disability Research*, 55(11): 1054–63.

Jinks, A., Cotton, A. and Rylance, R. (2010) Obesity interventions for people with a learning disability: an integrative literature review. *Journal of Advanced Nursing*, 67(3): 460–71.

McCarthy, H.D., Ellis, S. and Cole, T. (2003) Central overweight and obesity in British youth aged 11–16: cross sectional surveys of waist circumference. *British Medical Journal*, 326(7390): 624–6.

Melville, C.A., Cooper, S.-A., Morrison, J., Allan, L., Smiley, E. and Williamson, A. (2008) The prevalence and determinants of obesity in adults with intellectual disabilities. *Journal of Applied Research in Intellectual Disabilities*, 21: 425–37.

Melville, C.A., Hamilton, S., Miller, S., Boyle, S., Robinson, N., Pert, C. et al. (2009) Carer knowledge and perceptions of healthy lifestyles for adults with intellectual disabilities, *Journal of Applied Research in Intellectual Disabilities*, 22: 298–306.

National Institute for Health and Care Excellence (NICE) (2006) *Obesity: Guidance on the Prevention, Identification, Assessment and Management of Overweight and Obesity in Adults and Children*. Clinical Guideline #43. London: National Institute for Health and Care Excellence.

Rimmer, J.H., Rowland, J.L. and Yamaki, K. (2007) Obesity and secondary conditions in adolescents with disabilities: addressing the needs of an underserved population. *Journal of Adolescent Health*, 41(3): 224–9.

Rimmer, J.H., Yamaki, K., Davis Lowry, B.M., Wang, E. and Voge, L.C. (2010) Obesity and obesity-related secondary conditions in adolescents with intellectual/developmental disabilities. *Journal of Intellectual Disability Research*, 54(9): 787–94.

Salaun, L. and Berthouze-Aranda, S. (2011) Obesity in school children with intellectual disabilities in France. *Journal of Applied Research in Intellectual Disability*, 24(4): 333–40.

Singh, A.N., Matson, J.L., Hill, B.D., Pella. R.D., Cooper, C.L. and Adkins, A.D. (2010) The use of clozapine among individuals with intellectual disability: a review. *Research in Developmental Disabilities*, 31: 1135–41.

Slevin, E., McConkey, R., Truesdale-Kennedy, M., Livingstone, B. and Fleming, P. (2008) *Prevalence, Determinants and Strategies for Countering Overweight and Obesity in School Aged Children and Adolescents: A Comparison of Learning Disabled and Non-learning Disabled Pupils*. Belfast: Research and Development Office, PHA/University of Ulster.

Stewart, L., Van de Ven, L., Katsarou V., Rentziou, E., Doran, M., Jackson, P. et al. (2009) High prevalence of obesity in ambulatory children and adolescents with intellectual disability. *Journal of Intellectual Disability Research*, 53(10): 882–6.

Thomas, G.R. and Kerr, M.P. (2011) Longitudinal follow-up of weight change in the context of a community-based health promotion programme for adults with an intellectual disability. *Journal of Applied Research in Intellectual Disabilities*, 24: 381–7.

Utter, J., Denny, S., Crengle, S., Ameratunga, S., Robinson, E., Clark, T. et al. (2010) Overweight among New Zealand adolescents: associations with ethnicity and deprivation. *International Journal of Pediatric Obesity*, 5: 461–6.

World Health Organization (WHO) (2008) *Waist Circumference and Waist–Hip Ratio*. Report of a WHO Expert Consultation. Geneva: WHO. Available at: http://whqlibdoc.who.int/publications/2011/9789241501491_eng.pdf [accessed 20 June 2013].

World Health Organization (WHO) (2011) *Obesity and Overweight*. Fact sheet #311. Updated March 2011. Geneva: WHO. Available at: http://www.who.int/mediacentre/factsheets/fs311/en/ [accessed 20 June 2013].

Zeller, M.H., Reiter-Purtill, J., Modi, A.C., Gutzwiller, J., Vannatta, K. and Davies, W.H. (2007) Controlled study of critical parent and family factors in the obesigenic environment. *Obesity*, 15(1): 126–36.

Diabetes

6

Laurence Taggart, Michael Brown, and Thanos Karatzias

Introduction

Diabetes is increasing worldwide; its growth is associated with lifestyle choices and an ageing population. Yet like many chronic secondary conditions, Type 2 diabetes can be prevented. Evidence indicates that people with intellectual disabilities are at a higher risk of developing both Type 1 diabetes, as a result of genetics, and Type 2 diabetes, as a consequence of obesity, leading to more sedentary lifestyles and poorer diets. Identifying people with intellectual disabilities who are at risk of developing Type 2 diabetes has been shown to be difficult and it has also been found that the management of the condition among this population is poor. This chapter focuses on the prevention of Type 2 diabetes and, for those people with the disorder, how to self-manage the condition.

What is diabetes?

Diabetes affects approximately 1 in 20 people across the world (International Diabetes Federation 2007). According to the WHO (2006), rates of diabetes worldwide will increase from 177 million in 2000 to 366 million by 2030, a global prevalence rate of 6.3 per cent. Blindness, renal failure, amputation and cardiovascular problems, such as stroke and myocardial infarction, which can lead to premature death, are the major complications if left undetected and untreated. Although both conditions are characterized by a raised blood sugar, the causes of Type 1 and Type 2 diabetes are different.

Type 1 diabetes is caused by an autoimmune disorder that develops when the body's immune system attacks and destroys the cells that produce insulin. In contrast, Type 2 diabetes develops when the body does not produce enough insulin to maintain a normal blood glucose concentration (called Hb1Ac), or when the body is unable to effectively use the insulin that is produced.

If blood glucose is high, called hyperglycaemia, individuals are likely to experience a range of physical symptoms such as increased thirst, headaches, difficulty concentrating, blurred vision, frequent urination, fatigue, erectile dysfunction, weight loss, and mental health symptoms, such as mood change, agitation, withdrawal, and verbal and physical aggression.

The risk factors relating to Type 2 diabetes

Specific risk factors for the development of Type 2 diabetes include:

- leading a sedentary lifestyle
- little exercise/activity

- poor nutrition resulting from a diet high in fat and sugar foods
- obesity, leading to an increased BMI and waist circumference
- high cholesterol
- high blood pressure
- smoking
- increasing age
- family history of diabetes
- ethnicity.

Diabetes treatment

Standard management of Type 1 diabetes always involves insulin. For Type 2 diabetes, diet and lifestyle modifications are always necessary with oral anti-glycaemic agents (tablets) and then insulin added according to recognized treatment algorithms. Type 1 diabetes is usually managed at specialist diabetes clinics in hospitals, while Type 2 diabetes is generally managed within general practice by the patient's GP, specialist diabetic nurse or practice nurse during three-monthly visits to the health centre. In relation to individuals with intellectual disability, diabetes has been found to be more common in women than men, with the prevalence increasing with age and being higher in those with mild to moderate intellectual disability (McCarron et al. 2011).

Type 1 diabetes and people with intellectual disabilities

Anwar et al. (2004) found that Type 1 diabetes was more prevalent in individuals with chromosomal syndromes such as Down syndrome, Klinefelter syndrome, Prader-Willi syndrome, Noonan syndrome, and Williams syndrome. Diabetes has also been associated with Down syndrome and Prader-Willi Sydrome because of the propensity for weight gain that is characteristic of these conditions. Extra weight has been identified as contributing to insulin resistance and the consequent development of diabetes (de Winter et al. 2009).

Type 2 diabetes and people with intellectual disabilities

People with intellectual disabilities are more likely to develop Type 2 diabetes than the non-disabled population (Havercamp et al. 2004; Shireman et al. 2010). The prevalence figures of diabetes vary from 7.1 per cent to 14 per cent across studies (McDermott et al. 2006; Shireman et al. 2010; Lunsky et al. 2011). Diabetes UK (2009) has estimated that 270,000 people with intellectual disabilities have Type 2 diabetes, and that the prevalence of Type 2 diabetes is two to three times higher in people with intellectual disabilities than among the non-disabled population. Reichard and Stolzle (2011) also reported that there is a significantly higher prevalence and earlier onset of diabetes among individuals with intellectual disabilities.

Many young people and adults with intellectual disabilities are more likely to have a higher number of risk factors for developing diabetes. These include leading a more sedentary lifestyle, undertaking low levels of activity and exercise, and consuming high fat diets, all of which can contribute towards greater obesity (Melville et al. 2006). As with the non-disabled population, people with intellectual disabilities are living longer, making them more susceptible to developing Type 2 diabetes. The incidence of this condition is therefore likely to increase if early detection and preventative measures are not put in place (Sohler et al. 2009; Emerson and Baines 2011; Taggart et al. 2012). The detrimental impact of diabetes may be greater for this population, due to the poor capacity to communicate effectively and self-manage the symptoms (Cardol et al. 2012).

Self-management of Type 2 diabetes in people with intellectual disabilities

Lennox et al. (2007) found that a considerable number of people with intellectual disabilities living in the community who had Type 2 diabetes and were obese were neither identified nor managed. Diabetes self-management, irrespective of the presence of an intellectual disability, should include an annual health check to screen for a range of chronic secondary conditions (for example, blindness, renal failure, amputation, and cardiovascular problems – stroke and myocardial infarction) that can lead to a premature death. However, adults with intellectual disabilities and diabetes are screened less often than is recommended in national clinical guidelines (Shireman et al. 2010; Taggart et al. 2012). The key healthcare essentials for effective diabetes management have been identified as follows:

1. Annual blood glucose monitoring.
2. Annual blood pressure monitoring.
3. Annual monitoring of cholesterol.
4. Annual screening for signs of retinopathy.
5. Annual monitoring and review of legs and feet, focusing on skin, circulation, and nerve supply.
6. Annual monitoring and review of kidney function, including protein as a sign of possible kidney disease.
7. Review and monitoring of weight to identify the need for weight loss.
8. Advice and support to quit smoking.
9. Attend for regular diabetes review to identify and manage conditions such as heart disease to minimize the risk of stroke.
10. Work with healthcare professionals to develop a clear care plan to support diabetes management to minimize risks and complications.
11. Make use of accessible information about the management of diabetes.
12. Provide for carers to enable the effective management of diabetes.
13. Access education programmes about diabetes and effective management.
14. Access information and specialist care when planning a family to ensure effective diabetes control and management.
15. Access healthcare professionals with knowledge and skills of diabetes to enable effective management.
16. Access emotional and psychological support from specialist healthcare professionals about issues and concerns about diabetes management and control.

(adapted from Diabetes UK 2011)

The principles of good diabetes management are globally relevant. National and international guidelines have been developed across western countries to enhance the prevention, early detection, and management of Type 2 diabetes. Within the UK, there are a number of documents that are important in setting the key performance indicators of good diabetes management (Department of Health 2001; Diabetes UK 2011; NICE 2011). While the reports and guidelines cited here relate specifically to the UK, many countries have comparable policy documents (e.g. American Diabetes Association 2006). Indeed, many standards are developed by international teams such as the International Diabetes Federation (Standl 2002), the European Association for the Study of Diabetes (Nathan et al. 2006), and WHO (2011).

Preventing Type 2 diabetes and promoting its self-management

We present a number of pro-active steps that can prevent Type 2 diabetes from developing. Many of these steps can also promote effective self-management.

Reducing obesity

Obesity is a well-established risk factor for many health conditions for the non-disabled population as well as for people with intellectual disabilities. In particular, it plays an important role in the development of Type 2 diabetes. As many young people and adults with intellectual disabilities are overweight/obese (BMI over 25), opportunities for targeting this high-risk group during annual health checks should be taken, and appropriate lifestyle and behaviour modifications suggested.

Diet control

Research indicates that a healthy diet among those with an intellectual disability is difficult to achieve. A detailed review of the literature on the health inequalities of people with an intellectual disability revealed that less than 10 per cent of this population in supported living/ residential accommodation ate a balanced diet, with an insufficient intake of fruit and vegetables (Emerson and Baines 2010). Some suggestions for improving diet include:

- reducing sugar intake
- reducing fats and saturated food intakes
- eating smaller portions of starchy carbohydrate foods, such as potatoes, rice, and bread, which are converted into glucose (sugar) when digested
- eating the five recommended daily portions of fruit and vegetables
- eating smaller portions of food – with a focus on portion control using the Eat Well Plate
- monitoring calorie intake
- increasing weekly intake of oily fish per week.

Promoting activity/exercise

Many people with intellectual disabilities do not engage in the recommended levels of physical activity. Those with a severe/profound disability and aged over 50 years are more likely to be inactive (Stanish and Draheim 2007; Melville et al. 2009). All people with intellectual disabilities should be educated on the benefits of physical activity and supported to engage in regular physical activity, taking into account their own capabilities and interests. Small steps such as walking short distances could be encouraged, building up to more strenuous activity such as taking longer walks and/or swimming.

Stopping/reducing smoking

There are a growing number of nicotine-replacement therapies commercially available such as patches, inhalers, and gum; the advice of the individual's medical practitioner should be sought before purchasing these alternatives. Many countries offer smoking cessation programmes: a family member or front-line member of staff could support individuals to attend such a programme. As with many non-intellectually disabled smokers, getting support from others to quit smoking is also beneficial.

Complying with medication regimes

Medication is a core part of the diabetes intervention plan whether for reducing blood glucose, high blood pressure or high cholesterol. Therefore, it is important to ensure that the medication regime is followed, as prescribed.

Reducing blood pressure and high cholesterol

Reducing obesity levels, being more active, and eating a healthy diet (such as reducing salt intake, changing from saturated to monounsaturated fats, and reducing alcohol intake) will, along with medication, all help to reduce hypertension and cholesterol.

Looking after the circulation and feet

A complication of Type 2 diabetes is poor circulation that is frequently observed in the feet and legs. To help prevent and diminish this, it is important to lose weight, reduce blood pressure, reduce cholesterol, and stop smoking. The medical practitioner may prescribe aspirin or statins for this condition. An annual feet examination and skin checks should be undertaken.

Diabetes education

Access to education for family careers and front-line staff regarding the prevention of Type 2 diabetes and appropriate self-management is vital. Several studies have found that front-line staff members in residential accommodation and day centres have limited knowledge regarding healthy dietary intake and undertaking health promotion activities (Melville et al. 2009; Hanna et al. 2011). Carers and front-line staff who are educated in these areas can help to educate and empower the person with intellectual disabilities to be aware of the risk factors for developing Type 2 diabetes and therefore modify their lifestyle behaviours. User-friendly accessible literature or DVDs can be used to supplement this explanation (see Useful Resources). Shoneye (2012) emphasized that role-modelling behaviour is important to foster a culture of peer and carer support for healthy eating and physical activity so that individuals with intellectual disability do not feel isolated and are supported and encouraged to engage in changing their lifestyle behaviours.

Diabetes health promotion information

A preliminary study of people with intellectual disabilities in England found that there was a lack of appropriate information on diabetes, diet management, and physical activity and that little emotional support was being offered (Diabetes UK 2009). A small amount of health promotion information has been targeted at people with intellectual disabilities, including easy-to-read picture booklets and leaflets for children ('Meet Pete the Pancreas', Diabetes Federation of Ireland) and adults with intellectual disabilities (Reading Community Team, England) (see Useful Resources).

There are a number of conceptual models that show how people with intellectual disabilities can successfully develop new knowledge and skills and therefore change their lifestyle behaviours (Wilson and Goodman 2011). Taggart et al. (2008) highlighted the importance of addressing the person's intrinsic motivation in changing their behaviour and engaging in self-help, possibly by using the techniques of motivational interviewing rather than enforcing motivation from external sources. Other successful techniques include offering both group and one-to-one sessions with more time flexibility, based on repetition, greater use of kinesic learning and role-play scenarios, and also utilizing family and paid carers to support the person with intellectual disability to maintain the behaviour changes over time.

Diabetes self-management programmes

People in the general population with either Type 1 or 2 diabetes are typically offered a structured education programme to improve their biomedical, psychosocial, and self-management strategies (for example, to maintain a healthy blood glucose, weight, blood pressure, cholesterol level). However, structured education programmes are not routinely offered to people with intellectual disabilities (Slowie et al. 2010; Taggart et al. 2012). These structured education programmes have neither recognized nor addressed the specific challenges posed by this population's cognitive deficits, communication difficulties, low levels of literacy skills, and learning styles. Wilson and Goodman (2011) found that in England adults with mild-to-moderate intellectual disability and co-morbid physical health conditions (for example, Type 2 diabetes, arthritis, hypertension) could successfully participate in appropriately modified chronic disease self-management programmes.

Type 2 diabetes screening

People with intellectual disabilities are rarely screened for Type 2 diabetes despite their high risk for developing this chronic condition. A number of countries are introducing annual health checks, although many do not include blood glucose monitoring.

Summary

- Type 2 diabetes is more common in people with intellectual disabilities and is on the increase, yet it is a condition that can be prevented.
- People with intellectual disabilities who are at high risk for Type 2 diabetes due to obesity and inactivity should be screened for the disease during their annual health check.
- A number of pro-active steps can be taken to prevent Type 2 diabetes from developing. Many of these steps can also promote better self-management:
  - reduce weight
  - reduce high sugar and starchy carbohydrate foods
  - increase fruit and vegetables in diet
  - smaller portions
  - increase activity
  - reduce blood pressure
  - reduce cholesterol
  - stop smoking.
- Self-management can prevent many of the complications of diabetes, including blindness, renal failure, amputation, and cardiovascular problems, such as stroke and myocardial infarction, as well as premature death.
- There are national guidelines for managing diabetes that should be adhered to.
- People with intellectual disabilities and diabetes, and their carers, should be routinely offered structured education programmes to promote their self-management strategies.
- Family carer and front-line staff education is important so that they can support and empower the person with Type 2 diabetes to make healthy lifestyle choices.

Useful resources

- DVD on diabetes for adults with intellectual disabilities and diabetes: http://www.diabetes.org.uk/About_us/News_Landing_Page/Diabetes-UK-launches-DVD-to-help-people-with-learning-disabilities/

- 'Pete the Pancreas': http://www.diabetes.ie/wp-content/uploads/2011/08/15-Jun-2011-Pete-for-children-FINAL-UPLOAD.pdf

- Type 2 Diabetes – Living a Healthier Life [DVD]. London: Speakup. Good clear information for people with learning disabilities about diabetes and living with the condition.

Web resources

- Diabetes: http://www.easyhealth.org.uk/listing/diabetes-(leaflets)

References

American Diabetes Association (2006) Standards of medical care in diabetes – 2006 (Position Statement). *Diabetes Care*, 29(suppl. 1): S4–S42.

Anwar, A., Walker, D. and Frier, B. (2004) Type 1 diabetes mellitus and Down syndrome: prevalence, management and diabetes complications. *Diabetic Medicine*, 15: 160–3.

Cardol, M., Rijken, M. and van Schrojenstein Lantman-de Valk, H. (2012) People with mild to moderate intellectual disability talking about their diabetes and how they manage. *Journal of Intellectual Disability Research*, 56(4): 351–60.

Department of Health (2001) *National Service Framework for Diabetes: Standards.* London: Department of Health. Available at: http://www.gov.uk/government/uploads/system/uploads/attachment_data/file/198836/National_Service_Framework_for_Diabetes.pdf [accessed 20 June 2013].

de Winter, C.F., Magilsen, K.W., van Alfen, J.C., Penning, C. and Evenhuis, H.M. (2009) Prevalence of cardiovascular risk factors in older people with intellectual disability. *American Journal of Intellectual and Developmental Disabilities*, 114(6): 427–36.

Diabetes UK (2009) Diabetes UK launches DVD to help people with learning disabilities, Press release, 23 April: Available at: http://tinyurl.com/cus6qd [accessed 27 November 2012].

Diabetes UK (2011) *The Care You should Receive: 15 Healthcare Essentials.* Available at: http://www.diabetes.org.uk/upload/About%20us/15%20measures%20checklist.pdf [accessed 12 December 2012].

Emerson, E. and Baines, S. (2010) *Health Inequalities and People with Learning Disabilities in the UK: 2010.* Improving Health and Lives: Learning Disability Observatory. London: Public Health England.

Emerson, E. and Baines, S. (2011) Health inequalities and people with intellectual disabilities in the UK. *Tizard Learning Disability Review*, 16(1): 42–8.

Hanna, L.M., Taggart, L. and Cousins, W. (2011) Cancer prevention and health promotion for people with intellectual disabilities: an exploratory study of staff knowledge. *Journal of Intellectual Disability Research*, 55(3): 281–91.

Havercamp, S., Scandlin, D. and Roth, M. (2004) Health disparities among adults with developmental disabilities, adults with other disabilities, and adults not reporting disability in North Carolina. *Public Health Reports*, 119(4): 418–26.

International Diabetes Federation (2007) *Diabetes Atlas*, 3rd edn. Brussels: IDF.

Lennox, N., Bain, C. and Rey-Conde, T. (2007) Effects of a comprehensive health assessment programme for Austrialian adults with intellectual disability: a cluster randomised trial. *International Journal of Epidemiology*, 36: 139–46.

Lunsky, Y., Timt, A., Robinson, S., Khodaverdian, A. and Jaskulski, C. (2011) Emergency psychiatric service use by individuals with intellectual disabilities living with family. *Journal of Mental Health Research in Intellectual Disabilities*, 4(3): 172–85.

McCarron, M., Swinburne, J., Burke, E., McGlinchey, E., Mulryan N., Andrews, V. et al. (2011) *Growing Older with an Intellectual Disability in Ireland 2011: First Results from The Intellectual Disability Supplement of The Irish Longitudinal Study on Ageing.* Dublin: School of Nursing and Midwifery, Trinity College.

McDermott, S., Moran, R., Platt, T. and Dasari, S. (2006) Variation in health conditions among groups of adults with disabilities in primary care. *Journal of Community Health*, 31: 147–59.

Melville, C., Hamilton, S., Hankey, C., Miller, S. and Boyle, S. (2006) The prevalence and determinants of obesity in adults with intellectual disabilities. *Obesity Review*, 8: 223–30.

Melville, C., Hamilton, S., Miller, S., Boyle, S., Robinson, N. and Pert, C. (2009) Carer knowledge and perceptions of healthy lifestyles for adults with intellectual disabilities. *Journal of Applied Research in Intellectual Disabilities*, 22: 298–306.

Nathan, D., Buse, J.B., Davidson, M.B., Heine, R.J., Holman, R.R., Sherwin, R.S. et al. (2006) Management of hyperglycemia in Type 2 diabetes: a consensus algorithm for the initiation and adjustment of therapy. A consensus statement from the American Diabetes Association and the European Association for the Study of Diabetes. *Diabetes Care*, 29: 1963–72.

National Institute for Health and Care Excellence (NICE) (2011) *Guidelines for Diabetes.* Available at: http://guidance.nice.org.uk/Topic/EndocrineNutritionalMetabolic/Diabetes [accessed 15th November 2012].

Reichard, A. and Stolzle, H. (2011) Diabetes among adults with cognitive limitations compared to individuals with no cognitive disabilities. *Intellectual and Developmental Disabilities*, 49(3): 141–54.

Shireman, T., Reichar, A., Nazir, N., Backes, J., Pharm, D. and Griener, A. (2010) Quality of diabetes care for adults with developmental disabilities. *Disability and Health Journal*, 3: 179–85.

Shoneye, C. (2012) Prevention and treatment of obesity in adults with learning disabilities. *Learning Disability Practice*, 15(3): 32–7.

Slowie, D., Warner, J. and Eaton, S. (2010) Diabetes and learning disability. *Diabetes Update*, Winter Edition, pp. 18–20.

Sohler, N., Lubetkin, E., Levy, J., Soghomonian, C. and Rimmerman, A. (2009) Factors associated with obesity and coronary heart disease in people with intellectual disabilities. *Social Work in Health Care*, 48: 76–89.

Standl, E. (2002) International Diabetes Federation European Policy Group's Standards for Diabetes. *Endocrine Practice*, 8(1): 37–40.

Stanish, H.I. and Draheim, C.C. (2007) Walking activity, body composition and blood pressure in adults with intellectual disabilities. *Journal of Applied Research in Intellectual Disabilities*, 20: 183–90.

Taggart, L., Huxley, A. and Baker, G. (2008) Alcohol and illicit drug misuse in people with learning disabilities: implications for research and service development. *Advances in Mental Health in Learning Disabilities*, 2(1): 11–21.

Taggart, L., Truesdale-Kennedy, M. and Coates, V. (2012) Management and quality indicators of diabetes mellitus in people with intellectual disabilities. *Journal of Intellectual Disability Research* (DOI: 10.1111/j.1365-2788.2012.01633.x).

Wilson, P. and Goodman, C. (2011) Evaluation of a modified chronic disease self-management programme for people with intellectual disabilities. *Journal of Nursing and Healthcare of Chronic Illness*, 3: 310–18.

World Health Organization (WHO) (2006) *The Global Burden: Diabetes and Impaired Glucose Tolerance.* Geneva: WHO. Available at: http://www.idf.org/sites/default/files/The_Global_Burden.pdf [accessed 18 September 2012].

World Health Organization (WHO) (2011) *Use of Glycated Haemoglobin (HbA1c) in the Diagnosis of Diabetes Mellitus.* WHO: Geneva.

7 Epilepsy

Penny Blake and Mike Kerr

Introduction

This chapter introduces the key issues of epilepsy relating to people with an intellectual disability. With regard to epilepsy there are several areas of health promotion that are particularly important. Specific application of high-quality intervention may lead to a reduction in morbidity and mortality. The following areas are explored in relation to health promotion and epilepsy: bone health, obesity, risk of falls and injury, risk of drowning, sudden unexplained death, mental health, hospitalization, and rescue medication. For each area we review the evidence that epilepsy or its treatment can have a negative impact on the health of the individual before discussing management changes that could improve the person's health.

Epilepsy and intellectual disability

Epilepsy is the most common serious co-morbidity in people with an intellectual disability. Recent community estimates for the prevalence of epilepsy in the intellectual disabilities population suggest a prevalence of approximately 18 per cent (Matthews et al. 2008), whereas in the general population the prevalence of epilepsy is less than 1 per cent (Linehan et al. 2010).

Epilepsy is a chronic neurological disorder that affects part or all of the brain and is characterized by a tendency to recurrent seizures. Seizures vary between patients and there are numerous different types ranging from slight changes in sensation with no impairment in consciousness (simple partial seizures), to complete loss of consciousness and convulsions of the entire body (tonic clonic seizures). The classification of seizures is complex and currently undergoing change. However, it is still appropriate to consider seizures by their presumed origin: focal, starting in one part of the brain, or generalized, starting all over the brain. These definitions help in classifying seizures for means of treatment choice and syndrome diagnosis but also a clear definition of seizures can help when considering risk. This is particularly true as seizures that have no warning, such as atonic (drop) seizures, can cause considerable damage to the individual, yet a seizure with warning (known as an aura) can occasionally let an individual find a place of safety before the seizure progresses.

Often persons with intellectual disabilities develop seizures early on in their childhood, but a first seizure can occur at any age. Many factors predispose individuals with intellectual disabilities to develop epilepsy; to cover them in detail here is beyond the scope of this chapter. Broadly they include:

- genetic disorders
- cerebral malformations
- cerebral infections
- cerebral trauma.

When a person with intellectual disabilities experiences a first seizure, they usually present to medical professionals urgently where a thorough history is taken from the patient and witnesses. Preliminary investigations to determine if there has been a trigger for the event, such as a concurrent illness or an electrolyte imbalance, may be done. An electrocardiogram (ECG) is usually also performed to see if an underlying cardiac cause made the person lose consciousness.

Once the patient is stabilized, they will usually be referred to a specialist as an outpatient (see Figure 7.1). This is likely to be a neurologist or other epilepsy specialist. The specialist will record a thorough history encompassing all aspects of the patient's general health. They will focus on possible risk factors within the history that may predispose the person to develop epilepsy, such as brain damage from a variety of causes (as is often seen in patients with intellectual disabilities), family history of epilepsy, history of severe infections of the brain such as meningitis or encephalitis, or specific genetic disorders.

Specific investigations will be undertaken to confirm a diagnosis of epilepsy and identify causation. There are two investigations of choice:

1. Magnetic resonance imaging (MRI) of the head that looks at the general structure of the brain and whether there are any specific abnormalities.
2. Electroencephalography (EEG), used to monitor the electrical activity within the brain and look for any signs of epileptic activity (NICE Clinical Guidelines 2012).

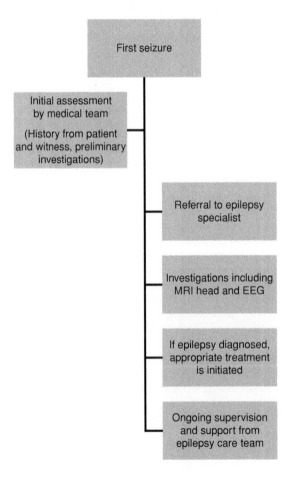

Figure 7.1 The epilepsy diagnostic pathway

Many patients with intellectual disabilities have difficulty with undergoing these investigations, particularly where patient participation is required, or if the investigation takes a significant length of time. The professional may therefore need to weigh up how important the investigation is to the management of the patient, compared with the distress it may cause.

When a diagnosis of epilepsy has been made, the initial treatment is anti-epileptic medication of which there are many types. The drug chosen will reflect the type of epilepsy, the age, the sex, and the other health problems of the individual. The aim is to prevent further seizures without causing intolerable side-effects. In intellectual disability patients, often several medications are needed to improve seizure control; this is known as polypharmacy. Unfortunately, complete freedom from seizures may not be achieved.

Obesity

Obesity is in itself a risk factor for other illnesses, most notably coronary artery disease (see Chapter 8), stroke, some cancers (see Chapter 9), diabetes mellitus, sleep disorders, and joint pathology. It is often associated with raised plasma cholesterol and triglyceride concentrations.

People with intellectual disability have a higher prevalence of obesity than the general population (Gazizova et al. 2012). Current estimates for obesity in the intellectual disability population range from 21 to 35 per cent (de Winter et al. 2012) (see Chapter 5). Reasons for the increase in obesity in the population as a whole are complex and multi-factorial, and this is also true for those with intellectual disabilities and epilepsy. Unfortunately, little research has been conducted into the impact of epilepsy and its treatment on rates of obesity in the intellectual disability population; much of the evidence comes from studies examining the non-disabled adult population.

Reasons for higher obesity rates

Some of the possible reasons for increased rates of obesity in the intellectual disability population who also have epilepsy are hypothesized below.

Anti-epileptic medications

Many regularly prescribed anti-epileptic medications have the potential to have an impact on weight. Increased weight has been reported in individuals on gabapentin (Antel and Hebebrand, 2012), sodium valproate (Biton et al, 2001), and pregabalin (Lee et al, 2009). However, some are weight neutral, such as leveteracetam (Lyseng-Williamson 2011) and lamotrigine (Biton et al. 2001), and some cause weight loss including topiramate and zonisamide (Antel and Hebebrand 2012). The mechanisms that lead to appetite and weight changes are complex and do not occur in all patients.

Lifestyle issues

Obesity and physical exercise are often linked. The possibility of participating in physical activity can be compromised in persons with severe epilepsy, severe intellectual disabilities, and/or physical disabilities (see Chapter 16). These conditions often co-exist, providing individuals with intellectual disability with less opportunity to participate in physical exercise than members of the non-disabled population. Ben-Menachem (2007) reported that several studies in the non-disabled adult population found lower levels of physical activity in people with epilepsy, even if their seizures were controlled compared with the general population.

Proposed health promotion interventions

Given the often already complex health needs of people with intellectual disabilities, obesity may complicate things further. Health interventions, which are relevant to the population as a whole and also to patients with intellectual disabilities and epilepsy, are set out below.

Weight monitoring

Regular monitoring of a patient's weight can be used to calculate that patient's BMI (see Chapter 5). However, specialist weighing equipment, such as wheelchair scales, may be required for persons with co-morbid physical disability. Any changes in weight can be reacted to and appropriate management taken (Ben-Menachem 2007).

Education

Many people with intellectual disability, particularly those with more severe disability, have help to choose their food and prepare their meals. Healthy eating education is essential for patients and also their carers (see Chapter 4). It is also necessary to educate patients and carers regarding types of exercise and activity in which the patient is able to participate. Healthy lifestyle groups where individuals can be educated, weighed, and seen by specialists such as dieticians to help them to achieve a stable, healthy weight could help facilitate this.

Choice of medication

When selecting a drug, it is important to consider weight-altering side-effects. If a medication is suspected to be responsible for a detrimental alteration in weight, alternatives should be considered (Ben-Menachem 2007). Notwithstanding the known association between weight gain and some anti-epileptic drugs, it is extremely important that weight gain is not purely attributed to the epilepsy treatment. It will be a rare patient whose weight gain is solely drug related and more frequently it is multi-factorial and the impact of prescription change, including its risk, should be thoroughly assessed.

Risks of falls

Reasons for increased risk of falls and injury

Often patients have little or no warning that they are about to have a seizure and therefore cannot get to a place of safety to minimize the risk of injury to themselves. Fractures can occur in these circumstances depending on where the individual is and in what way they fall. Often people with an intellectual disability also have co-morbid physical disabilities and hence may have an increased susceptibility to falls and injury. Some falls can be due to clumsiness, tripping, and falling (Koppel et al. 2005), which are all problems that can also occur with anti-epileptic drug toxicity and with the neurological disorder leading to the epilepsy.

Proposed health promotion interventions

In patients with intractable epilepsy and frequent falls due to seizures, it may be necessary to adapt frequently used environments to minimize injury, such as soft padding around furniture and cushioning the floor.

In all patients with unsteadiness or falls who also have epilepsy and intellectual disabilities, an assessment should be made for the potential for anti-epileptic drug side-effects. Unsteadiness is particularly common for patients on high doses of carbamazepine and also where phenytoin toxicity is present. Drug levels can be valuable in particular if the individual is unable to articulate side-effects such as dizziness. Further drug effects, such as when two sodium blocking drugs are co-prescribed (for example, lamotrigine and carbamazepine), or drug-induced hyponatraemia, should also be explored.

Bone health

Bone is a tissue that responds to changes both within and outside the body. It alters in structure and architecture throughout life. Bone strength can be altered by factors such as changes in body weight, exercise or changes in calcium homeostasis. A person whose bone strength is reduced is more susceptible to fractures (Sheth and Harden 2007). The fracture rate in people with epilepsy is two to six times that seen in the non-disabled population without epilepsy (Souverin et al. 2005).

There is specific evidence of increased fracture rates in people with intellectual disabilities compared with their peers without epilepsy (Jancar and Jancar 1998). The risk of fracture from falls is further complicated by the association of intellectual disabilities and being on anti-epileptic drugs and osteoporosis.

Reasons for poorer bone health

There are two main factors that may have an impact on bone health in people with epilepsy and intellectual disabilities: decreased mobility and anti-epileptic medications. Physical activity is well known to have a positive effect on bone health. Inactivity, particularly lack of weight-bearing exercise, is a risk factor for osteoporosis. Osteoporosis puts people at greater risk of fractures. As noted above, people with epilepsy tend to be less physically active than the non-disabled population. This can be for a variety of reasons, but include co-morbid physical problems, difficulty in accessing activities that are at an appropriate level for them, or a lack of awareness of the benefits of exercise.

Anti-epileptic medications can affect the bone density, particularly if they act on liver enzymes. They can lower vitamin D concentrations, which alters calcium metabolism and hence impacts on bone density. This can lead to the development of osteoporosis where bones are weakened and at a higher risk of fracture. This is particularly the case in post-menopausal women taking anti-epileptic drugs.

Proposed health promotion interventions

Recent research has found that bone health in people with epilepsy has the potential to be improved by several lifestyle modifications and health interventions (Sheth and Harden 2007):

- avoidance of cigarettes and excessive alcohol
- increase in weight-bearing exercises
- calcium and vitamin D supplementation
- evaluation of anti-epileptic drugs in individuals who have had a fracture and consideration of changing to a drug that has less impact on bone density
- specialist referral for consideration of hormone replacement therapy/bisphosphonates/calcitonin
- improved seizure control to reduce the risk of injury and fracture during a seizure.

Regular monitoring of bone health in patients at risk of developing osteoporosis is recommended. Also, before starting anti-epileptic treatment in a newly diagnosed patient, an evaluation of their risk of developing osteoporosis should be made so that an appropriate anti-epileptic drug can be selected (Svalheim et al. 2011). There may be some difficulties with people with intellectual disabilities adhering to all of the above lifestyle modifications. In particular, the strategy of increasing weight-bearing exercise may be slightly more difficult to achieve, as there is great variation between the mobility levels of individuals.

Risk of drowning

People with epilepsy suffer an increased risk of drowning. A range of locations are possible including large areas of water such as the sea, a lake or a swimming pool, and also in smaller areas such as a bath or paddling pool.

Reasons for increased risk of drowning in patients with epilepsy

The increased risk of drowning in persons with epilepsy was thought to be less in children than in adults. It was hypothesized that this might be due to increased supervision of children in situations involving water. It has also been found that many of the deaths in childhood are due to inadequate supervision. There is a scarcity of studies looking specifically at drowning in persons with epilepsy and intellectual disabilities. If the decreased number of deaths in children is solely due to supervision, it is possible to hypothesize that individuals with increasingly severe intellectual disability are more likely to be supervised both when bathing and when participating in water-based activities. This may therefore reduce their risk of drowning to that of children with epilepsy. A lower incidence of drowning was also found by Klenerman et al. (1993), who examined all causes of death in severe epilepsy patients in long-term residential care. Again it was hypothesized that this could be due to increased supervision during bathing and a relatively sheltered living environment. It was reported that this might not apply to more able people living more independently in the community.

Proposed health promotion interventions

Despite some suggestion that there has been a small decrease in recent years in the number of deaths by drowning in epilepsy, the number is still far greater than in the non-disabled population (Bell et al. 2008). This emphasizes the need to educate people with epilepsy and their carers. Advice should be given about the use of showers instead of baths, where possible, and also the risks associated with water-based activities, such as swimming. People with ongoing seizures are at greater risk of drowning than those that have been seizure free for several years. We recommend that specific bathing risk plans that usually recognize the risk of scalding should include specific risk assessment for drowning.

Sudden unexplained death in epilepsy

Sudden unexplained death in epilepsy (SUDEP) is defined as 'sudden, unexpected, witnessed or unwitnessed, non-traumatic and non-drowning death in patients with epilepsy, with or without evidence for a seizure and excluding documented status epilepticus, in which post mortem examination does not reveal a toxicological or anatomic cause for death' (Nashef 1997: 7). Several hypotheses have been postulated as to its cause, including respiratory arrest, cardiac arrhythmias or ictally determined neurological shut down. People with intellectual disabilities appear to be at an increased risk of SUDEP; the causes of this are discussed below but in the main it appears to be related to the severity of epilepsy in people with intellectual disabilities.

Reasons for the increased risk of SUDEP in people with epilepsy and intellectual disabilities

Some potential risk factors for people with epilepsy in general include young age, early onset of seizures, refractory epilepsy, generalized tonic seizures, being male, and being in bed at the time of death (Jehi and Najm 2008). Several of these risk factors are more commonly seen in the intellectual disability population and therefore these patients are at increased risk of SUDEP.

Proposed health promotion interventions

Shorvon and Tomson (2011) have suggested that the key areas of prevention of SUDEP in people with intellectual disabilities are seizure reduction and seizure management. Sudden unexplained death in epilepsy is usually associated with a high frequency of generalized tonic clonic seizures. Studies have found that reducing this through appropriate use of anti-epileptic drugs reduces the risk of SUDEP. Any individual with epilepsy and intellectual disabilities who has continued seizures should be considered to be at risk of SUDEP. In such cases, it is crucial that specialist assessment of seizure control is accessed. Epilepsy surgery can also have a positive effect on SUDEP if, as a result of surgery, the individual experiences fewer convulsive seizures.

Shorvon and Tomson (2011) recommend improving post-ictal surveillance whereby there is close observation of the patient after a tonic clonic seizure until the patient has regained consciousness. This would enable any complications from the seizure to be seen and treated at the earliest opportunity. This is more easily achieved in a hospital setting and also for patients who have 24-hour family or social support where seizures are more likely to be witnessed.

Mental health

Mental illness in individuals with intellectual disabilities is common, and the rate is higher than that seen in the general population (see Chapter 11). Levels of mental illness increase with increasing severity of intellectual disabilities. It is also known that individuals with epilepsy within the non-disabled population are at increased risk of mental illness. Turky et al. (2011) found that the risk for developing a common psychiatric disorder among adults with intellectual disabilities and epilepsy was more than seven times that among those with intellectual disabilities only. The main single disorder was anxiety.

Reasons for increased mental illness in patients with epilepsy and intellectual disabilities

There has been little consensus as to whether there is an associated risk of mental illness in people with intellectual disabilities and epilepsy compared with those with intellectual disabilities alone. Patients can also develop psychiatric disorders at the time of their seizures. This is usually in the form of a psychosis and can be classified as peri-ictal (occurring at the time of the seizure). These can be further classified into pre-ictal (before), ictal (during) or post-ictal (after) psychoses. The timing of their seizures in relation to the psychosis is important in classification and management. Peri-ictal psychoses usually occur for a short duration and can be managed with a combination of good epilepsy control and psychotropic medication. There is a high chance of these events occurring in a susceptible individual each time they have a seizure (Gonzalez et al. 2013). Evidence in the non-disabled population has found that treating a mental illness may also have a positive impact on seizure control.

Anti-epileptic drugs can also have an effect on mood, behaviour, and cognition depending on their mechanism of action within the brain (Cavanna et al. 2010). Some drugs can cause sedation, which can lead to cognitive slowing, and other drugs are thought to cause anxiety, agitation, irritability or depression in some individuals. People with a history of mental illness should be monitored in case their symptoms recur.

Proposed health promotion interventions

Recent studies indicate the need for everyone involved in the care of adults with intellectual disabilities and epilepsy to be educated about mental illness and to be vigilant for the signs and symptoms (Turky et al. 2011) (see Chapters 11 and 15). There should also be support for carers, if a person for whom they care develops a mental illness. Early identification of mental illness and prompt treatment is important. In addition, an improvement in seizure control should be aimed for where possible. Both pharmacological and non-pharmacological modes of treatment should be tried depending on the nature and severity of the mental illness. Clinicians treating individuals need to bear in mind the potential for drug interactions between psychotropic medications and anti-epileptic drugs. They should also be alert to the fact that some psychotropic drugs can cause an alteration in seizure threshold.

Hospitalization

Persons with intellectual disabilities have more hospital admissions than the non-disabled population. In the UK, it is estimated that 26 per cent of people with intellectual disabilities are admitted to general hospitals every year, compared with 14 per cent of their non-disabled peers (Band, 1998).

Reasons for increased rates of hospitalization

People with intellectual disabilities have an increased risk of co-morbid illness compared with the non-disabled population, and consequently have higher rates of admission to hospital. These admissions may frequently be the result of seizures, particularly if they have severe, poorly controlled epilepsy. Usually, people who are known to have epilepsy can be managed at home following a seizure. However, if a person has a prolonged seizure, clusters of seizures or goes into status epilepticus, it may be necessary for them to receive emergency hospital treatment.

Proposed health promotion interventions

Often hospital admissions can be avoided if a patient is able to achieve better seizure control in the first place. Referral to a specialist is therefore essential for any patient who is having ongoing seizures, particularly if they are convulsive seizures. The specialist can optimize anti-epileptic drug therapy to improve seizure control. Often it will not be possible to completely eliminate seizures, and therefore alternative 'rescue' medications may be needed to prevent prolonged seizures. In recent years, the introduction of buccal midazolam has made the administration of rescue medication easier and more dignified compared with rectal diazepam that was used in the past. The rescue medication is given either because of a prolonged seizure, or several seizures close together, with the aim of making the seizure(s) cease. This can minimize morbidity and mortality associated with the seizure.

Families and care staff require specialist training on managing the individual they care for with regard to their epilepsy. They should be able to recognize when the patient is having a seizure and the type of seizure. They should also be able to administer rescue medication and recognize when the individual is deteriorating and requires additional medical intervention by a medical practitioner.

Often patients will have a care plan that has been individually designed to reflect the type of seizures experienced and indicate when to administer rescue medication. It will also outline to carers when they should contact the emergency services in order for the patient to receive hospital care. If a patient is admitted to hospital, it is essential that they have someone with them who can explain to the medical team about the individual, if they themselves are unable to do so. This will help the medical team fully assess the situation and provide good quality care.

To conclude, we provide an illustrative example of developing a health promotion plan.

Case study

John is a 34-year-old man with complex epilepsy: generalized tonic clonic seizures and drop attacks. He has frequent head injuries and hospitilization for prolonged seizures.

A multi-professional and multi-dimensional plan is needed to improve John's wellbeing. His medication needs to be reviewed to assess whether it is appropriate for his seizures and whether it may produce bone disease. A dietician needs to be involved in John's diet regarding this. A specialist epilepsy nurse needs to work with the consultant and the carer to develop a rescue medication plan that reduces hospitalization. An occupational therapy assessment is needed to minimize the risk from injury in the environment and the possibility of using a helmet in certain environments. A detailed discussion on night-time monitoring is needed to assess means to reduce the risk of SUDEP. Finally, it is likely that a best interest meeting will need to be called to discuss least restrictive means, especially the use of night monitoring and the possibility of a helmet.

Summary

The main risks associated with epilepsy and appropriate health interventions are identified in Table 7.1.

Table 7.1 Risks associated with epilepsy and proposed health interventions

Risk	Suggested health promotion measures
Obesity	Weight monitoring Education Medication choice
Falls and injury	Environmental measures Review side-effects of medication and monitor closely for signs of toxicity
Fractures	Avoidance of cigarettes and excessive alcohol Increase in weight-bearing exercise Evaluation of anti-epileptic medication Specialist referral to bone specialist Improved seizure control
Drowning	Education Use of showers instead of baths Open water/pool safety
SUDEP	Improve seizure control Post-ictal surveillance
Mental health	Education Early identification Appropriate treatment and management
Hospitalization	Improve seizure control Referral to a specialist Rescue medication Epilepsy care plans

---

Useful resources

- Prasher, V. and Kerr, M. (2008) *Epilepsy and Intellectual Disabilities*. London: Springer-Verlag.

Web resources

- Epilepsy Society (Canada): http://www.epilepsyontario.org/
- Epilepsy and Learning Disability Society (UK): http://www.epilepsysociety.org.uk/AboutEpilepsy/Epilepsyandyou/Epilepsyandlearningdisability-1
- Leaflets about epilepsy from the Easy Health website www.easyhealth.org.uk/listing/epilepsy-(leaflets)
- Videos about epilepsy from the Easy Health website http://www.easyhealth.org.uk/listing/epilepsy-(videos)

References

Antel, J. and Hebebrand, J. (2012) Weight reducing side effects of the antiepileptic agents topiramate and zonisamide [review]. *Handbook of Experimental Pharmacoogy*, 209: 433–66.

Band, R. (1998) *The NHS: Health for All? People with Learning Disabilities and Health Care*. London: Mencap.

Bell, G., Gaitatzis, A., Bell, C., Johnson, A. and Sander, J. (2008) Drowning in people with epilepsy: how great is the risk? *Neurology*, 71: 578–82.

Ben-Menachem, E. (2007) Weight issues for people with epilepsy – a review. *Epilepsia*, 48(suppl. 9): 42–5.

Biton, V., Mirza, W., Montouris, G., Vuong, A., Hammer, A.E. and Barrett, P.S. (2001) Weight change associated with valproate and lamotrigine monotherapy in patients with epilepsy. *Neurology*, 56(2): 172–7.

Cavanna, A., Ali, F., Rickards, H. and McCorry, D. (2010) Behavioural and cognitive effects of anti-epileptic drugs. *Discovery Medicine*, 9(45): 138–44.

de Winter, C.F., Bastiaanse, L.P., Hilgenkamp, T.I.M., Evenhuis, H.M. and Echteld, M.A. (2012) Overweight and obesity in older people with intellectual disability. *Research in Developmental Disabilities*, 33: 398–405.

Gazizova, D., Puri, B., Singh, I. and Dhaliwal, R. (2012) The overweight: obesity and plasma lipids in adults with intellectual disability and mental illness. *Journal of Intellectual Disability Research*, 56(9): 895–901.

Gonzalez Mingot, C., Gil Villar, M.P., Calvo Medel, D., Corbalan Sevilla, T., Martinez Martinez, L., Iniguez Martinez, C. et al. (2013) Epileptic peri-ictal psychosis, a reversible cause of psychosis. *Neurologia*, 28(2): 81–7.

Jancar, J. and Jancar, M.P. (1998) Age-related fractures in people with intellectual disability and epilepsy. *Journal of Intellectual Disability Research*, 42(5): 429–33.

Jehi, L. and Najm, M.D. (2008) Sudden unexpected death in epilepsy: impact, mechanisms, and prevention. *Cleveland Clinic Journal of Medicine*, 75(2): 66–70.

Klenerman, P., Sander, J.W.A.S. and Shorvon, S.D. (1993) Mortality in patients with epilepsy: a study of patients in long term residential care. *Journal of Neurology, Neurosurgery and Psychiatry*, 56: 149–52.

Koppel, B.S., Harden, C.L., Nikolov, B.G. and Labar, D.R. (2005) An analysis of lifetime fractures in women with epilepsy. *Acta Neurologica Scandinavica*, 111(4): 225–8.

Lee, B.I., Yi, S., Hong, S.B., Kim, M.K., Lee, S.A., Lee, S.K. et al. (2009) Pregabalin add-on therapy using a flexible, optimized dose schedule in refractory partial epilepsies: a double-blind, randomized, placebo-controlled multicentre trial. *Epilepsia*, 50(3): 464–74.

Linehan, C., Kerr, M.P., Walsh, P.N., Brady, G., Kelleher, C., Delanty, N. et al. (2010) Examining the prevalence of epilepsy and delivery of epilepsy care in Ireland. *Epilepsy*, 51(5): 845–52.

Lyseng-Williamson, K.A. (2011) Spotlight on Levetiracetam in epilepsy. *CNS Drugs*, 25(10): 901–5.

Matthews, T., Weston, N., Baxter, H., Felce, D. and Kerr, M. (2008) A general practice-based prevalence study of epilepsy among adults with intellectual disabilities and of its association with psychiatric disorder, behavioural disturbance and carer stress. *Journal of Intellectual Disability Research*, 52(2): 163–73.

Nashef, L. (1997) Sudden unexpected death in epilepsy: terminology and definitions. *Epilepsia*, 38(suppl. 11): s6–s8.

National Institute for Health and Care Excellence (NICE) (2012) *The Epilepsies: The Diagnoses and Management of the Epilepsies in Adults and Children in Primary and Secondary Care*. NICE Clinical Guideline #137. London: NICE.

Sheth, R.D. and Harden, C.L. (2007) Screening for bone health in epilepsy. *Epilepsia*, 48(9): 39–41.

Shorvon, S. and Tomson, T (2011) Sudden unexpected death in epilepsy. *The Lancet*, 378(9808): 2028–38.

Souverin, P.C., Webb, D.J., Petre, H., Weil, J., Van Staa, T.P. and Egberts, T. (2005) Incidence of fractures among epilepsy patients: a population-based retrospective cohort study in the general practice research database. *Epilepsia*, 46: 304–10.

Svalheim, S., Røste, L.S., Nakken, K.O. and Taubøll, E. (2011) Bone health in adults with epilepsy. *Acta Neurologica Scandinavica*, 124(suppl.): s89–s95.

Turky, A., Felce, D., Jones, G. and Kerr, M. (2011) A prospective case control study of psychiatric disorders in adults with epilepsy and intellectual disability. *Epilepsia*, 52(7): 1223–30.

8 Cardiovascular disease

Jim Blair and Cathy Ross

Introduction

Living a healthy active lifestyle can lead to a long and fulfilling life; however, making the right choices and breaking habits of a lifetime can be difficult. Having an intellectual disability, which can vary considerably among individuals, means making the right choices is even more difficult. The lack of appropriate health information, health promotion initiatives, and health screening facilities to support understanding of the key messages further hinders change.

This chapter focuses on helping people with intellectual disabilities and their carers to understand what heart disease is, what the risk factors for coronary heart disease (CHD) are, and how lifestyle choices can impact on that risk.

What is cardiovascular disease?

Cardiovascular disease (CVD) – which includes CHD, diseases of the circulatory system, and stroke – is the largest cause of premature death in the world, with deaths expected to rise to 23.4 million by 2030 (WHO 2008). Coronary heart disease is the single biggest cause of premature death in the UK. There are currently over 2.7 million people living with the condition (Scarborough et al. 2010). While the number of deaths from CHD is falling due to improved risk prediction and early intervention and treatment, the number of people living with it is rising.

For people with intellectual disabilities, CHD is the second biggest cause of premature death. People with an intellectual disability are more likely to have high blood pressure, be overweight or obese, and be inactive, all of which are risk factors for CHD (Royal College of Nursing [RCN] 2011).

How the heart works

The heart is a muscle that pumps blood around the body, delivering oxygen and nutrients to all the cells. It has two small collecting chambers at the top of the heart, one on the left and one on the right, called the atria, and two larger pumping chambers at the bottom called ventricles. De-oxygenated blood leaves the right ventricle via the pulmonary artery where it is delivered back to the lungs to become enriched with oxygen again. The aorta on the left side of the heart delivers freshly oxygenated blood to the rest of the body (see Figure 8.1).

The heart needs its own supply of oxygen and nutrients so that it can pump blood around the body. It receives its own blood supply from the coronary arteries. There are three main coronary arteries: the left and right coronary arteries and the circumflex artery, on the outside of the heart (see Figure 8.2). These divide many times so that the blood reaches all the parts of the heart's muscular wall.

Right side

Left side

From the head and arms

To the head and arms

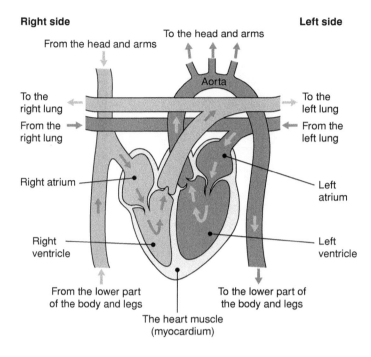

To the right lung

To the left lung

From the right lung

From the left lung

Aorta

Right atrium

Left atrium

Right ventricle

Left ventricle

From the lower part of the body and legs

To the lower part of the body and legs

The heart muscle (myocardium)

Figure 8.1 Diagram of the heart

Coronary heart disease

The coronary arteries are very small, with the largest ones being only the diameter of the inside of a biro (see Figure 8.3). They do, however, play an essential role in keeping the heart muscle healthy and pumping properly. Making the right lifestyle choices will help to keep these healthy

The heart

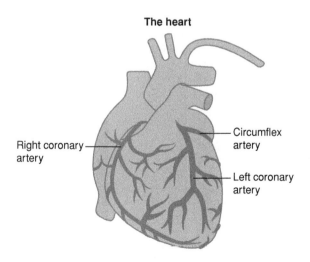

Right coronary artery

Circumflex artery

Left coronary artery

Figure 8.2 Diagram of the three arteries of the heart

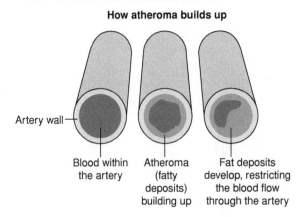

How atheroma builds up

Artery wall

Blood within   Atheroma   Fat deposits
the artery   (fatty   develop, restricting
                      deposits)   the blood flow
                      building up   through the artery

Figure 8.3 Diagram of the thickening of the arteries

and functioning properly. Coronary heart disease occurs when the coronary arteries become narrowed because fatty deposits called atheroma build up within the artery walls: this process is called atherosclerosis.

Angina and heart attacks

The atheroma that builds up in one or more coronary arteries may make the arteries so narrow that not enough blood reaches the heart muscle. This usually happens when someone is increasing their level of exertion, for example, walking briskly or running, but can also happen at rest. As there is not enough blood reaching the heart muscle, an individual may experience discomfort or pain in the chest. This pain is called angina. The pain may also present down the left arm, in the neck or jaw, and the amount of pain or discomfort felt does not always reflect how badly the coronary arteries are affected. Other symptoms such as feeling light-headed, sick, dizzy, sweaty, and slightly breathless may also be present.

The atherosclerotic process takes years to develop and is often the result of a lifetime of poor lifestyle choices. The onset of symptoms may be gradual or may not be present at all. Left untreated, however, and if lifestyle changes are not made, CHD can lead to a heart attack.

A heart attack occurs because the atheroma in the artery wall has become fragile and a piece may break off. A clot forms around the atheroma and can block the artery, cutting off the blood supply to the heart muscle. If the clot is not cleared, the heart muscle affected will be starved of oxygen and nutrients and will become severely damaged or will die. This could eventually lead to heart failure.

What increases the risk of coronary heart disease?

Risk factors for CHD are things about you or your lifestyle that increase the chances of getting CHD. There are some things that we can change and some that we cannot but there are always modifications that we can make to our lives that will make a difference and reduce the risk. The main risk factors for CHD are as follows:

- smoking any form of tobacco
- having high blood pressure
- having high blood cholesterol

- not taking enough physical activity
- being overweight or obese
- having diabetes
- having a family history of heart disease.

People with intellectual disabilities often have other medical conditions associated with being overweight and many have multiple co-morbidities or complex medical needs making them more susceptible to CHD. For example, research has shown that inflammatory conditions such as rheumatoid arthritis or having metabolic syndrome also increase the risk of CHD. A study in the Netherlands found that people with intellectual disabilities are 14 times more likely to have musculo-skeletal impairments, making taking part in physical activity difficult (van Schrojenstein Lantman-de Valk et al. 2000).

Metabolic syndrome, as defined by the International Diabetes Federation (IDF 2006), has been associated with a significant increase in risk of CHD and is used by practitioners as a marker point for intervention. Appropriate interventions include vigorous lifestyle modifications and, for some, prescribing medication to reduce the risk of developing the disease.

Using the IDF criteria, metabolic syndrome is defined as having:

- Central obesity (defined as waist circumference ≥94 cm for Europid men and ≥80 cm for Europid women, with ethnicity-specific values for other groups).
- Plus any two of the following four factors:
  - raised triglyceride level: ≥150 mg/dL (1.7 mmol/L), or specific treatment for this lipid abnormality
  - reduced high-density lipoproteins (HDL) cholesterol: <40 mg/dL (1.03 mmol/L) in males and <50mg/dL (1.29 mmol/L) in females, or specific treatment for this lipid abnormality
  - raised blood pressure: systolic BP ≥130 or diastolic BP ≥85 mmHg, or treatment of previously diagnosed hypertension
  - raised fasting plasma glucose (FPG) ≥100 mg/dL (5.6 mmol/L), or previously diagnosed Type 2 diabetes.

(If above 5.6 mmol/L or 100 mg/dL, an oral glucose tolerance test is strongly recommended but is not necessary to define the presence of the syndrome.)

What does being at risk actually mean?

Understanding risk can be a challenge. For some, a 25 per cent risk may seem less or greater than a risk presented as 1:4 or 25 out of 100. Expressing risk over time complicates matters further. For example, the risk of developing CHD is normally expressed as a risk occurring over a ten-year period. To some this could mean a risk at the end of ten years and to others a risk each year for a ten-year period. Understanding how risk affects the chances of developing a condition or risk of dying is not an easy concept.

It is important to choose the most appropriate method for communicating risk so as to ensure an understanding of the effects of risk factors on health and of the long-term lifestyle changes that need to be made. Pictorial charts are often used to emphasize the impact of risk, and how changes can improve the outcome or development of a disease.

Smiley face risk chart

The chart in Figure 8.4 displays the risk of developing CVD over a ten-year period, calculated using a cardiovascular risk score, for a fictional 52-year-old non-smoking male.

Note the difference in risk when our fictional person becomes a smoker. The risk rises to 31.4 per cent (see Figure 8.5). Pictorial charts can be used effectively to encourage lifestyle changes such as giving up smoking.

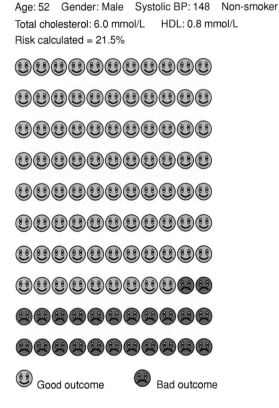

Age: 52   Gender: Male   Systolic BP: 148   Non-smoker
Total cholesterol: 6.0 mmol/L   HDL: 0.8 mmol/L
Risk calculated = 21.5%

Good outcome   Bad outcome

Figure 8.4 Example of risk for a non-smoker

How is risk assessed?

Most countries have a comparative cardiovascular risk assessment protocol similar to that used in the United Kingdom (UK). In the UK, everyone over the age of 40 years or who is assessed to be at high risk of CVD should be offered a cardiovascular risk assessment or health check (see Chapter 18). The health check will include:

- measurement of height, weight, and blood pressure
- blood tests for cholesterol and glucose (sugar) concentrations
- questions about family history, any prescribed medicines, diet, levels of physical activity, and smoking habits.

The health check looks at all the risk factors associated with CVD and not just at one risk factor in isolation. The more risk factors someone has, the greater the chance of getting CVD.

The combined results of the health check provide the practitioner with a better picture of the individual's general health as well as the risk of CVD, and inform the decision-making process about lifestyle changes to reduce the risk of heart disease, stroke, Type 2 diabetes, and kidney disease. If an individual's cholesterol or blood pressure is thought to significantly increase the risk of disease, medication may be prescribed to reduce that risk. While introducing medication may not be welcomed, especially for people who are often taking many other medications, it is essential to reduce the impact of the risk factors identified.

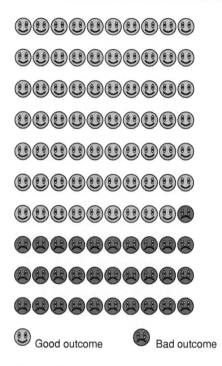

Good outcome   Bad outcome

Figure 8.5 Example of risk for a smoker

Understanding fully the impact of the risk factors will help individuals to identify lifestyle changes for themselves, which are more likely to be sustained, rather than having them imposed by others. This is particularly important where additional medication is prescribed so that compliance is successful.

How do the risk factors increase the risk of heart disease?

Each individual risk factor increases the risk of getting heart disease in a different way. However, while tackling them one at a time may make understanding them easier, many of them are interrelated with the result that addressing one issue could very well have an advantageous impact on several risk factors. For example, being physically active can reduce weight, increase the level of protective cholesterol (HDL), and decrease the risk of getting diabetes and having high blood pressure. Focusing on increasing the level of physical activity can have a positive impact on several risk factors in one go. Using this approach, where one lifestyle change has multiple impacts, can be highly motivating when used properly to encourage individuals to maintain their change. The impact of each of the risk factors is examined below.

Giving up smoking

Giving up smoking is probably the single most important thing that can be done to protect heart health. A 50-year cohort study found that mortality from cigarette smoking was 60 per cent higher for an average smoker compared with non-smokers (Doll et al. 2004). In the UK, 21 per cent of adults in the non-disabled population smoke (Scarborough et al. 2010).

While fewer adults with an intellectual disability smoke tobacco or drink alcohol compared with the non-disabled population, rates of smoking among adolescents with a mild intellectual disability are higher than their peers (Yusef et al. 2004) (see Chapter 12). Whatever the reason, quitting smoking is a challenge; using professional organizations and the advice of experienced helpers will help clients to address and understand the reasons why they started smoking and be more successful in their attempts to quit. The British Heart Foundation DVD (2009) *Live with a Healthy Heart* has a series of case studies that show how people with intellectual disabilities tackle the risk factors for CHD (see Useful Resources).

Controlling blood pressure

Over 12 million people in the UK are currently being treated for high blood pressure and it is suspected that a further 5 million are undiagnosed with the condition. High blood pressure brings with it a substantial health burden and risk of having a heart attack or stroke (Scarborough et al. 2010). The INTERHEART study estimates that 22 per cent of heart attacks in Western Europe are attributed to high blood pressure and that individuals with high blood pressure are nearly twice as likely to be at risk of a heart attack as those with a normal blood pressure (Yusef et al. 2004). The WHO report of 2002 estimated that 11 per cent of general disease burden in developed countries is due to raised blood pressure (WHO 2002), which further emphasizes the need for individuals to be aware of, and understand, their blood pressure readings.

Often it is only when blood pressure is extremely high that it presents with symptoms, thus earning it the reputation of being a silent killer. The only way to know if blood pressure is raised is to have it measured.

Screening is an important factor in identifying individuals at risk. With many people with intellectual disabilities requiring regular visits to health practitioners, it is good practice to ensure blood pressure measurements are done as part of a health check; this would limit the impact of white-coat hypertension (a condition where blood pressure is raised based on the anxiety surrounding the procedure but has no clinical significance).

Other risk factors that increase the likelihood of having high blood pressure include being overweight, eating food high in salt, and being physically inactive. Educating clients to cook with herbs rather than salt, not to add salt at the table, and to begin to understand the basics of food labelling will help to minimize the risk of high blood pressure.

Reducing blood cholesterol

Cholesterol is a fatty substance that is mainly produced by the liver and found in the blood. Cholesterol plays an essential role in how every cell in the body works. However, too much cholesterol in the blood can increase the risk of developing CVD.

Cholesterol is carried around the body by lipoproteins, which are a combination of cholesterol and proteins. There are two main types:

- LDL (low-density lipoproteins) is the *harmful* type of cholesterol
- HDL (high-density lipoproteins) is a *protective* type of cholesterol.

Triglycerides are another type of fatty substance in the blood, which are raised in people with a diet that contains lots of fatty and sugary foods and excessive amounts of alcohol. Raised triglycerides increase the risk of CHD.

There is no such thing as a 'normal' cholesterol reading, although most doctors would not treat otherwise healthy individuals without other risk factors if their cholesterol reading is around 5 mmol/L. However, for an accurate measurement and assessment of risk, a full cholesterol screening that measures HDL and allows for the calculation of LDL and triglycerides should be done. It is estimated that over 60 per cent of CHD and around 40 per cent of strokes are due to total blood cholesterol over 3.8 mmol/L (WHO 2002).

Understanding food labels and what is meant by 'good' and 'bad' fat can be difficult, but its importance should not be ignored. Like blood pressure, high cholesterol does not have any warning signs but can lead to the development of atheroma, resulting in angina and eventually a heart attack.

Health education programmes should explain the nutritional and health benefits of food groups with particular reference to protecting heart health. Embedding true understanding of the benefits of healthy eating without having to change a lifetime's eating habits can have more impact than just focusing on the negative attributes of food described as 'treats'. Identifying times when 'treats' can be enjoyed and sticking to these can help to reduce fat and sugar intake.

However, some people have high blood cholesterol even though their diet and lifestyle are healthy. For example, they may have inherited a condition called 'familial hypercholesterolaemia'. This condition will always require medical treatment as well as strict dietary control. It can be difficult to diagnose, and anyone suspected of having familial hypercholesterolaemia should be referred to a specialist.

Being physically active

Over 80 per cent of adults with intellectual disabilities take part in less physical activity than the minimum recommended by the Department of Health, and this is a much lower level of physical activity than among the non-disabled population (Robertson et al. 2000). People with intellectual disabilities take part in irregular physical activities, partly due to a lack of money and transport, in addition to a lack of motivation (see Chapter 16). Greater access to leisure and sporting facilities can promote community integration, physical, and mental wellbeing (Hallawell et al. 2012). Involvement in major sporting events such as Paralympics and Special Olympics enhances a person's social, psychological, and physical outcomes as well as increasing general awareness of the abilities of people with intellectual disabilities.

Introducing physical activity or increasing an activity in a daily routine can have a significant effect. Encouraging an individual to walk for part of their normal journey to work or to do their shopping can help them to lose weight, reduce their cholesterol and blood pressure, help control diabetes, and improve their sense of wellbeing.

To achieve the maximum benefit, physical activity should be regular and aerobic. People should aim to be active for some part of each day: benefits are seen when activity levels reach around 150 minutes a week. Encouraging varied activity everyday is likely to result in clients remaining engaged and wanting to take part. Organizations such as Special Olympics encourage physical activity and also reinforce lifestyle messages, including weight management and healthy eating.

Setting up group schemes and participating in local events can help to promote enjoyment and benefits. A wall progress chart can be used to document activity levels.

Maintaining a healthy body weight and shape

People with intellectual disabilities often have other health problems, many metabolic, which are commonly associated with being overweight. However, being overweight is a serious risk for CHD and can increase the risk of having high cholesterol, high blood pressure, and getting diabetes.

The incidence of obesity is greatest in people with mild intellectual disability, particularly women (RCN 2011). Fewer than 10 per cent of adults with intellectual disabilities residing in supported accommodation eat regular balanced diets, with the appropriate intake of fruit and vegetables (Robertson et al. 2000). Using charts to reflect progress with weight loss along with 'rewards' for achieving goals and making positive changes to eating habits can increase self-esteem and promote achievement. Helping an individual to chose their reward or aim for a specific target can be more effective in helping them stick to their goal rather than having a target or 'treat' selected for them.

When goals are achieved, rewarding success will maintain the journey through to the ultimate goal. Rewards should be appropriate and chosen with the individual. Rewards should not encourage reverting to habits that may encourage weight gain, such as eating sugary or fatty foods. Rewards could include buying a piece of clothing or a trip to a bowling alley or cinema. Joining a weight loss group such as Weightwatchers or Slimming World with friends, or starting your own can also help people to support and encourage each other to stick to their goal. Using BMI charts, tape measures or other visual aids, and keeping them prominent will also help them to achieve their goals (see Figure 8.6). Body shape is important, as excess weight around the middle significantly increases the risk of developing Type 2 diabetes (see Figure 8.7).

Having diabetes

Almost three million people in the UK have been diagnosed with diabetes and it is more common in men than women (Joint Heath Surveys Unit 2008). Many people with intellectual disabilities have diabetes due to other pre-existing metabolic disorders. They are more likely to develop diabetes than people who do not have an intellectual disability. This could be attributed to greater obesity, poor diet, and a less active lifestyle (RCN 2011). Diabetes significantly increases the risk of CVD. People from a South Asian or African Caribbean background are more likely to develop diabetes than the general population (Joint Heath Surveys Unit 2008).

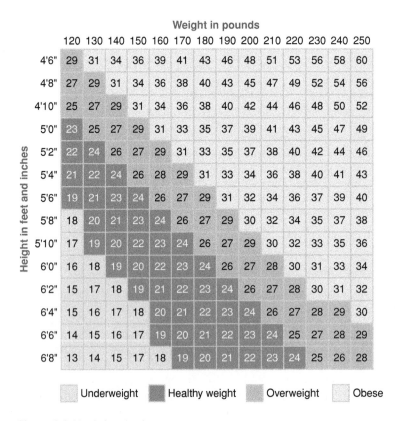

Figure 8.6 Height/weight chart

Note: 'Normal' height and weight vary depending on race/ethnicity and muscular build.

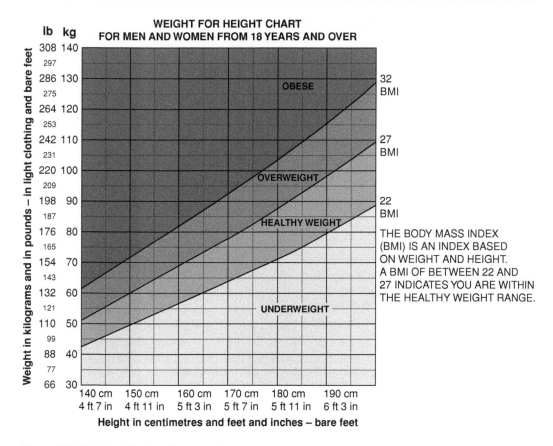

Figure 8.7 Height/weight chart for men and women

Having diabetes also increases the effect of some of the other risk factors for CVD, such as smoking and being overweight. There is a greater risk of having a high cholesterol and high blood pressure if you have diabetes.

Having a family history of heart disease

There is often confusion about who in the family is included in the term 'family history'. For someone to be considered as having a family history of CVD, they should have:

- a father or brother under the age of 55 who is diagnosed with angina, a stroke or having had a heart attack, or
- a mother or sister under the age of 65 who is diagnosed with angina, a stroke or having had a heart attack.

While it is important to acknowledge other family members who may have developed or died from CVD, the above definition focuses the risk on the immediate family. Although it is not possible to change a family history, anyone who has a first-degree relative with CVD who falls into one of these categories can make changes to their lifestyle that could reduce their risk of developing the disease at an early age.

How do we encourage good lifestyle choices?

Encouraging people with intellectual disabilities to understand the basics around food labelling and having easy-to-understand food groups that will benefit their general health will help them to make healthier choices. Tools such as the Healthy Eating Pate and traffic light labelling systems can enhance healthy decision making around food (see Chapter 5).

It is important to know what has worked for other people: peer support and encouragement can be extremely positive. The British Heart Foundation publication *Live with a Healthy Heart* (2009) is a very easy to use DVD and booklet (see Useful Resources). It uses animation and pictures to explain how the heart works, what CHD is, and how each of the risk factors can affect your chance of getting CHD. There are real-life case studies of people with intellectual disabilities who talk about changes they have made to their lives to try to reduce their risk of heart disease. Some of the changes they made centred on setting small achievable goals.

Summary

It is evident that there is much work to be done to ensure that CHD, a largely preventable condition, is no longer the second biggest cause of premature death among people with an intellectual disability. We recommend the following:

1. *Screen for heart disease*. Coronary heart disease is rarely seen as a first cause of illness in people with intellectual disabilities and is often not included in screening activities by general practitioners (GPs). Health screening programmes should incorporate cardiovascular risk assessment with appropriate recommendations for lifestyle changes.
2. *Accessible heart information*. Such information should be provided as photographs, pictures, signs, and symbols that will greatly benefit many people in society for whom words, regardless of their first language, are not the best way of relaying health messages. When created and used appropriately, these materials prove effective in reducing the ever-rising cost of heart disease.
3. *Diet and exercise*. To ensure a healthy life, individuals need a healthy diet and accessible information/guidance alongside exercise that is tailored to the individual's likes, needs, and abilities (Books Beyond Words have been shown to be extremely useful; Hollins and Flynn 2003). It may be that individuals walk a little further, do some sitting exercises, or start cycling – all of which will enhance their mental, emotional, and physical wellbeing. Joining a gym, a local walking group or Special Olympics group can improve a person's wellbeing and provide the peer support to keep going with healthy lifestyle choices.

Useful resources

- British Heart Foundation (2009) *Live with a Healthy Heart*. London: British Heart Foundation. Easy to use DVD and accompanying interactive booklet that shows what people with a learning disability can do to change their lifestyles to improve their heart health.

- British Heart Foundation (2009) *I'm Going to Go for It*. London: British Heart Foundation. Tracking the experience of a learning-disabled man's journey through heart surgery.

- Hollins, S., Cappuccio, F. and Adeline, P. (2005) *Looking After My Heart*. London: Gaskell and St. George's University of London. This is in the widely acclaimed 'Books Beyond Words' series and charts the story of Jane and her experiences of having heart problems and what she did to become healthier.

Risk factors

Genetics and lifestyle factors (for example, sedentary behaviour, poor diet, obesity, smoking, alcohol consumption) are widely seen as the two major leading causes of cancer worldwide. People with intellectual disabilities are also exposed to these two causes, but to a greater extent. It is well established that people with Down syndrome have a significantly higher rate of leukaemia than the general population, and that men with Down syndrome have a higher rate of testicular cancer; Satge et al. (2006) have identified a possible genetic basis for this.

Research has shown that people with intellectual disabilities are more likely to lead a sedentary lifestyle (McGuire et al. 2007), engage in low levels of exercise (Temple and Walkley 2003), and consume high fat diets (Ewing et al. 2004), all of which can contribute towards obesity, a significant risk factor for certain cancers including gastrointestinal and breast cancer (Magnusson et al. 1998). Another important risk factor associated with increased gastrointestinal and oesophageal cancer is *Helicobacter pylori* infection (Hogg and Tuffrey-Wijne 2008). The risk factors for developing stomach cancers are:

- *Helicobacter pylori* infection
- severe chronic atrophic gastritis (i.e. inflammation of the lining of the stomach)
- smoking and excessive use of alcohol
- diet: few fruits/vegetables, low fibre and high salt content
- medical conditions such as GORD, acid reflux and Barrett' oesophagus, which are more common in people with intellectual disabilities
- overweight/high BMI
- family history of gastrointestinal cancer
- low levels of physical activity and sedentary lifestyle (adapted from Cancer Research UK 2012).

In the case of cervical cancer Patja et al. (2001) has reported that women with intellectual disability are also more likely to develop cancer as a result of sexual inactivity, nulliparity (not having children), loss of menstruation with low oestrogen levels, and a shorter menstrual life. The risk factors are as follows:

- being between 50 and 69 years of age
- smoking
- nulliparity (not having children)
- age at menarche and at menopause
- oral contraceptives
- hormone replacement therapy
- breast density
- previous breast disease (proliferative breast disease without atypia)
- family history of breast cancer (adapted from Cancer Research UK 2012).

However, the low level of oestrogen seen in women with Down syndrome seems to act as a protective factor. It is also worth noting that sexual activity associated with both consensual sex or sexual abuse in women with intellectual disability is often underestimated if not completely denied.

The risk factors for testicular cancer are as follows:

- being of white origin
- being between 20 and 49 years of age
- previous history of testicular cancer
- cryptorchidism or undescended testes

- medical conditions such as an inguinal hernia and hypospadias
- family history of testicular cancer
- smoking (adapted from Cancer Research UK 2012).

Signs and symptoms of cancer

There is growing evidence to indicate that people with intellectual disabilities receive little information about the risk factors, and signs and symptoms of cancer. Furthermore, people with intellectual disabilities receive little health education and health promotion material regarding cancer prevention (Evenhuis et al. 2000; Disability Rights Commission 2006). Therefore, many people with intellectual disabilities are dependent upon family carers and front-line staff to advocate on their behalf to recognize the signs and symptoms of cancer and refer for medical attention. This includes family carers and front-line staff supporting the person with intellectual disabilities to make informed decisions, and subsequently engage in a healthier lifestyle to prevent certain cancers from developing. However, several studies have shown that front-line staff have not received specific education and therefore have limited knowledge regarding the signs and symptoms of gastrointestinal, breast and cervical cancers, and testicular cancer (Mencap 2004; Hanna et al. 2011).

Lindsey (2002) stated that one of the barriers to the access of people with intellectual disabilities to appropriate cancer health care is a lack of family carer and front-line staff awareness, as these carers may not be aware of the importance of a healthy lifestyle and may misinterpret behavioural and physical changes that point to underlying health problems. Additionally, Young et al. (2007) argue that proactive methods of supporting staff learning and development are urgently required among staff working with people with intellectual disability who may develop cancer.

The many barriers that have been documented in relation to breast and cervical cancer screening are related to women's characteristics (Poulos et al. 2006; Lalor and Redmond 2009; Proulx et al. 2009, 2012; Lin et al. 2010; Truesdale-Kennedy et al. 2011; McIlfatrick et al. 2011; Taggart et al. 2011):

- level of intellectual disability
- associated physical disabilities such as cerebral palsy
- challenging behaviours
- reactions to discomfort
- lack of understanding, embarrassment, and fears
- communication barriers
- negative attitudinal barriers from medical staff
- perception that screening is not in the best interest of the woman
- women are unable to consent
- women would be unable to cooperate
- systemic environmental setting issues (i.e. transportation barriers, lack of accessibility for a wheelchair, complexity of the service system).

The signs and symptoms of stomach cancer are:

- indigestion, acidity, and burping
- feeling full
- loss of appetite
- loss of weight
- bleeding of stomach ulcers and vomiting blood
- feeling tired or breathless as a result of loss of blood
- blood clots: pain or swelling in a leg, or sudden chest pain
- pain, sickness or some difficulty swallowing

- fluid in the abdomen
- blood in your stool (adapted from Cancer Research UK 2012).

The signs and symptoms of breast cancer are:

- breast lumps (but most are benign)
- a lump thickening in an area of breast
- change in size or shape of a breast
- dimpling of the skin
- change in the shape of the nipple (particularly if it turns in, sinks into the breast, or has an irregular shape)
- blood-stained discharge from the nipple
- rash on a nipple or surrounding area
- swelling or lump in the armpit (adapted from Cancer Research UK 2012).

The signs and symptoms of testicular cancer are:

- a lump in the testicle or swelling in part of one testicle
- discomfort or pain or a dull ache in the affected testicle or in the lower abdomen
- a heavy scrotum
- hormones in the blood: many testicular cancers make hormones that can be detected by blood tests
- sometimes testicular cancer cells can spread into lymph glands at the back of the abdomen; this can cause backache, which is usually constant and there will be a need to take painkillers
- having a cough, difficulty breathing, difficulty swallowing, and a swelling in the chest
- if testicular cancer has spread, there may be lumps in other parts of the body, around the collarbone, or in the neck for example; these lumps are affected lymph glands (adapted from Cancer Research UK 2012).

Cancer health education material

There have been a small number of educational initiatives targeted at this population involving the development of easy-to-read picture booklets and leaflets targeting certain cancers (see Useful Resources):

- *Cancer*: 'Common types of cancer'; 'Getting on with cancer'; 'Treatments for cancer'; 'Change cancer booklets'
- *Gastrointestinal and oesophageal cancers*: 'Bowel cancer'; 'Bowel screening'; 'Telling you about oesophageal cancer'
- *Breast and cervical cancers*: 'Be breast aware'; 'Looking after your breasts'; 'My boobs and me'; 'Having a mammogram'; 'Cervical cancer'; 'Cervical screening'
- *Testicular and prostate cancers*: 'Testicular awareness'; Testicular screening'; 'Looking after my balls'; 'Prostate cancer'; Prostate awareness', 'Your prostate examination'.

Cancer health promotion initiatives

Breast and cervical

In the UK, Symonds and Howsam (2004) developed a teaching pack for residential staff working with women with intellectual disabilities that focuses on breast awareness and how to prepare these women for breast screening. Evaluation of the educational resource was well received; however, no comment was made about whether uptake has improved or whether referrals for breast screening have increased.

The Women Be Healthy curriculum

This programme (Lunsky et al.) was developed in the USA to enable women with intellectual disabilities to become more active participants in their health care. Its primary emphasis is on teaching women about reproductive health and breast/cervical cancer screenings. The topics covered are relevant to any woman interested in increasing her knowledge about, and becoming more comfortable with, women's health issues. The curriculum focuses on three components to help women become better health advocates: health education, anxiety reduction, and assertiveness and empowerment training. The curriculum includes psycho-education, coping skills training, exposure to the medical setting, and assertiveness training. The programme offers a group-based intervention that helps women with intellectual disabilities become more knowledgeable and eventually more comfortable with healthcare procedures. The curriculum was first assessed in 2003 with 22 women, who completed assessments of health knowledge, health behaviour beliefs, and coping strategies before and after participation in the eight-week curriculum, which took place in a group setting at a clinic for people with intellectual disabilities.

More recently, Parish et al. (2012) conducted a randomized control trial to test the effectiveness of the curriculum (on a sample of 175 women). The trial showed that women's knowledge about both cervical and breast cancer screening can be improved. The programme is particularly effective in reference to breast cancer screening. It is a promising short-term intervention addressing fairly complex health care procedures.

Cancer health screening

Evidence-based data, as well as evolving investigation techniques and treatment options, have demonstrated the importance of early diagnosis in dealing with breast cancer. Many industrialized countries have implemented organized breast cancer screening programmes. Such programmes generally target segments of women more at risk: those aged 50–79 years. Those public health measures are usually offered in accordance with the principle of equity of access. However, accessibility and utilization of screening has been identified as a major issue for population sub-groups such as women living with disabilities, especially those with intellectual disabilities (McIlfatrick et al. 2011; Taggart et al. 2011; Truesdale-Kennedy et al. 2011).

Organized breast cancer screening programmes generally consist of a step-by-step process involving different actions to be taken by the woman or those who support her. Women may receive an invitation letter or a prescription from their doctor. They then need to make an appointment and find their way to where the mammogram will take place. Depending on the programme, they may be asked to sign a consent form. Even if there is no consent form, professionals need to be sure the woman is sufficiently informed in order to consent. Women have to undergo the mammogram and then wait for their results. If abnormal results are found, additional tests might be necessary. If some cancer cells are detected, women need to be informed about, and give their consent to, relevant treatment. To understand and negotiate the different stages, facilitators involved in access to organized breast cancer screening programmes need to explore existing issues at different entry points to breast cancer screening programmes (Poulos et al. 2006; Truesdale-Kennedy et al. 2011; Proulx et al. 2012).

Summary

Identification of those at risk

- Identify those at risk of developing gastrointestinal (i.e. stomach and gallbladder) and oesophageal cancers, breast and cervical cancers, and testicular and prostate cancers.
- Recognize the genetic risk factors: family history age, gender, ethnicity.

- Recognize the lifestyle risk factors: obesity, high BMI, poor diet, sedentary lifestyle, smoking, alcohol consumption.
- Recognize medical associated conditions: *Helicobacter pylori* infection, GORD, reflux, nulliparity, other medical conditions, change in appetite/weight, vomiting, blood in stools.

Health education

All front-line staff to be offered training on gastrointestinal (i.e. stomach and gallbladder) and oesophageal cancers, breast and cervical cancers, and testicular and prostate cancers.

Educational and resource materials for front-line staff need to be made available, so they can educate and empower people with intellectual disabilities about the risk factors, signs and symptoms, and lifestyle choices, as well as uptake of screening opportunities.

Ensure that women with intellectual disabilities understand the importance of breast checks and attending for a mammogram; likewise for cervical awareness, and cervical smears should be encouraged.

Ensure men with intellectual disabilities are taught about the importance of testicular examinations and that they seek medical advice early.

Health screening and annual health checks

- Family carers and front-line staff should be proactive, observing for changes and making referrals to the GP.
- Ensure adults with intellectual disabilities engage in yearly annual health checks.
- Women with intellectual disabilities need to be supported to check for breast cancer.
- Men with Down syndrome need to be supported to check for testicular cancer signs and symptoms.
- Screen for *Helicobacter pylori* infection.

Useful resources

- Taggart, L. (2010) *Me and my Boobs? Breast Cancer What does it Mean to Me?* An information booklet for women with learning disabilities. University of Ulster and Compass Advocacy Network. http://www.science.ulster.ac.uk/inr/public/pdf/Me_and_my_boobs.pdf

- *Pap Test: The Plain Facts*, a booklet for people with intellectual disability: www.cddh. monash.org/assets/paptestbooklet.pdf

- *Being a Healthy Woman – An Educational Resource for Women with Intellectual Disability, their Families, Health Care Providers, Carers and Support Workers*: http://www.health.nsw.gov.au/pubs/2010/pdf/being_a_healthy_woman.pdf

- *Preventative Women's Health Care for Women with Intellectual Disabilities*: www.cds.org.au/publications-home/cat_view/50-health-publications

- Queensland Centre for Intellectual and Developmental Disability: www2.som.uq.edu.au/som/Research/ResearchCentres/qcidd/Pages/Resources.aspx

---

Web resources

- Cancer: http://www.easyhealth.org.uk/listing/cancer-(leaflets)
- Cervical screening: http://www.easyhealth.org.uk/listing/cervical-screening-(leaflets)
- Looking after your breasts: http://www.easyhealth.org.uk/listing/breasts-(leaflets)
- Testicular awareness: http://www.easyhealth.org.uk/listing/testicles-(leaflets)

References

Bonell, S. (2010) System disorders: neoplasms, in J. O'Hara, J. McCarthy and N. Bouras (eds.) *Intellectual Disability and Ill Health: A Review of the Evidence.* Cambridge: Cambridge University Press.

Boyle, P. and Levin, B. (2008) *World Cancer Report 2008.* Geneva: WHO. Cancer Research UK (2012) Available at: http://info.cancerresearchuk.org/cancerstats/types

Disability Rights Commission (DRC) (2006) *Equal Treatment: Closing the Gap. A Formal Investigation into Physical Health Inequalities Experienced by People with Learning Disabilities and/or Mental Health Problems.* London: DRC.

Duff, M., Scheepers, M., Cooper, M., Hoghton, M. and Baddeley, P. (2001) *Helicobacter pylori*: has the killer escaped from the institution? A possible cause of increased stomach cancer in a population with intellectual disability. *Journal of Intellectual Disability Research,* 45: 219–25.

Durvasula, S. and Beange, H. (2002) Mortality of people with intellectual disability in northern Sydney. *Journal of Intellectual and Developmental Disability,* 27: 255–64.

Evenhuis, H., Henderson, C.M., Beange, H., Lennox, N. and Chicoine, B. (2000) *Healthy Ageing – Adults with Intellectual Disabilities: Physical Health Issues.* Geneva: WHO. Available at: http://www.who.int/mental_health/media/en/21.pdf [accessed 29 November 2012].

Ewing, G., McDermott, S., Thomas-Koger, M., Whitner, W. and Pierce, K. (2004) Evaluation of a cardiovascular health program for participants with mental retardation and normal learners. *Health Education and Behaviours,* 31: 77–87.

Hanna, L.M., Taggart, L. and Cousins, W. (2011) Cancer prevention and health promotion for people with intellectual disabilities: an exploratory study of staff knowledge. *Journal of Intellectual Disability Research,* 55(3): 281–91.

Hogg, J. and Tuffrey-Wijne, I. (2008) Cancer and intellectual disability: a review of some key contextual issues. *Journal of Applied Research in Intellectual Disabilities,* 21: 509–18.

Hollins, S., Attard, M.T., von Fraunhofer, N., McGuigan, S. and Sedgwick, P. (1998) Mortality in people with learning disability: risks, causes, and death certification findings in London. *Developmental Medicine and Child Neurology,* 40: 50–6.

Jaffe, J.S., Esinberg, A.M. and Chambers, J.T. (2002) Low prevalence of abnormal cervical cytology in an institutionalised population with intellectual disability. *Journal of Intellectual Disability Research,* 46(7): 567–74.

Lalor, A. and Redmond, R. (2009) Breast screening for post-menopausal women. *Learning Disability Practice,* 12(9): 28–33.

Lin, J., Lin, P., Lin, L., Wu, S. and Wu, L. (2010) Physical activity and its determinants among adolescents with intellectual disabilities. *Research in Developmental Disabilities,* 31(1): 263–9.

Lindsey, M. (2002) Comprehensive health care services for people with learning disabilities. *Advances in Psychiatric Treatment,* 8: 138–48.

Lunsky, Y., Straiko, A., & Armstrong, S.C. (2002). *Women Be Healthy: A curriculum for women with mental retardation/developmental disabilities.* Revised by SM Havercamp, C. Kluttz-Hile, & Dickens, P. Chapel Hill, NC: North Carolina Office on Disability and Health.

Magnusson, C., Baron, J., Persson, I., Wolk, A., Bergström, R. and Trichopoulous, D. (1998) Body size in different periods of life and breast cancer risk in post-menopausal women. *International Journal of Cancer,* 76: 29–34.

McGuire, B.E., Daly, P. and Smyth, F. (2007) Lifestyle and health behaviours of adults with an intellectual disability. *Journal of Intellectual Disability Research,* 51: 497–510.

McIlfatrick, S.J., Taggart, L. and Truesdale-Kennedy, M.N. (2011) Supporting women with intellectual disabilities to access breast cancer screening: a health care professional perspective. *European Journal of Cancer Care,* 20: 412–20.

Mencap (2004) *Treat me Right! Better Healthcare for People with a Learning Disability.* Available at: http://www.mencap.org.uk/sites/default/files/documents/2008-03/treak_me_right_easyread.pdf [accessed 5 July 2013].

Parish, S.L., Rose, R.A., Luken, K., Swaine, J.G. and O'Hare, L. (2012) Cancer screening knowledge changes results from a randomized control trial of women with developmental disabilities. *Research on Social Work Practice,* 22: 43–53.

Patja, K., Eero, P. and Livanainen, M. (2001) Cancer incidence among people with intellectual disability. *Journal of Intellectual Disability Research,* 45: 300–7.

Poulos, A.E., Balandin, S., Llewellyn, G. and Dew, A.H. (2006) Women with cerebral palsy and breast cancer screening by mammography. *Archives of Physical Medicine and Rehabilitation,* 87(2): 304–7.

Proulx, R., Lemétayer, F., Mercier, C., Jutras, S. and Major, D. (2009) *Proposals to Facilitate Access to the Quebec Breast Cancer Screening Program for Women with Activity Limitations*. Montréal: Intellectual Disability, Pervasive Developmental Disorders and Intersectorality Research Team.

Proulx, R., Mercier, C., Lemétayer, F., Jutras, S. and Major, D. (2012) Access to breast cancer screening programs for women with disabilities. *Journal of Health Care for the Poor and the Underserved*, 23(4): 1609–19.

Satge, D., Sasco, A.J., Vekemans, M.J., Portal, M.L. and Flejou, J.F. (2006) Aspects of digestive tract tumours in Down syndrome: a literature review. *Digestive Diseases and Sciences*, 51(11): 2053–61.

Sullivan, S., Hussain, R., Slack-Smith, L.M. and Bittles, A.H. (2003) Breast cancer uptake of mammography screening services by women with intellectual disabilities. *Preventive Medicine*, 37: 507–12.

Sullivan, S., Hussain, R., Threlfall, T. and Bittles, A. (2004) The incidence of cancer in people with intellectual disabilities. *Cancer Causes and Control*, 15: 1021–5.

Symonds, D. and Howsam, K. (2004) Breast awareness in learning disabilities. *Cancer Nursing Practice*, 3: 8–10.

Taggart, L., Truesdale-Kennedy, M.N. and McIlfatrick, S.J. (2011) The role of community and residential staff in supporting women with intellectual disabilities to access breast screening services. *Journal of Intellectual Disability Research*, 55(1): 41–52.

Temple, V.A. and Walkley, J.W. (2003) Physical activity of adults with intellectual disability. *Journal of Intellectual and Developmental Disability*, 28: 323–34.

Truesdale-Kennedy, M.N., Taggart, L. and McIlfatrick, S.J. (2011) Breast cancer knowledge among women with intellectual disabilities and their experiences of breast mammography. *Journal of Advanced Nursing*, 67(6): 1294–1304.

Young, A.F., Chesson, R.A. and Wilson, A.J. (2007) People with learning disabilities, carers and care workers awareness of health risk and implications for primary care. *Family Practice*, 24: 576–84.

10 Sexual health

Gillian Eastgate and Judith Moyle

Introduction

People with intellectual disabilities commonly experience opposition to sexual activity and difficulty expressing their sexuality in a safe and healthy way. Those supporting them face complex challenges. Lack of acceptance of the sexuality of people with intellectual disabilities also has implications for access to sexuality-related health promotion, screening, and health care. The key areas in sexual health promotion for people with intellectual disabilities include: relationship formation; sexual abuse and relationship violence; appropriate sexual behaviour; contraception, sterilization, and menstrual management; pregnancy and parenting; and screening in sexual and reproductive health. This chapter outlines the challenges, practice issues, and potential solutions for promoting the sexual health of people with intellectual disabilities.

Sexual health for people with intellectual disabilities

The sexuality of people with intellectual disabilities has been the object of fear, stigma, and doubt. People with intellectual disabilities may be viewed as asexual 'innocents' in need of protection or as oversexed 'degenerates' from whom the rest of society needs protection (Brown 2003). When sexual activity is acknowledged, attitudes may be negative and even punitive.

Since the 1970s, de-institutionalization and 'normalization' have led to greater recognition of the sexual rights of people with intellectual disabilities (Stokes and Kaur 2005; Sullivan and Caterino 2008; Hosseinkhazadeh et al. 2012). However, as with other health issues, people with intellectual disabilities have suboptimal sexual and reproductive health. The main areas of concern are discussed below.

Relationship formation

People with intellectual disabilities express interest in and longing for intimate relationships. However, a person with intellectual disabilities may experience difficulty negotiating the complexities of forming a sexual relationship due to limited social opportunities and poor social skills. Permission or privacy for sexual activity may be limited; this may lead to unsafe or illegal activity such as sex in parks or other public places (Healy et al. 2009). Capacity to consent to sexual activity may be difficult for caregivers to assess, and legislation regarding consent is confusing (Murphy and O'Callaghan 2004).

Sexual abuse and relationship violence

People with intellectual disabilities are at high risk of sexual abuse (McCarthy and Thompson 1997). Perpetrators include family members, caregivers, and other people with intellectual disabilities. Vulnerability to abuse is related to a poor understanding of appropriate behaviour, difficulty negotiating equal relationships, susceptibility to manipulation, lack of awareness of one's rights, and difficulty in reporting abuse (O'Hara and Martin 2001; Valenti-Hein 2002). Long-term sequelae of sexual abuse include maladjustment, poor sexual and relationship function, risky sexual activity, and repeated victimization (Polusny and Follette 1995). People with intellectual disabilities may also be at increased risk of violence in their relationships (Ward et al. 2010).

Appropriate sexual behaviour

Concerns are frequently raised regarding inappropriate sexual behaviours, including public masturbation or soliciting sex inappropriately, such as from minors or in public places (Charman and Clare 1992). A person with intellectual disabilities may be charged with a sexual offence, sometimes with no idea why (Lindsay 2002). Men with intellectual disabilities may be given androgen suppressant medication such as cyproterone (which has multiple adverse health effects) in response to inappropriate sexual behaviour, sometimes without appropriate education or behavioural support.

Contraception, sterilization, and menstrual management

Despite the availability of a range of contraceptive methods, women with intellectual disabilities are very likely to be treated with depot medroxyprogesterone acetate (DMPA) (McCarthy 2011), which is associated with weight gain and osteoporosis (Westhoff 2003). DMPA is often used for 'menstrual suppression' even though most women with intellectual disabilities can learn basic menstrual hygiene. Sterilization (Dorozynski 2000) or hysterectomy (Pandya 1997) may be sought for a girl or woman with intellectual disabilities without her knowledge or consent (Chou and Lu 2011). Legal restrictions may be circumvented (Stansfield et al. 2007); in some countries, they may be non-existent.

Pregnancy and parenting

Most people with intellectual disabilities have normal fertility, and many desire children. However, when a woman with intellectual disabilities becomes pregnant, the news is often met with dismay, and some women report pressure to terminate the pregnancy. Opposition to pregnancy and childbearing may limit access to preconception care (Harelick et al. 2011) and support after the birth (Walsh-Gallagher et al. 2012). Parents with intellectual disabilities face multiple challenges related to their disability and to associated socio-economic disadvantage. Their children may be at increased risk of having intellectual disabilities as well. Children without intellectual disabilities may outgrow their parents' ability at a young age and are over-represented in the child protection system (McConnell et al. 2000). Appropriate support may be limited or difficult to access. Even with support in place, children may need alternative caregivers (Willems et al., 2007).

Screening in sexual and reproductive health

Screening for sexually transmitted infections

Information regarding sexually transmitted infections (STIs) for people with intellectual disabilities is limited (Servais 2006). Adolescents with intellectual disabilities, like all adolescents, are prone to sexual risk behaviours, and are at similar or greater STI risk as other young people (Mandell et al. 2008). Clandestine relationships, sexual abuse and exploitation increase the risk of unrecognized STIs and failure to provide screening (Horner-Johnson and Drum 2006).

Screening for breast and cervical cancer

Women with intellectual disabilities are less likely to receive breast and cervical cancer screening than other women, due to lack of awareness of the need for screening, lack of support, and an inability to tolerate the required procedure (McIlfatrick et al. 2011) (see Chapter 9).

Screening for prostate and testicular cancer

For men in general, the evidence regarding prostate and testicular cancer screening is inconsistent. There is little information regarding screening of men with intellectual disabilities. Men with intellectual disabilities appear to have less prostate cancer but more testicular cancer than men in the general population (Hogg and Tuffrey-Wijne 2008) (see Chapter 9).

Practice issues relevant to sexual health

Like other health issues, the sexual health of people with intellectual disabilities is affected not only by the disability itself but by the commonly associated negative health determinants of poverty, poor education, inadequate accommodation, unemployment, discrimination, limited social integration, and poor access to health services. Many people with intellectual disabilities need ongoing support and supervision. These needs are most often met by living with family members or in group situations with other people with disabilities. Where a person with intellectual disabilities is housed and with whom is vitally important and may have lifelong implications: the wellbeing of the person must always be the priority. The housing situation of a person with intellectual disabilities may limit privacy and permission for sexual relationships (Kelly et al. 2009). People may also be at risk of sexual abuse and assault from family members, support staff or co-residents (McCarthy and Thompson 1997).

The design of shared housing must address issues of both privacy and safety. Rules and policies need to be clarified and reviewed regularly to ensure both respect for appropriate couple relationships and the safety and comfort of other residents. Staff training and permission to discuss sexuality is important. Informal discussion about sexual issues may help to overcome some of the subtle but powerful environmental and systemic barriers to learning.

Many incidents of sexual assault in shared housing can be averted by strong, enforceable policies governing decisions about placement of vulnerable individuals in shared residential services. Equally important is a robust system for screening accommodation support staff before and during employment, and a commitment to thorough investigation of complaints about staff behaviour.

Sexual violence, abuse, and offending

People with intellectual disabilities may find it difficult to protect themselves against relationship violence (Ward et al. 2010), sexual abuse, and exploitation (Eastgate et al. 2011). Teaching of self-protection skills is inconsistent; furthermore, it is not always followed by frequent reinforcement, which is needed by this group (Eastgate et al. 2012). There are few services providing sexual assault services tailored to the needs of people with intellectual disabilities (Barger et al. 2009). There is a need for recognition of the problem and for the provision of appropriate ongoing education, prevention, and support services.

Responses to inappropriate sexual behaviour and offending must include adequate education and intensive behavioural reinforcement. Some people with intellectual disabilities may have absorbed the message that any sexual expression is unacceptable (Hingsburger et al. 1999). Others may have absorbed mistaken understandings about sexual behaviours from television or other media. These misconceptions need to be addressed before more acceptable behaviours can be taught.

Menstrual management, contraception, and sterilization

People with intellectual disabilities have the same right to choice in menstrual and fertility management as other people in the community. It is important to ensure the 'least restrictive alternative'. For example, women should be given the opportunity to learn menstrual hygiene measures before 'menstrual suppression' is considered. Good educational resources exist, and should be promoted and made freely available.

It is important to consider the full range of contraceptive and menstrual management options available, the suitability of each for the person, the person's ability to use each method, and any possible interactions with other medications. Education and awareness-raising exercises among people with disability, support workers, and health professionals is needed to improve the range of choices offered.

Most 'developed' countries have laws governing the sterilization of people with intellectual disabilities. In general, sterilization must be approved by relevant agencies, usually only after the failure of less restrictive alternatives. However, sterilizations still occur outside these guidelines (Stansfield et al. 2007; Brady et al. 2001). It is important to ensure understanding of, and adherence to, the law. There is also a need for community and professional education about alternatives to sterilization, and promotion of attitudinal change to reduce pressure for sterilization. It is also essential to emphasize that prevention of pregnancy is no substitute for prevention of sexual abuse. In countries with less legal protection, it is important to involve people with intellectual disabilities in the decision-making process, and to encourage the development of protective legislation (Pandya 1997).

Pregnancy care for women with intellectual disability

Preconception care has an important role in reducing health risks before and during pregnancy, and improving pregnancy outcomes (Van Der Zee et al. 2011). Women of low socio-economic status experience more risk factors and are less likely to receive preconception care (Harelick et al. 2011); most women with intellectual disabilities also experience socio-economic disadvantage. While attitudes towards pregnancy and childbirth for women with intellectual disabilities remain negative (Walsh-Gallagher et al. 2012), such women are likely to face opposition to their intention to have children, making preconception care unlikely (Quilliam et al. 2001).

Although women with disabilities have reported pressure to terminate their pregnancies (Walsh-Gallagher et al. 2012), the extent of this phenomenon is not known. It is likely that such terminations occur, possibly without the women's full informed consent, but are not openly discussed.

Women with intellectual disabilities experience a lack of support and isolation during and after pregnancy (McConnell et al. 2008). There is a need for education and attitudinal change among families, support workers, and health professionals to enhance these women's experiences before, during, and after pregnancy.

Parents with intellectual disability

Less than 2 per cent of people with intellectual disabilities are parents. Most of these have border-line to mild disability. Many are able to care for their children with minimal support (McConnell et al. 2000; Willems et al. 2007). However, parents with intellectual disabilities may have difficulty understanding and responding to their children's needs, and may find it difficult to access important developmental activities due to social exclusion or lack of money. When support is needed, there is a shortage of appropriate services (McConnell et al. 2000). Even where these exist, people with intellectual disabilities may experience difficulty accessing them.

Should a parent need supported accommodation, it may be difficult or impossible to place parents and children together. There appears to be little research or policy regarding this issue, but there are anecdotal accounts of parents being placed in supported accommodation while their children are placed in foster care.

Children of parents with intellectual disabilities are much more likely to be removed from the care of their parents than the children of other parents who come to the notice of child protection authorities (McConnell and Llewellyn 1998). In some cases, the children are removed shortly after birth, suggesting a presumption of inability to care for children. Parents with intellectual disabilities may be marginalized by the court system and their children removed without a trial of added support within the family. Children may even be removed due to lack of appropriate support services (McConnell and Llewellyn 1998). Difficulties may be attributed to the parents' disabilities without reference to the multiple associated disadvantages faced by these parents, including financial difficulty, housing instability, and stigma. There is a need for education and attitudinal change for professionals within the child protection system (McConnell et al. 2000).

Sexual health screening

The value of annual health checks is discussed elsewhere in this book (see Chapter 18). Sexual health should be integrated into health checks for all adolescents and adults. When considering screening for STIs, it is important to acknowledge that a person with intellectual disabilities may not speak readily about sexual activity, and his or her family or support carers and front-line staff may be unaware of such activity. When considering the need for STI screening, it is important to consider the possibility of clandestine relationships and sexual abuse.

Increasing the level of screening for sexual health issues for this population requires education and awareness-raising among people with intellectual disabilities, their families, support staff, and health professionals (Hanna et al. 2011). Educational material needs to be available in forms that people with intellectual disabilities can understand. People with intellectual disabilities may need support to undergo the often uncomfortable examinations and procedures required for screening such as cervical smears and mammograms.

Sexuality education

Understanding of the body, sexual function, relationships, and appropriate behaviour is fundamental to healthy sexual expression, safe, mutual relationships, and resistance to abuse (Walker-Hirsch 2007a). Appropriate education is essential to achieve this. People with intellectual disabilities have difficulty retaining information, so education needs to be reinforced throughout the lifespan (Walker-Hirsch 2007b). It is also important to be able to assess understanding of sexuality. Tools such as the Assessment of Sexual Knowledge (ASK) tool (Galea et al. 2004) facilitate individual support and inform training programmes. People with intellectual disabilities may lack basic sexual knowledge: this has been associated with vulnerability to abuse, inappropriate behaviour, and sexual offending (Healy et al. 2009; Eastgate et al. 2011).

Most sexuality and relationship education is provided to adolescents at school. It is often not compulsory, and may exclude students with intellectual disabilities due to perceived lack of need, poor awareness of the need to learn protective behaviours, or to misplaced fears of increased sexual interest or arousal. Well-designed programmes, adequate training of teachers, and awareness-raising exercises among families are needed to ensure that all adolescents receive adequate sexuality education (see Chapter 15).

For adults, there is even less access to education. There are few structured long-term programmes and limited resources. Although most adults access information informally from books, television or the Internet, adults with intellectual disabilities may have low literacy, poor access to resources or difficulty synthesizing information. They may misunderstand what they see on television or online, or be exploited by pornographic or 'dating' sites (Eastgate et al. 2012).

Consistent, effective sexuality education and support for people with intellectual disabilities requires suitable curricula, adequate funding, inclusion in all education and employment services, and appropriate training and support for families and professionals.

Case study: Samuel and Paulette

Samuel and Paulette attend the same day activity programme. They live in different community residential units. Samuel, aged 28, has autism spectrum disorder and intellectual disabilities. Paulette, aged 35, has mild intellectual disability. Both have epilepsy. After some months of friendship they have indicated that they are 'in a relationship'. They go on dates (with a support worker) and visit each other's houses for meals and private (unsupervised) time together. Both have indicated that they are 'having sex'.

Paulette and Samuel have previously attended sexuality training programmes. However, their support workers are concerned about their knowledge of STIs and contraception, and refer them for counselling. The counsellor is not sure that they are describing sexual intercourse when they discuss 'having sex' with each other, or that they understand the use of condoms.

The counsellor completes the Assessment of Sexual Knowledge tool with Samuel and Paulette separately. Results indicate that neither understands many of the words they use to describe their times of intimacy. Both have limited understanding of sexual intercourse and no knowledge of STIs, contraception, or pregnancy. For example, the word 'condom' seems to have been used to describe a male erection. In addition, Paulette says that she wants to have babies, but Samuel indicates that he does not like children and would not cope with crying babies 'because of his seizures'. The counsellor recommends comprehensive education about the reproductive system, relationships, and contraception. Samuel and Paulette will also need to address their disagreement about prospective parenthood.

If Paulette and Samuel wish to progress their relationship, further consideration will need to be given to:

- *Housing*: considerable negotiation may be needed if the couple wants to move in together, as both will continue to need accommodation support.
- *Medical assessment*: which may include contraception, preconception care, and genetic counselling.
- *Parenting support*: if they do have a child.

Summary

- People with intellectual disabilities experience similar sexual needs to those of people without disabilities.
- People with intellectual disabilities experience inadequate sexuality education, difficulty forming relationships, obtaining sexual health care and screening, and barriers to family formation and parenting. There is a large unmet need for education, support, and skill development for people with intellectual disabilities, their support people, and health and legal professionals.
- Many of these difficulties experienced by people with intellectual disabilities are compounded by social disadvantage, including poverty, poor housing, restriction of rights, and stigmatization.
- Strong policies and the necessary funding are required for provision of adequate accommodation, sexuality education, relationship and parenting support, and health care.

Useful resources

- Health Scotland (2008) *Sexual Health and Relationships: A Review of Resources for People with Intellectual Disabilities*. Glasgow: Health Scotland. Provides a list of resources: http://www.healthscotland.com/documents/1185.aspx

- International Online Resource Centre on Disability and Inclusion. Links to relevant articles: http://asksource.ids.ac.uk/cf/keylists/keylist2.cfm?topic=az&search=QL_DISSEX05

- United Nations Population Fund (2007) *Emerging Issues: Sexual and Reproductive Health of Persons with Disabilities*. New York: United Nations: http://www.unfpa.org/upload/lib_pub_file/741_filename_UNFPA_DisFact_web_sp-1.pdf

- World Health Organization (WHO) (2009) *Promoting Sexual and Reproductive Health for Persons with Disabilities*, WHO/UNFPA Guidance Note. Geneva: WHO/United Nations Population Fund: http://whqlibdoc.who.int/publications/2009/9789241598682_eng.pdf

- The President and Fellows of Harvard College (2008) *We Have Human Rights: A Human Rights Handbook for People with Developmental Disabilities*. Harvard Project on Disability. Accessible-language document on human rights for people with disabilities: http://hpod.pmhclients.com/pdf/we-have-human-rights.pdf

- The Assessment of Sexual Knowledge (ASK) is a new test that aims to provide workers within disability services and other health professionals with a tool to assess the sexual knowledge and attitudes of people with an intellectual disability: http://www.cddh.monash.org/assets/ask-order-form.pdf

Web resources

- Maternity: http://www.easyhealth.org.uk/listing/maternity-(leaflets)

- Menopause: http://www.easyhealth.org.uk/listing/menopause-(leaflets)

- Parenting: http://www.easyhealth.org.uk/listing/parenting-(leaflets)

- Pregnancy: http://www.easyhealth.org.uk/listing/pregnancy-(leaflets)

- Puberty: http://www.easyhealth.org.uk/listing/puberty-(leaflets)

References

Barger, E., Wacker, J., Macy, R. and Parish, S. (2009) Sexual assault prevention for women with intellectual aisabilities: a critical review of the evidence. *Intellectual and Developmental Disabilities*, 47: 249–62.

Brady, S., Briton, J. and Grover, S. (2001) *The Sterilisation of Girls and Young Women in Australia: Issues and Progress*. Sydney, NSW: Human Rights and Equal Opportunity Commission.

Brown, H. (2003) 'An ordinary sexual Life?' A review of the normalisation principle as it applies to the sexual options of people with learning disabilities. *Disability and Society*, 9: 123–44.

Charman, T. and Clare, I. (1992) Education about the laws and social rules relating to sexual behaviour. *Mental Handicap*, 20: 74–80.

Chou, Y.C. and Lu, Z.Y.J. (2011) Deciding about sterilisation: perspectives from women with an intellectual disability and their families in Taiwan. *Journal of Intellectual Disability Research*, 55: 63–74.

Dorozynski, A. (2000) Sterilisation of 14 mentally handicapped women challenged. *British Medical Journal*, 321(7263): 721.

Eastgate, G., Van Driel, M.L., Lennox, N.G. and Scheermeyer, E. (2011) Women with intellectual disabilities – a study of sexuality, sexual abuse and protection skills. *Australian Family Physician*, 40: 226–30.

Eastgate, G., Scheermeyer, E., Van Driel, M.L. and Lennox, N. (2012) Intellectual disability, sexuality and sexual abuse prevention: a study of family members and support workers. *Australian Family Physician*, 41: 135–9.

Galea, J., Butler, J. and Iacono, T. (2004) The assessment of sexual knowledge in people with intellectual disability. *Journal of Intellectual and Developmental Disability*, 29: 350–65.

Hanna, L.M., Taggart, L. and Cousins, W. (2011) Cancer prevention and health promotion for people with intellectual disabilities: an exploratory study of staff knowledge. *Journal of Intellectual Disability Research*, 55: 281–91.

Harelick, L., Viola, D. and Tahara, D. (2011) Preconception health of low socioeconomic status women: assessing knowledge and behaviors. *Women's Health Issues*, 21: 272–6.

Healy, E., McGuire, B.E., Evans, D.S. and Carley, S.N. (2009) Sexuality and personal relationships for people with an intellectual disability. Part I: Service-user perspectives. *Journal of Intellectual Disability Research*, 53: 905–12.

Hingsburger, D., Chaplin, T., Hirstwood, K., Tough, S., Nethercott, A. and Roberts-Spence, D. (1999) Intervening with sexually problematic behaviour in community environments, in J.R. Scotti and L.H. Meyer (eds.) *Behavioural Intervention: Principles, Models and Practice*. Baltimore, MD: Paul H. Brookes.

Hogg, J. and Tuffrey-Wijne, I. (2008) Cancer and intellectual disability: a review of some key contextual issues. *Journal of Applied Research in Intellectual Disabilities*, 21: 509–18.

Horner-Johnson, W. and Drum, C.E. (2006) Prevalence of maltreatment of people with intellectual disabilities: a review of the recently published research. *Mental Retardation and Developmental Disabilities Research Reviews*, 12: 57–69.

Hosseinkhazadeh, A.A., Tahare, M. and Esapoor, M. (2012) Attitudes to sexuality in individuals with mental retardation from ferspectives of their parents and teacher. *International Journal of Sociology and Anthropology*, 4: 134–46.

Kelly, G., Crowley, H. and Hamilton, C. (2009) Rights, sexuality and relationships in Ireland: 'It'd be nice to be kind of trusted'. *British Journal of Learning Disabilities*, 37: 308–15.

Lindsay, W. (2002) Research and literature on sex offenders with intellectual and developmental disabilities. *Journal of Intellectual Disability Research*, 46: 74–85.

Mandell, D.S., Eleey, C.C., Cederbaum, J.A., Noll, E., Hutchinson, M.K., Jemmot, L.S. et al. (2008) Sexually transmitted infection among adolescents receiving special education services. *Journal of School Health*, 78: 382–8.

McCarthy, M. (2011) Prescribing contraception to women with intellectual disabilities: general practitioners' attitudes and practices. *Sexuality and Disability*, 29: 339–49.

McCarthy, M. and Thompson, D. (1997) A prevalence study of sexual abuse of adults with intellectual disabilities referred for sex education. *Journal of Applied Research in Intellectual Disabilities*, 10: 105–24.

McConnell, D. and Llewellyn, G. (1998) Parental disability and the threat of child removal. *Family Matters*, 51: 33–6.

McConnell, D., Llewellyn, G. and Ferronato, L. (2000) *Parents with a Disability and the NSW Children's Court*. Report to the Law Foundation of NSW. Sydney, NSW: University of Sydney.

McConnell, D., Mayes, R. and Llewellyn, G. (2008) Pre-partum distress in women with intellectual disabilities. *Journal of Intellectual and Developmental Disability*, 33: 177–83.

McIlfatrick, S., Taggart, L. and Truesdale-Kennedy, M. (2011) Supporting women with intellectual disabilities to access breast cancer screening: a healthcare professional perspective. *European Journal of Cancer Care*, 20: 412–20.

Murphy, G.H. and O'Callaghan, A. (2004) Capacity of adults with intellectual disabilities to consent to sexual relationships. *Psychological Medicine*, 34: 1347–57.

O'Hara, J. and Martin, H. (2001) A learning-disabled woman who had been raped: a multi-agency approach. *Journal of the Royal Society of Medicine*, 94: 245–6.

Pandya, S. (1997) Medical Council of India on hysterectomy in the mentally retarded. *The National Medical Journal of India*, 10: 36.

Polusny, M.A. and Follette, V.M. (1995) Long-term correlates of child sexual abuse: theory and review of the empirical literature. *Applied and Preventive Psychology*, 4: 143–66.

Quilliam, S., Dalrymple, J. and Whitmore, J. (2001) A low-IQ couple wanting children. *The Practitioner*, 245: 359–74.

Servais, L. (2006) Sexual health care in persons with intellectual disabilities. *Mental Retardation and Developmental Disabilities Research Reviews*, 12: 48–56.

Stansfield, A.J., Holland, A.J. and Clare, I.C.H. (2007) The sterilisation of people with intellectual disabilities in England and Wales during the period 1988 to 1999. *Journal of Intellectual Disability Research*, 51: 569–79.

Stokes, M.A. and Kaur, A. (2005) High functioning autism and sexuality: a parental perspective. *Autism*, 9: 266–89.

Sullivan, A. and Caterino, L.C. (2008) Addressing the sexuality and sex education of individuals with autism spectrum disorders. *Education and Treatment of Children*, 31: 381–94.

Valenti-Hein, D. (2002) Use of visual tools to report sexual abuse for adults with mental retardation. *Mental Retardation*, 40: 297–303.

Van Der Zee, B., De Beaufort, I., Temel, S., De Wert, G., Denktas, S. and Steegers, E. (2011) Preconception care: an essential preventive strategy to improve children's and women's health. *Journal of Public Health Policy*, 32: 367–79.

Walker-Hirsch, L. (2007a) *The Facts of Life – and More: Sexuality and Intimacy for People with Intellectual Disabilities*. Baltimore, MD: Paul H. Brookes.

Walker-Hirsch, L. (2007b) Sexuality across the lifespan, in L. Walker-Hirsch (ed.) *The Facts of Life – and More: Sexuality and Intimacy for People with Intellectual Disabilities*. Baltimore, MD: Paul H. Brookes.

Walsh-Gallagher, D., Sinclair, M. and McConkey, R. (2012) The ambiguity of disabled women's experiences of pregnancy, childbirth and motherhood: a phenomenological understanding. *Midwifery*, 28: 156–62.

Ward, K., Bosek, R. and Trimble, E. (2010) Romantic relationships and interpersonal violence among adults with developmental disabilities. *Intellectual and Developmental Disabilities*, 48: 89–98.

Westhoff, C. (2003) Depot-medroxyprogesterone acetate injection (Depo-Provera): a highly effective contraceptive option with proven long-term safety. *Contraception*, 68: 75–87.

Willems, D.L., De Vries, J.N., Isarin, J. and Reinders, J.S. (2007) Parenting by persons with intellectual disability: an explorative study in the Netherlands. *Journal of Intellectual Disability Research*, 51: 537–44.

Mental health

Eddie Chaplin and Jane McCarthy

Introduction

Mental health is an important component of wellbeing, but there is still no agreement of what it means. The WHO's (2010) definition states that mental health is 'a state of well-being in which every individual realizes his or her own potential, can cope with the normal stresses of life, can work productively and fruitfully, and is able to make a contribution to her or his community'.

The National Health Service (NHS) and Social Services expenditure for mental disorder in England is around 23 per cent, costing £22.5 billion, compared with 16 per cent each for cancer and cardiovascular disease, and is expected to rise to £47.5 billion by 2026 (McCrone et al. 2008). Currently, mental health expenditure is biased towards existing problems rather than on prevention and early intervention, even though 50 per cent of cases occur by the age of 14 (Knapp et al. 2011). This chapter examines the principles of promoting good mental health for people from the wider population and the implications from this evidence for people with intellectual disabilities. The chapter concludes with a summary of key issues in promoting mental health across the lifespan of people with intellectual disability.

Policy and mental health promotion

For mental health promotion to work to help reduce the discrimination and social exclusion experienced by those with mental health problems, it should be integral to mental health policy rather than something that is done in isolation.

In 2005, the WHO published *Promoting Mental Health: Concepts, Emerging Evidence, Practice* (Herrman et al. 2005). Among its messages were:

- to recognize the link between the protection of basic civil, political, economic, and social rights and mental health, and
- the need for promoting healthy behaviours to reduce the international disease burden.

This was followed in 2010 by a publication that included some key facts on mental health (WHO 2010):

- More than 450 million people suffer from mental disorders. Many more have mental problems.
- Mental health is an integral part of health; indeed, there is no health without mental health.
- Mental health is more than the absence of mental disorders.
- Mental health is determined by socio-economic, biological, and environmental factors.
- Cost-effective inter-sectoral strategies and interventions exist to promote mental health.

Health promotion across the lifespan

The implementation of mental health promotion programmes varies from childhood to old age. This is true not only in terms of the materials and media used to promote good mental health, but also by the underpinning philosophy that drives current practice. For example, for children and young people there is the resilience model that includes school-based programmes for social and emotional learning (see Chapter 15), while in adult mental health services there is the recovery model and an industry based on self-help tools designed to promote good mental health (SLAM/SWLSTG 2010). For older adults, the focus is on factors that promote good mental health for those at risk for dementia.

Children

Central to mental wellbeing in children is the concept of resilience – that is, the better the resilience of the young person, the better their mental health will be. Resilience in young people can be increased by protective factors such as good schools, communities, and supportive families (see Chapters 14 and 15). However, this can also be negatively affected when other factors such as abuse and poor socio-economic status are present. Resilience works to increase the self-esteem and self-worth of the young person. To achieve this, a wide support network is necessary, the role of which is to offer praise and positive reinforcement for tasks, actions, behaviours, and so on, which have been completed well. As well as promoting the person's strengths, it is also necessary to help tackle any weaknesses, thereby helping to provide small steps for the person to reach achievable goals and reach their potential rather than fail by placing unrealistic aspirations. The person should be a part of this and be involved in choices, be treated as an individual and not just part of a family group. As well as positive support, there is also a need to anticipate stressors and what impact these may have on the person.

In the UK, *Every Child Matters* (Department for Education and Skills 2005) identified five desirable outcomes for every child and young person, including to be healthy, to be safe, and to enjoy and achieve. Resilience refers to a child's positive adaptation to difficult circumstances: for the individual, this could be their specific disability; at the family level, it could be ill health in a parent or an environmental difficulty such as poverty. Resilience seeks to focus on the strengths of the individual and the key protective factors for development.

Families supporting a child with intellectual disability are at increased risk of experiencing poverty due to the financial and social impact of caring. The association between poverty and intellectual disability accounts in part for the health and social inequalities experienced by people with intellectual disability, including those with mental health problems (Emerson and Baines 2010). It has been shown that social economic disadvantage accounts for a significant proportion of the increased risk for poor mental health of children and adolescents with intellectual disability (Emerson et al. 2007).

A study of more than 18,000 children across England found that embedding mental health support in schools led to improvements in self-report of behavioural problems. Part of the initiative saw schools provide the children with self-help leaflets explaining what to do if they were feeling stressed or troubled. This initiative is part of a wider study of Targeted Mental Health in Schools (Department for Education 2011). The impact of such school-based interventions on the mental health of young people across the range of abilities from mild to severe intellectual disability requires further evaluation. Most of the research to date is on school-based interventions on developing social skills in young people with autism spectrum disorders (Machalicek et al. 2008) rather than on mental health promotion for the wider population of young people with intellectual disability. Research needs to be undertaken that evaluates interventions for those with severe intellectual disability and also into what works for those with mild intellectual disability in addressing their behavioural and emotional problems.

Older adults

At the other end of the lifespan are older adults. For this group there are a number of issues, with 'Dementia being one of the most distressing and devastating disorders we face' (Department of Health 2009: 16). There are approximately 700,000 people with dementia and the cost is £17 billion to the UK economy (Knapp and Prince 2007). The risk of dementia in people with intellectual disability is increased in specific groups such as those with Down syndrome, in whom onset may occur 30–40 years earlier than in the general population (Holland et al. 1998). Currently, research is in progress on how early interventions may reduce this risk (Dementia in Down's Syndrome study, DiDS: http://www.psychiatry.cam.ac.uk/research/groups/ciddrg/dids/). Preventing recurrent cerebrovascular disease is recognized to be essential for the whole population in terms of dementia risk (Department of Health 2009). Therefore, good management of blood pressure and blood glucose with a healthy lifestyle, such as a good dietary intake of fish and vegetables with moderate alcohol intake, is important.

It is important for people to remain mentally, physically, and socially active, as this may postpone the onset of dementia (Fratiglioni and Henderson 2009). The study of these factors has not yet been reported for people with intellectual disability in promoting mental health in later life (see Chapter 13).

Intellectual disability

It is widely accepted that people with intellectual disability are at risk of increased co-morbidity from both physical and mental illness across the lifespan. The WHO (2001) estimates prevalence rates of up to 3 per cent for this population. In England, there are estimated to be 1.2 million people with mild to moderate intellectual disability and 210,000 have severe to profound intellectual disability, using a population estimate of 2.5 per cent (Department of Health 2001). The severe and profound group are uniformly distributed geographically in terms of socio-economic status, while the mild group are predominantly found in urban areas, due to deprivation and lifestyle factors (Department of Health 2001). Compared with the general population, people with intellectual disability have a lower life expectancy, increased mortality, and higher levels of physical co-morbidity (Michaels 2008; McCarthy and O'Hara 2011). People with intellectual disability are also less likely to be in employment and to access health services, and have little awareness of what is available in terms of assistance with mental health promotion (Kerr 2004).

To promote positive mental health, we need to understand the factors that can make an individual vulnerable and to target these. Mental illness can affect anyone but it has a greater impact on the more disadvantaged (Marmot 2010). People with intellectual disability have significantly poorer lives (Disability Rights Commission 2006). Rates of mental illness are estimated at 22.4 per cent for a clinical diagnosis of mental ill health; when problem behaviours and autistic spectrum disorders are added, this increases to 40.9 per cent (Cooper et al. 2007). The aetiology of mental illness is a matter of debate, although it is widely recognized that a combination of biological, psychological, and social factors can be responsible (see Table 11.1).

Keeping mentally well

Good mental health is not only the absence of stress, poverty, trauma, and other destabilizing factors, but it is what we do to keep well and look after ourselves, such as taking exercise, socializing, finding time for self, and so on. All too often these areas are neglected because of stigma or they are thought to be unnecessary, as individuals are unable to see that physical and mental health are interlinked (British Medical Journal 2000). Most people will have, or at

Table 11.1 Risk factors for mental illness

Biological	Psychological	Social
Hereditary conditions	Stress	Economic pressures
Trauma	No stabilizing relationships	Poverty
Genetic	Lack of support	Poor education
Poor physical condition and lifestyle	Low self-esteem	Risk of violence
Neurochemical	Disempowerment	Poor housing
		Racism

least know of, strategies that can promote wellbeing, for example a healthy diet (see Chapter 4 and 5), exercise (see Chapter 16), and regular check-ups (see Chapter 18). People need to have the same understanding about mental wellbeing, as something that affects us all. In terms of people with intellectual disability, this will mean a fundamental shift in the way they are supported on a daily basis.

Promoting mental health involves any action that enhances the wellbeing of individuals, families, and communities. Taggart and McKendry (2009) identified three barriers to health promotion for people with intellectual disabilities:

- *Individual barriers*: people with intellectual disabilities may lack the knowledge required of what to do when feeling unwell, and where to go to get help.
- *Carer barriers*: many people with intellectual disabilities are dependent upon family carers and front-line staff to identify symptoms when they are unwell and make a prompt referral to a GP. However, many of these carers may not recognize the early indications/triggers of mental ill health.
- *Professional barriers*: primary healthcare professionals may have limited experience in working with people with intellectual disabilities and have less knowledge about the needs of this population who have mental health problems.

The Department of Health (2001) highlighted a two-stage model of promoting mental health:

1. *Reducing risk factors*: poverty, deprived communities, high unemployment, financial difficulties, poor educational opportunities, high crime rates, emotional/physical/sexual abuse, high stress levels, social exclusion, family break-up, long-term caring.
2. *Increasing protective factors*: quality environments, increasing self-esteem and empowerment, self-management skills, social participation.

Black and Devine (2008) developed a mental health promotion booklet for parents, teachers, and front-line staff who care for children and young people with intellectual disabilities, entitled *Head Start*. The booklet identifies those factors that make young people resilient or protect against them developing mental ill health, as well as highlighting potential risk factors. The following is a list of key factors to help build resilience; although each factor is important in itself, they all overlap, interact, and reinforce each other:

- good physical health
- exercise and activity
- success and achievement
- self-awareness
- positive family connections
- friendships and relationships
- meaningful social activity
- support during changes and transitions

- involvement in making choices and decisions
- care and support.

In *Head Start* (Black and Devine 2008), each one of these ten factors is discussed individually and practical tips are offered for the carer to achieve this optimal goal. For example, young people with an intellectual disability who have some understanding and awareness of themselves and the challenges they face are more likely to have stronger emotional resilience. It is important that, from an early age, children and young people are helped to see and regard their intellectual disability as being only one aspect of themselves. This helps to build confidence and enables them to recognize their strengths as much as their limitations. Examples include:

- Children and young people should be given opportunities to talk about the limitations imposed by their disability.
- It is important to be open and honest about the disability and to help them understand more about their particular condition. Many organizations provide useful leaflets, videos, and DVDs to explain particular conditions and the likely effects on daily living and lifestyle.
- Group work with peers is one way of helping children and young people with learning disabilities understand that everyone is unique and that everyone has their own limitations.
- Involve the young person in activities and pursuits that provide the best match with their abilities. Focus on activities where participation is not going to draw attention to their disability.
- Emphasize and focus your energy on their talents and abilities.

Recovery

In adults, mental health provision is centred on the recovery model. Recovery principles are about personalized networks to support individuals to realize their potential and reduce stigma. A recovery-orientated system of care:

- focuses on people rather than services
- monitors outcomes rather than performance
- emphasizes strengths rather than deficits or dysfunction
- educates service providers, schools, employers, the media, and the public to combat stigma
- fosters collaboration between people who need support and the people who support them as an alternative to coercion
- promotes autonomy through enabling and supporting self-management and, as a result, decreases the need for people to rely on formal service and professional supports.

(National Institute for Mental Health in England 2005).

The effectiveness of any health promotion intervention will be measured by its impact on the outcomes for, and wellbeing of, individual service users. Recovery is not an intervention but a description of the processes to ensure people with severe mental health problems are able to achieve meaningful and satisfying lives, which could include successful employment and the ability to self-manage their own condition. The relationship between the professional and service user is one of partnership. The core concepts of recovery are key in the lives of people with intellectual disability who present to mental health services. The opportunity to have more inclusive lives, be active members of the community, and contribute socially through work opportunities all fit with the wider aspirations and policy for people with intellectual disability (SLAM/SWLSTG 2010).

The reality is that recovery principles are already integral to intellectual disability services through person-centred working. Banks et al. (2008) identified seven issues that need to be addressed for the recovery model to work for people with intellectual disability and mental health problems:

1. Better understand the interplay between vulnerabilities and resilience to identify their relative contribution and encourage resilience in professionals' approaches.
2. Develop techniques to assess the impact of psychosocial stressors in the lives of people with intellectual disability, to inform diagnostic protocols, treatment strategies and service systems, and to determine protective factors and methods to quantify an individual's resilience.
3. Social and neuro-developmental perspectives should both be considered so that service users with intellectual disability can benefit from the study of interaction between genes and environment.
4. Acquire/modify tools to evaluate recovery in people with intellectual disability. These can be instruments to quantify quality of life and clinical and social recovery, as well as techniques such as neuro-imaging, which may measure the impact of interventions.
5. Focus on treatment as an on-going process rather than as cure.
6. Involve the service users and their carers more in designing appropriate service provision and expand the role of the 'expert patient'.
7. Evaluate complex interventions with rigour, build inter-agency partnerships, and local and flexible treatment options.

Mental health promotion

For people with intellectual disability, there are a number of examples of mental health promotion resources in the form of training packs and booklets, including *How are you Today? Mental Health . . . What does it Mean to Me?* (Hardy and Woodward 2004; Hardy et al. 2004, 2008; Taggart and McKendry 2009).

Groups

The 'Tuesday Group' is a specialist mental health promotion group for people with intellectual disability (Hardy et al. 2004). The aim of the group is to promote positive mental health by helping people to understand about mental health and teaching coping strategies in an attempt to reduce vulnerability of group members. This is done in a number of ways: participants talk about their own experiences, what they understand by mental health and how it affects them personally. In terms of keeping well, the group also talk about what helps them and what they like doing to promote a healthy lifestyle. The group identifies activities weekly. These have included going out, learning to be independent, and being treated as an adult and having a life of their own. The members of the group also provide each other with a social network. Local groups like this are invaluable, as people with intellectual disability have found mainstream health promotion programmes inaccessible, so even in priority areas that attract high investment, such as drug awareness programmes, there has been no impact for the overwhelming majority of people with intellectual disability.

Strategies for keeping safe

It is estimated that nine out of ten people with intellectual disability will have experienced a hate crime. Given the damage and devastation it brings to people, there is a duty not only to stamp it out, but also to provide people with strategies for keeping safe until that is a reality. One campaign by Mencap in the UK, 'Stand by Me', has been set up to help people understand more about hate crime and how to stop it. The case study that follows is of Jack, a 48-year-old man, who attended staying safe sessions.

Case study

Jack has been troubled by a number of negative and abusive experiences that make him not want to go out. These experiences include being robbed and assaulted, receiving nasty comments and teasing from school children, and being bothered by people for money or possessions. As well as being terrifying, these experiences have caused Jack to have panic attacks.

Jack attends a mental health promotion group. The group dedicated a number of sessions to keeping safe. These were held over several weeks and the following themes were discussed.

1 Talking about bullying/hate crime, sharing common experiences
2 Exploring ways to cope with difficult situations:
   a) Talking about thoughts and feelings
   b) Using role play to practise what to say
3 Recognizing how we feel: how do we know when we are anxious or feeling depressed?
4 Coping strategies: using general coping strategies to promote good mental health and to relieve stress
5 Keeping safe – invite the local policeman:
   a) Tips to stay out of trouble:
     • walk away
     • avoid doing things at certain times if possible, like getting on the bus when the children have just finished school
   b) What to do if the worst happens:
     • how to report crime and get leaflets about how to do this, which we could share with others
6 Threats to our mental health: how to cope with anxiety and panic attacks
7 Helping others: being supported to write articles and attend conferences.

Following the sessions, Jack still occasionally gets unwanted attention from people. However, he feels that the group has helped him to cope better with this type of situation. He has learned to make changes to his routine at high-risk times. For example, he does not get the bus after the local schools have finished for the day, or he travels with someone else. The group has become a network of support based upon common experience. What Jack found most useful was that the group repeats staying safe sessions from time to time to discuss current problems and to reinforce what he has learned to keep safe.

Guided self-help

With more responsibility, people have become aware of the importance of good mental health. This has led to interventions that are aimed at the promotion of healthy lifestyles. One such intervention where people are at the centre of their treatment and which promotes positive mental health is the technique of guided self-help. Although this is of growing interest within general psychiatry and primary care, there is limited literature on this approach for people with intellectual disability. The Self Intervention Assessment (SAINT) is a guided self-help booklet (Chaplin 2012; Chaplin et al. 2013). The SAINT was developed by both service users and clinicians. It consists of a diary to record emotions and feelings along with what coping strategies have been used. There is a list of feelings and coping strategies (all with examples), so that, when recorded, they can be used as a chronology to monitor the person's mental health and what coping strategies the person uses to best effect. The use of the SAINT is reviewed at weekly sessions with a health professional whose role is to reinforce positive aspects from the previous week and help the person look at how they might handle anticipated stressful situations. The SAINT also encourages positive comment, so it is not associated with negative feelings. Training is provided on the SAINT for users and those supporting them. An example of the text of one of the vignettes from the training manual is given in Box 11.1.

Box 11.1 SAINT example

Jesoda was finding it hard to do things, so she looked at her SAINT book.

Jesoda was not a good reader, so she asked a friend she knew well to help her.

Together they looked at the SAINT book and her friend helped to explain it to her.

After looking through the list of feelings with her friend, Jesoda chose number **4: I find it difficult to do things** to describe how she was feeling.

Jesoda put the number 4 in the diary part of the SAINT.

Her friend suggested that they should both look at the coping part of the SAINT book to see if there was something that Jesoda could choose to do to help her feel better.

Jesoda's friend explained to her about the ideas in the coping list and what she might choose to do to help herself.

Jesoda remembered how well she had done in the past and chose **number 12: positive thoughts.**

Jesoda then put the number 12 in her diary after telling herself how well she had done previously when she had felt like this and how it had helped her.

Finally, Jesoda's friend wrote a note in her diary, to say what Jesoda had done to help herself and that thinking positive thoughts had worked.

Summary

- Mental health is essentially concerned with how individuals, families, organizations, and communities think and feel.
- Mental health promotion for adults is about individual health behaviours and wider support by society for individuals who are socially and economically disadvantaged.
- The recovery model has developed across mental health services with an emphasis on autonomy and supporting self-management.
- The recovery model can work for people with intellectual disability in promoting mental health through increasing social inclusion and independence.
- For children with intellectual disability, the concept of resilience is important in developing their self-esteem and mental health.
- It is important that older people with an intellectual disability have similar opportunities as the wider population in living healthy lifestyles so as to foster their mental health in later life.

Useful resources

- *Accessible Information about Mental Health Medication*. A series of leaflets using pictures and simple English to describe 18 different types of psychotropic medication. The Elfrida Society: www.elfrida.com

- *All About Feeling Down*. Foundation for People with Learning Disabilities: www.learningdisabilities.org.uk

- Black, L.A. and Devine, M. (2008) *Head Start: Promoting Positive Mental Health for Children and Young People with a Learning Disability*. South Eastern Health and Social Care Trust: http://www.wellnet-ni.com/publications.php

- 'Books Beyond Words'. A series of picture books that provide information and address the emotional aspects of different events such as bereavement, going into hospital, being a victim of crime, and feeling depressed.

- Dodd, K., Turk, V. and Christmas, M. (2002) *Down's Syndrome and Dementia Resource Pack*. Kidderminster: British Institute of Learning Disabilities.

- Edwards, N., Lennox, N., Holt, G. and Bouras, N. (2003) *Mental Health in Adult Developmental Disability: Education and Training Kit for Professionals and Service Providers*. Brisbane, QLD: QICIDD, University of Queensland.

- Foundation for People with Learning Disabilities (FPLD) (2006) *Well-being Workshop: Recognising the Emotional and Mental Well-being of People with Profound and Multiple Learning Disabilities*. London: FPLD.

- Gregory, M., Newbigging, K., Cole, A. and Pearsall, A. (2003) *Working Together: Developing and Providing Services for People with Learning Disabilities and Mental Health Problems*. London: Mental Health Foundation.

- Hollins, S. and Curran, J. (1997) *Understanding Depression in People with Learning Disabilities*. Brighton: Pavilion.

- Holt, G., Gratsa, A., Bouras, N., Joyce, T., Spiller, M.J. and Hardy, S. (2004) *Guide to Mental Health for Families and Carers of People with Intellectual Disability*. London: Jessica Kingsley.

- Holt, G., Hardy, S. and Bouras, N. (2005) *Mental Health in Learning Disabilities: A Training Resource*. Brighton: Pavilion.

- Wertheimer, A., Hewitt, A. and Morgan, H. (2003) *Meeting the Emotional Needs of Young People with Learning Disabilities*. London: Mental Health Foundation: www.learningdisabilities.org

Web resources

- Check out the Mental Health and People with Intellectual Disabilities blog: http://intellectual-disabilities.blogspot.co.uk

- Estia Centre: Web: www.estiacentre.org

- International Association for the Scientific Study of Intellectual Disabilities: www.iassid.org

- Mental health: http://www.easyhealth.org.uk/listing/mental-health-(leaflets)

- National Association of Dual Diagnosis: www.nadd.org. This is a very good site regarding mental health issues in people with learning disabilities.

References

Banks, R., Hassiotis, A., Kellas, A., Ruedrich, S. and Weissman, S. (2008) Recovery and resilience in intellectual disabilities. *Learning Disability Psychiatry, Newsletter of the Psychiatry of Learning Disability*, 10: 5–7.

Black L.A. and Devine, M. (2008) *Head Start: Promoting Positive Mental Health for Children and Young People with a Learning Disability*. South Eastern Health and Social Care Trust. Available at: http://www.wellnet-ni.com/publications.php

British Medical Journal (2000) Editorial: Depression in Parkinson's disease. *British Medical Journal*, 320: 1287.

Chaplin, E. (2012) *Promoting mental well being: developing a guided self help package (SAINT) for people with intellectual disability,* PhD draft, Kings College Institute of Psychiatry, London.

Chaplin, E., Chester, R., Tsakanikos, E., McCarthy, J., Craig, T. and Bouras, N. (2013) Reliability and validity of the SAINT: a guided self help tool for people with intellectual disabilities. *Journal of Mental Health Research in Intellectual Disabilities*, 6(3): 245–53.

Cooper, S.A., Smiley, E., Morrison, J., Williamson, A. and Allan, L. (2007) Mental ill-health in adults with intellectual disabilities: prevalence and associated factors. *British Journal of Psychiatry*, 190: 27–35.

Department for Education (DfE) (2011) *Me and My School: Findings from the National Evaluation of Targeted Mental Health in Schools 2008–2011*. Research Report DFE-RR177. London: DfE.

Department for Education and Skills (DfES) (2005) *Common Assessment Framework*. London: DfES.

Department of Health (2001) *Valuing People: A New Strategy for Learning Disability for the 21st Century*. London: Department of Health.

Department of Health (2009) *Living Well with Dementia: A National Dementia Strategy*. London: Department of Health.

Disability Rights Commission (DRC) (2006) *Equal Treatment: Closing the Gap*. Stratford-Upon-Avon: DRC.

Emerson, E. and Baines, S. (2010) *Health Inequalities and People with Learning Disabilities in the UK: 2010*. Improving Health & Lives: Learning Disabilities Observatory. London: Public Health England.

Emerson, E., Hatton, C. and MacLean, W.E., Jr. (2007) Contribution of socioeconomic position to health inequalities of British children and adolescents with intellectual disabilities. *American Journal on Mental Retardation*, 112(2): 140–50.

Fratiglioni, L. and Henderson, S. (2009) The ageing population and epidemiology of mental disorders among the elderly, in. M. Gelder, N. Andreasen, J. Lopez-Ibor and M. Geddes (eds.) *New Oxford Textbook of Psychiatry*. Oxford: Oxford University Press.

Hardy, S. and Woodward, P. (2004) Vulnerability to protection: promoting the positive mental health of people with learning disabilities. *Living Well*, 4(1): 22–7.

Hardy, S., Essam, V. and Woodward, P. (2004) The Tuesday Group: promoting mental health. *Learning Disability Practice*, 7(8): 20–3.

Hardy, S., Woodward, P., Halls, S. and Creet, B. (2008) *Mental Health Promotion for People with Learning Disabilities: Supporting People with Learning Disabilities to Stay Mentally Well*. Brighton: Pavilion.

Herrman, H., Saxena, S. and Moodie, R. (2005) *Promoting Mental Health: Concepts, Emerging Evidence, Practice*. A Report of the World Health Organization, Department of Mental Health and Substance Abuse in Collaboration with the Victorian Health Promotion Foundation and the University of Melbourne. Geneva: WHO.

Holland, A.J., Hon, J., Huppert, F.A., Stevens, F. and Watson, P. (1998) Population-based study of the prevalence and presentation of dementia in adults with Down's syndrome. *British Journal of Psychiatry*, 172: 493–8.

Kerr, M. (2004) Improving the general health of people with learning disabilities. *Advances in Psychiatric Treatment*, 10(3): 200–6.

Knapp, M. and Prince, M. (2007) *Report. Dementia UK*. London: London School of Economics, King's College London and the Alzheimer's Society.

Knapp, M., McDaid, D. and Parsonage, M. (2011) *Mental Health Promotion and Mental Illness Prevention: The Economic Case*. London: Department of Health.

Machalicek, W., Davis, T., O'Reilly, M., Beretvas, S.N., Sigafoos, J., Lancioni, G. et al. (2008) Teaching skills in school settings, in J.K. Luiselli, D. Russo, W. Christian and S. Wilczynski (eds.) *Effective Practices for Children with Autism: Educational and Behavioural Support Interventions that Work*. Oxford: Oxford University Press.

Marmot, M. (2010) *Fair Society, Healthy Lives: Strategic Review of Health Inequalities in England Post 2011*. London: The Marmot Review.

McCarthy, J. and O'Hara, J. (2011) Ill-health and intellectual disabilities. *Current Opinion in Psychiatry*, 24(5): 382–6.

McCrone, P., Dhanasiri, S., Patel, A., Knapp, M. and Lawton-Smith, S. (2008) *Paying the Price: The Cost of Mental Health Care in England to 2026*. London: Kings Fund.

Michaels, J. (2008) *Healthcare for All: Report of the Independent Inquiry into Access to Healthcare for People with Learning Disabilities*. London: Aldridge Press.

National Institute for Mental Health in England (2005) *NIMHE Guiding Statement on Recovery*. London: Department of Health.

South London and Maudsley NHS Foundation Trust and South West London and St. George's Mental Health Trust (SLAM/SWLSTG) (2010) *Recovery is for All: Hope, Agency and Opportunity in Psychiatry. A Position Statement by Consultant Psychiatrists*. London: SLAM/SWLSTG.

Taggart, L. and McKendry, L. (2009) Developing a mental health promotion booklet for young people with learning disabilities. *Learning Disability Practice*, 12(10): 27–32.

World Health Organization (WHO) (2001) *The World Health Organisation Report 2001 – Mental Health: New Understanding, New Hope*. Geneva: WHO.

World Health Organization (WHO) (2010) *Mental Health: Strengthening our Response*. Fact sheet #220. Available at: http://www.who.int/mediacentre/factsheets/fs220/en/ [accessed 2 January 2013].

12 Substance abuse

Laurence Taggart and Beverley Temple

Introduction

Smoking, alcohol abuse, and use of illicit drugs are known to be leading causes of premature and preventable deaths worldwide. Heart disease, various cancers, chronic obstructive pulmonary disease, periodontal disease, asthma, and other diseases have been frequently associated with smoking. Similarly, alcohol abuse can lead to insomnia, memory problems, increased injury, liver disease, depression, hypertension, stroke, and CHD. Illicit drug use can lead to twitching, sleep disturbance, over- or under-eating, depression, anxiety and paranoia, and social withdrawal. Despite the substantive evidence for the impact that these substances have on the individual's health, their families, communities, and health services, there is limited evidence of the effect in people with intellectual disabilities.

In this chapter, we examine health promotion with regards to smoking, alcohol, and illicit drug use. There is growing concern about the number of people with intellectual disabilities who have access to such substances and the impact that these have upon their health as more people are supported to live in the community. This chapter identifies the risk factors for using such substances and examines the health promotion strategies that can be used to prevent people with intellectual disabilities from smoking, abusing alcohol, and using illicit drugs.

Prevalence rates of smoking, alcohol use/abuse, and illicit drug use

Prevalence rates for smoking, alcohol use/abuse, and illicit drug use in both the non-disabled and intellectual disabilities populations vary depending upon age, gender, where they live, socio-economic group, ethnic group, geographical variations, and methods of report (i.e. self versus proxy informant).

Across many westernized countries, smoking is gradually declining from over 70 per cent of the population in the 1960s to 19 per cent today. Within the UK and USA, around 21 per cent of men and 17 per cent of women (aged 18 and over) continue to smoke (Centre for Disease and Prevention Control 2011; Cancer Research UK 2012). In a review of the literature, Steinberg et al. (2009) reported that there were no large-scale surveys of smoking among people with intellectual disabilities, thus obtaining accurate figures is difficult. A number of studies have examined the prevalence of smoking in this population, with some reporting that young people with intellectual disabilities are less likely to use tobacco whereas others have reported higher use compared with their non-disabled peers (Emerson and Turnbull 2005; McGillicuddy 2006; McCrystal et al. 2007; McGuire et al. 2007; Shawna et al. 2012). Overall, smoking appears to be more common among people with mild-to-moderate intellectual disabilities, as they are more independent in their decision making and other settings may create external restrictions on their activities, such as in institutions or community shift staffed homes.

It is estimated that over 60 per cent of the non-disabled population uses alcohol within safe limits, but 10 per cent of men and 5 per cent of women misuse or abuse alcohol (Grant et al.

2004; NHS 2009). Most studies cite that alcohol use in both teenagers and adults with intellectual disabilities is lower compared with their non-disabled peers as a result of limited choice, access, and living in restrictive environments. Prevalence rates of alcohol abuse in people with intellectual disabilities appear to be slightly lower compared with their non-disabled peers. Studies in the UK suggest a 1–2 per cent prevalence rate of substance abuse in people with intellectual disabilities (McGillicuddy 2006; Taggart et al. 2006; Cooper et al. 2007), whereas in the USA it is reported to be between 1 and 2.6 per cent (Shawna et al. 2012). However, these figures may be an underestimate, as many people with mild intellectual disabilities who are at risk of abusing such substances do not use intellectual disabilities services or are not known to addiction services (Cocco and Harper 2002; Taggart et al. 2006; Shawna et al. 2012).

Prevalence rates of illicit drug use in the USA indicate that approximately 21 per cent of older adolescents and young people have experimented with marijuana, 8–9 per cent with amphetamines and inhalants, and about 2–3 per cent with hallucinogens (National Institute on Drug Abuse 2012). These figures are similar across other countries. Illicit drug use in people with intellectual disabilities has been reported to be lower than in the non-disabled population. Living in supervised accommodation and having limited money restricts the ease of obtaining and using these drugs (Snow et al. 2001; Sturmey et al. 2003).

It is often difficult to identify the amounts of alcohol and drugs that are misused by people with intellectual disabilities because of lack of consistency of definition in the literature and small sample sizes of studies. It is not known if there are differences in patterns of usage and if there are different physiological responses, based on the consumption and potential medications being taken, compared withn the non-disabled population.

Impact of substance misuse in people with intellectual disabilities

Of those studies exploring the impact of substance misuse in people with intellectual disabilities, a number of other physical and mental health conditions, as well as behaviours, have been identified. These include problems such as cardiovascular, respiratory tract, and gastrointestinal conditions; sexual diseases and HIV; increased epileptic activity; increased risk of violent behaviour and links with offending behaviour; greater likelihood of having a co-morbid mental health problem; higher levels of risk-taking behaviour (including suicide attempts); being exploited by others (including sexually); and greater likelihood of admission into a specialist hospital (Taggart et al. 2006; Slayter 2010; Shawna et al. 2012). It appears from the literature that such substances may also exacerbate these co-existing conditions.

Risk factors

Risk-taking behaviour and substance use among the general population of adolescents has generated studies that have identified some factors that increase the risk of substance abuse (Iacono et al. 2008). Since many more young people with intellectual disabilities are being encouraged and supported to integrate into schools, it seems likely that these adolescents would be at risk for substance abuse when similar conditions are present for them. Table 12.1 provides readers with a list of intra- and inter-personal risk factors for people with intellectual disabilities to abuse substances.

Many of these core risk factors have also been identified in the non-disabled population who abuse a range of substances. There is also growing research exploring the factors that predispose young people with and without intellectual disabilities to engage in alcohol abuse and illicit drug use. These include biological factors, low self-esteem, social isolation, personality, mental health, behaviours, perceived environment, and social environment. On the other hand, there is

Table 12.1 Risk factors for substance abuse in people with intellectual disabilities

Intra-personal variables	Inter-personal variables
Having a borderline to mild intellectual disability	Living in the community with low levels of supervision
Being young and male	Poverty
Having a specific genetic condition	Parental alcohol-related neuropsychiatric disorders
Adolescents with conduct disorders, ADHD, and anti-social personality disorders	Presence of negative role models with punitive child management practices
Compromised tolerance to drugs	Family dysfunction
Coming from an ethnic minority group	Negative life events (i.e. neglect, abuse, bereavement)
Co-existence of a mental health problem	Unemployment
Low self-esteem	Limited educational and recreational opportunities
Disempowerment	Excessive amounts of free time
Inadequate self-control/regulatory behaviour	Deviant peer group pressure
Impulsivity	Limited relationships/friends
Cognitive limitations (i.e. illiteracy, short attention span, memory deficits, poor problem-solving skills, tendencies to distort abstract cognitive concepts, overly compliant dispositions)	Lack of meaning in life Lack of routine
Frustration	Loneliness Desire for social acceptance/method for 'fitting in'

ADHD, attention-deficit hyperactivity disorder.
Source: Reproduced from Taggart et al. (2008).

some literature pertaining to factors that protect young people from abusing such substances, such as perceived closeness to parents and perceptions of parental expectations for school. In the USA, Gress and Boss (1996) identified several characteristics that might be related to why young people with intellectual disabilities turn to alcohol and illicit drugs. They included the inability to:

- establish self-identity
- develop social attachment
- project affective social images within their own peer groups
- experience immediate gratification of beliefs or desires.

Taggart et al. (2007) interviewed ten adults with intellectual disabilities about their reasons for using alcohol and illicit drugs. They found that many people with intellectual disabilities abused alcohol and used illicit drugs to 'self-medicate against life's negative experiences' and 'psychological trauma' associated with such negative life events as mental health problems, domestic violence, bereavement, and physical and/or sexual abuse. Another main reason for abuse of substances includes both adolescents/young people and adults with intellectual disabilities wanting to 'fit in', citing that smoking and drinking alcohol with their non-disabled friends helps them to 'fit in' and avoids being different (Cocco and Harper 2002; Taggart et al. 2007) (see the Case Study below). Adults with intellectual disabilities report similar reasons as non-disabled adults for abusing such substances in order to cope with stressful events in their lives, such as loss of job and strained relationships with friends and families (Walters and Rotgers 2012).

Case study

John is a 24-year-old man with mild intellectual disability. He lives with his mother and father and two older brothers and one sister; John's father has a history of heavy drinking. He attended a mainstream primary school and was supported to attend a mainstream secondary school. His parents found it difficult to accept that John had an intellectual disability and was different from his other brothers and sister, although they were content with his progression through school. John recalls numerous accounts of being bullied and having no friends during his schools years and feeling different. It was not until John's late teens that his behaviour changed. After leaving secondary school he obtained a place at a college of further education where his attendance was sporadic. He became uncommunicative, isolating himself from his family, wanting to remain in his bedroom, and not wanting to go out of the house. He was using his money for his lunch to buy beer. His parents have stated that he has stolen money from them to buy more beer, and more recently he has been buying vodka. As a result of these behaviours he was referred to the community intellectual disability team, where he told his nurse that he was drinking to null the pain of being lonely and to hide how he was really feeling about being called names when at school. He very much wanted to be like his brothers to have friends and also he wanted a girlfriend.

There are difficulties recognizing the signs and symptoms of substance abuse disorder in people with intellectual disabilities (Taggart and Chaplin 2013). Slayter and Steenrod (2009) reported that some of the behavioural problems displayed by people with intellectual disabilities may mask the substance-related problems. Recognizing and assessing these risk factors in people with intellectual disabilities is not well developed, and few studies have assessed motivation to use such substances with regards to trauma, isolation, and acceptance. Social exclusion can often result when there is family breakdown, poor housing, poor health, unemployment, and greater criminal activity in the general population (Neale 2008). All of these risk factors are often present for people with mild intellectual disability. When places of work are being considered, it would be important to avoid placing people with intellectual disabilities where consumption of substances was part of the normal work environment (such as in bars).

Health education and health promotion interventions

Offering a smoking cessation programme or an alcohol or drug programme to a person with an intellectual disability can be complex, as some individuals can be 'unwilling' about engaging fully in the therapeutic process. Huxley et al. (2005) highlighted that this 'uncooperativeness' should not be interpreted as poor motivation, as it can be partly due to their lack of understanding, communication difficulties, illiteracy, short attention span, memory deficits, low self-esteem, and inadequate self-control/regulatory behaviour. Individuals with intellectual disabilities have also been found to have poorer understanding regarding units of alcohol and the impact of such substances. Therefore, any successful treatment package must be adapted to reflect the learning style of the person with intellectual disabilities.

Many people with intellectual disabilities express an interest in quitting smoking or reducing their alcohol intake but need to be offered appropriate education, emotional and practical supports to enable them to be successful (McGillicuddy 2006; Kerr et al. 2012; Taggart and Chaplin 2013). Educational materials need to be developed that are accessible and appropriate for this population. Traditional programmes for smoking cessation and alcohol reduction may not incorporate the time that is required to make them effective for people with intellectual disabilities. Healthcare providers and family attitudes must also make this a priority – they need to suggest regularly that people with intellectual disabilities should stop smoking or using other tobacco products (Steinberg et al. 2009). Support workers will need to be educated as well, since much of the emotional and practical support provided in community homes may be provided by people with low educational backgrounds who may smoke and use alcohol themselves, which in turn influences the people with intellectual disabilities.

Treatment for any addiction may be more likely to occur in settings where other services are being provided (Slayter and Steenrod 2009). Staff within these settings may not be well versed in how to communicate and work with people with intellectual disabilities with cognitive deficits and communication difficulties and they may have differing values for the treatment of people with addictions (McLaughlin et al. 2007). People with intellectual disabilities may require more careful assessment of their support staff or sponsors and require more repetition of messages in accessible language, such as 'one day at a time' philosophy. Group sessions may need to be shorter in duration and the place of the treatment may need to be more focused on the current set of supports in place, such as the family home, group home or day programmes. Often addiction treatments are in places mandated by the penal system or in isolated environments in an effort to control the environment (Taggart et al. 2007; Slayter and Steenrod 2009).

Smoking cessation programmes

Tracy and Hosken (1997) undertook a small smoking education programme for 11 adults with intellectual disabilities in a community setting in Australia, and found that on completion of the programme half of the participants quit smoking. Chester et al. (2011) undertook a smoking cessation programme with an emphasis on health education and nicotine replacement within a forensic hospital for 48 adults with intellectual disabilities in England. The authors reported that one-third of these smokers stopped smoking and over half reduced the number of cigarettes smoked. Singh et al. (2011) conducted a mindfulness-based smoking cessation programme for a man with intellectual disabilities who had smoked for 17 years. The programme focused upon three areas: (1) intention, (2) mindful-observation of thoughts, and (3) meditation. Three months after completion of the programme, the man stopped smoking and at 12-month and 3-year follow-up the man was still abstaining from smoking. Medications or nicotine replacement would need to be carefully prescribed considering all other medications that are being taken by people with intellectual disabilities, who may have epilepsy or other conditions requiring regular medication use (Kerr et al. 2012). Other interventions could be used such as nicotine patches, nicotine replacement therapies, as well as electronic cigarettes; however, no studies have examined these interventions with this population.

Alcohol treatment programmes

In conjunction with the individual with intellectual disabilities, it is important to establish goals that they would like to achieve. This process will help gain an understanding of the person's knowledge and also reasons/motivation for drinking. This information will help to identify key priority areas for the person with intellectual disabilities (for example, trauma, family issues, loneliness, offending behaviours) and allow structure to be built into the treatment programme, thereby promoting a person-centred approach to the therapeutic process (Taggart et al. 2008; Kerr et al. 2012). These person-centred targets can act as evaluation and progress markers, and further motivate the person with intellectual disabilities to monitor their own improvement.

Degenhardt (2000) has indicated that 'abstinence' might be a more appropriate treatment goal than 'controlled drinking'. 'Controlled drinking' involves understanding the rules about 'units of alcohol', 'when' and 'where' to drink, and what 'not' to drink, and gives the individual responsibility for managing their own consumption, whereas 'abstinence' requires the individual to abstain totally from alcohol. Nevertheless, other interventions have been developed and adapted for this population.

There are a number of robust alcohol treatment programmes that have been developed for the non-disabled population. However, although some of these interventions have been adapted for people with intellectual disabilities, no systematic evaluation of these has been conducted (Kerr et al. 2012).

Detoxification

The first step in any treatment plan for those individuals dependent upon alcohol is to detoxify both physically and psychologically from the alcohol.

Psychopharmacology

Various medications are used depending on the substance used. Some work by reducing craving (e.g. bupropion for smoking, naltrexone for alcohol), while others such as disulfiram (Antabuse) work on the metabolism to produce unpleasant and potentially dangerous side-effects, if the person consumes alcohol during treatment (e.g. nausea and dizziness).

Education programmes

Brown and Coldwell (2006) developed an alcohol awareness programme for adults with intellectual disabilities within a medium secure hospital in England; this programme was adapted from a mainstream alcohol programme. The eight-week programme, two hours per week, aimed to increase the knowledge of the participants regarding the positive and negative effects of using alcohol, and therefore develop an understanding of using alcohol in a safe and controlled pattern. A variety of methods were employed that included videos, quizzes, work files, assignments, posters, group work, discussions, observations, role plays, drink tests, and practical visits to the pub. Hospital staff were trained within this programme and then they had to deliver the programme to the participants.

Modifications of Alcoholics Anonymous and the Twelve Step Programme

The Twelve Steps, originated by Alcoholics Anonymous (AA), is the spiritual foundation for personal recovery from the effects of alcoholism, not only for the alcoholic, but also for their friends and family in Al-Anon Family Groups. Many members of the 12-step recovery programmes have found that these steps were not merely a way to stop drinking, but they became a guide to a new way of life. This programme may suit people with borderline/mild intellectual disabilities but they will need support to work through the programme (Miller and Whicher 2009).

Skills training

Both building upon existing and developing new skills to manage everyday life including pressures and stresses can prevent relapse and a return to abusing alcohol. These skills include social skills training, communication skills training, refusal skills training (i.e. saying 'no', suggesting an alternative) and structured problem solving.

Behavioural and cognitive approaches

These can be used for alcohol and other substances and involve assertiveness skills, and distinguishing between positive and negative role models within substance abuse situations.

Motivational interviewing

Motivational interviewing has been used to address both alcohol and other substance use. It uses an empathetic approach designed to motivate the person to change by taking their perspective as to the pros and cons of their substance use by exploring their goals and associated ambivalence towards it. Mendel and Hipkins (2002) used motivational interviewing techniques in assisting seven people with intellectual disabilities and alcohol-related problems within a forensic hospital in England through the Stages of Change (Prochaska and DiClemente 1986).

Relapse prevention programmes

This type of programme focuses on self-regulation of thinking and feeling, accepting past relapses, identifying the causes of relapse, and learning to prevent and interrupt relapses.

Drug treatment programmes

Within all schools today, young people receive information and education on the dangers of illicit drugs. While debate surrounds the effectiveness of this type of education as many teenagers experiment with illicit drugs, some authors have also questioned the efficacy of this type of education for young people with intellectual disabilities. In a review of drug education for young people with intellectual disabilities, Snow et al. (2001) question how such cognitively based alcohol and drug education programmes could be appropriate for this population. Such programmes do not utilize material in a format that is accessible to young people with cognitive deficits and communication difficulties, instead relying on group education.

Prevention of substance abuse

There has been some discussion about the benefits of the current public health prevention and education programmes that promote the cessation of smoking, drinking in moderation, and deterrence of illicit drug use within schools and in local communities across some countries for teenagers and adults with intellectual disabilities (Taggart and Chaplin 2013). However, the impacts of such national campaigns have not been examined. Many people with intellectual disabilities will struggle to understand the importance and implications of such written campaigns and programmes, as a result of their cognitive and communication limitations (Burtner et al. 1995). Snow et al. (2001) found that children and teenagers with intellectual disabilities were often excluded from school smoking, alcohol, and drug education programmes and other preventative measures. McCrystal et al. (2007) have argued that, as a result of a lack of a strong evidence base in substance abuse in young people and adults with intellectual disabilities, this has had serious implications for policy initiatives such as targeted smoking, alcohol, and drug prevention programmes in schools and at the community level. As many countries are supporting people with intellectual disabilities to engage in their local communities and mainstream activities and services today, this is also an opportunity to educate and inform people with intellectual disabilities about the consequences of substance use and abuse. However, such opportunities are not being availed of and people with intellectual disabilities are not being educated about substance use and abuse (McGillicuddy 2006).

Summary

- Recognize the risk factors and triggers for developing substance problems (see Table 12.1).
- Improve family networks and develop friendships and community connectedness.
- Educate young people in schools at an early stage, using accessible information about the health risks associated with smoking, alcohol, and illicit drug use.
- Promote smoke-free environments.
- Use media to educate and encourage people with intellectual disabilities to abstain from using substances (e.g. Kramer on the Case DVD).
- If tobacco, alcohol, and drugs are used for stress relief, assist the person to identify healthy strategies to relieve stress.
- Identify individuals who have experienced trauma and negative life experiences (e.g. bereavement, mental health problems, domestic violence, physical/sexual abuse), and offer counselling to manage their pain.
- Provide educational, emotional, and practical support for people with intellectual disabilities to attend smoking cessation, alcohol control, and drug programmes within their local health centre and local communities.
- People with intellectual disabilities may have greater difficulty in generalizing knowledge and skills acquired in one setting to another setting, thus more simplification, repetition, and opportunities for mastery are required.

Useful resources

- Kramer on the Case DVD: Drug awareness for people with learning disabilities: www.bild. org.uk

Web resources

- Centre for Addiction and Mental Health, Nicotine Dependence Clinic, Toronto: https://www.nicotinedependenceclinic.com/English/CANADAPTT/Pages/Tools%20and%20Resources/Guideline-Tools.aspx

- Smoking: http://www.easyhealth.org.uk/listing/smoking-(leaflets)

- Alcohol: http://www.easyhealth.org.uk/listing/alcohol-(leaflets)

- Smoking cessation programme for people with intellectual disabilities: http://www.cddh.monash.org/quit-manual.pdf

References

Brown, G. and Coldwell, B. (2006) Developing a controlled drinking programme for people with learning disabilities living in conditions of medium security. *Addiction Research and Theory*, 14(1): 87–95.

Burtner, A.P., Wakham, M.D., McNeal, D.R. and Garvey, T.P. (1995) Tobacco and the institutionalised mentally retarded: usage choices and ethical consideration. *Special Care in Dentistry*, 15(2): 56–60.

Cancer Research UK (2012) *Smoking Statistics*. Available at: http://info.cancerresearchuk.org/cancerstats/types/lung/smoking/lung-cancer-and-smoking-statistics [accessed 30 November 2012].

Centre for Disease and Prevention Control (2011) *Current Cigarette Smoking Prevalence Among Working Adults: United States, 2004–10*. Available at:http://www.cdc.gov/mmwr/preview/mmwrhtml/mm6038a2.htm [accessed 31 October 2012].

Chester, V., Fatima, N. and Alexander, R.T. (2011) An audit of a smoking cessation programme for people with intellectual disability resident in a forensic unit. *Advances in Mental Health and Intellectual Disabilities*, 5(1): 33–41.

Cocco, K. and Harper, D. (2002) Substance use in people with mental retardation: assessing potential problem areas. *Mental Health Aspects of Developmental Disabilities*, 5(4): 101–8.

Cooper, S.A., Smiley, E., Morrison, J., Williamson, A. and Allan, L. (2007) Mental ill-health in adults with intellectual disabilities: prevalence and associated factors. *British Journal of Psychiatry*, 190: 27–35.

Degenhardt, L. (2000) Interventions for people with alcohol use disorders and a learning disability: a review of the literature. *Journal of Intellectual and Developmental Disability*, 25(2): 135–46.

Emerson, E. and Turnbull, L. (2005) Self-reported smoking and alcohol use among adolescents with intellectual disabilities. *Journal of Intellectual Disabilities*, 9(1): 58–69.

Grant, B., Dawson, D., Stinson, F., Chou, P., Dufour, M. and Pickering, R. (2004) The 12-month prevalence and trends in DSM-IV Alcohol Abuse and Dependence United States, 1991–1992 and 2001–2002. *Alcohol Research and Health*, 29(2): 79–91.

Gress, J.R. and Boss, M.R. (1996) Substance abuse differences among students receiving special education school services. *Child Psychiatry and Human Development*, 26: 235–46.

Huxley, A., Copelo, A. and Day, E. (2005) Substance misuse and the need for integrated services. *Learning Disability Practice*, 8(6): 14–17.

Iacono, W., Malone, S. and McGue, M. (2008) Behavioral disinhibition and the development of early-onset addiction: common and specific influences. *Annual Review of Clinical Psychology*, 4: 325–48.

Kerr, S., Lawrence, M., Darbyshire, C., Middleton, A.R. and Fitzsimmons, L. (2012) Tobacco and alcohol-related interventions for people with mild/moderate intellectual disabilities: a systematic review of the literature. *Journal of Intellectual Disability Research*, 56: 7–8.

McCrystal, P., Percy, A. and Higgins, K. (2007) Drug use amongst young people attending emotional and behavioural difficulty units during adolescence: a longitudinal analysis. *Emotional and Behavioural Difficulties*, 12(1): 49–68.

McGillicuddy, N. (2006) A review of substance use research among those with mental retardation. *Mental Retardation and Developmental Disabilities*, 12: 41–7.

McGuire, B., Daly, P. and Smyth, F. (2007) Lifestyle and health behaviours of adults with an intellectual disability. *Journal of Intellectual Disability Research*, 1: 497–510.

McLaughlin, D., Taggart, L., Quinn, B. and Milligan, V. (2007) The experiences of professionals who care for people with intellectual disabilities who have substance-related problems. *Journal of Substance Use*, 12(2): 133–43.

Mendel, E. and Hipkins, J. (2002) Motivating learning disabled offenders with alcohol-related problems: a pilot study. *British Journal of Learning Disabilities*, 30(4): 153–8.

Miller, H. and Whicher, E. (2009) Substance misuse, in A. Hassiotis, D.A. Barron and I. Hall (eds.) *Intellectual Disability Psychiatry: A Practical Handbook*. Chichester: Wiley-Blackwell.

National Health Service (NHS) (2009) *Statistics on Alcohol, England 2009*. Available at: http://www.hscic.gov.uk/pubs/alcohol/9 [accessed 21 June 2013].

National Institute on Drug Abuse (2012) *Drug Facts: USA Nationwide Trends*. Available at: http://www.drugabuse.gov/publications/drugfacts/nationwide-trends [accessed 31 July 2012].

Neale, J. (2008) Homelessness, drug use and hepatitis C: a complex problem explored within the context of social exclusion. *Science Direct*, 19: 429–35.

Prochaska, J.O. and DiClemente, C. (1986) Toward a comprehensive model of change, in W.R. Miller and N. Heather (eds.) *Treating Addictive Behaviors: Processes of Change*. New York: Plenum Press.

Shawna, L., Chapman, C. and Wu, L.-T. (2012) Substance abuse among individuals with intellectual disabilities. *Research in Developmental Disabilities*, 33(4): 1147–56.

Singh, N.H., Lancioni, G.E., Winton, A.S.W., Singh, A.N., Singh, J. and Singh, A.D. (2011) Effects of a mindfulness-based smoking cessation programme for adults with mild intellectual disabilities. *Research in Developmental Disabilities*, 32: 1180–5.

Slayter, E. (2010) Demographic and clinical characteristics of people with intellectual disabilities with and without substance abuse disorders in a medicaid population. *Intellectual and Developmental Disabilities*, 48(6): 417–31.

Slayter, E. and Steenrod, S. (2009) Addressing alcohol and drug addiction among people with mental retardation in non-addiction settings: a need for cross-system collaboration. *Journal of Social Work Practice in the Addictions*, 9: 71–90.

Snow, P.C., Wallace, S.D. and Munro, G.D. (2001) Drug education with special needs populations: identifying and understanding the challenges. *Drugs, Education, Prevention and Policy*, 8(3): 261–73.

Steinberg, M., Heimlich, L. and Williams, J. (2009) Tobacco use among individuals with intellectual or developmental disabilities: a brief review. *Intellectual and Developmental Disabilities*, 47(3): 197–207.

Sturmey, P., Reyer, H., Lee, R. and Robek, A. (2003) *Substance-Related Disorders in Persons with Mental Retardation*. New York: NADD Press.

Taggart, L. and Chaplin, E. (2013) Substance abuse disorder, in E. Tsakanikos and J. McCarthy (eds.) *Handbook of Psychopathology in Intellectual Disability*. New York: Springer.

Taggart, L., McLaughlin, D., Quinn, B. and Milligan, V. (2006) An exploration of substance misuse in people with intellectual disabilities. *Journal of Intellectual Disability Research*, 50(8): 588–97.

Taggart, L., McLaughlin, D., Quinn, B. and McFarlane, C. (2007) Listening to people with intellectual disabilities who misuse alcohol and drugs. *Health and Social Care in the Community*, 15(4): 360–8.

Taggart, L., Huxley, A. and Baker, G. (2008) Alcohol and illicit drug misuse in people with learning disabilities: implications for research and service development. *Advances in Mental Health in Learning Disabilities*, 2(1): 11–21.

Tracy, J. and Hosken, R. (1997) The importance of smoking education and preventative health strategies for people with intellectual disability. *Journal of Intellectual Disability Research*, 41(5): 416–21.

Walters, S. and Rotgers, F. (2012) *Treating Substance Abuse: Theory and Technique*, 3rd edn. New York: Guilford Press.

Ageing

Tamar Heller, Dora Fisher, and Beth Marks

Introduction

Health promotion is of crucial importance for older adults, both with intellectual disabilities and without. About 80 per cent of older adults have one chronic condition, and 50 per cent have at least two (Centers for Disease Control and Prevention 2010), thus making their health behaviours of public health import. As adults with intellectual disabilities are living longer than ever before, these issues are a particular matter of concern for this population (Slevin et al. 2011). People with intellectual disabilities have a higher risk of contracting health conditions at younger ages than the general population due to access to care, and biological and lifestyle factors (Bittles et al. 2002). As adults with intellectual disabilities age, they experience chronic health conditions related to the interaction of the ageing process with their disability.

Advances in health promotion research are increasingly focused on ways to incorporate interventions in communities by making them a part of everyday life instead of only in clinical settings. Researchers try to identify successful translational strategies to bring interventions to places where participants naturally congregate. While this kind of research is more established in ageing, translational strategies for intellectual disability interventions are still in their early stages, with only a few recent initiatives demonstrating a programme brought to a community setting. Gerontological researchers have come up with unique ways to incorporate different target populations of older adults, different interests and ways to motivate and engage older adults, and ways to bring health promotion to the context of daily life. Because this research is more established, intellectual disability researchers can look to ageing for new ideas and strategies.

Due to the ageing of adults with intellectual disabilities, efforts must be made to learn from the advances in the ageing field, and thus improve the lives of people ageing with intellectual disabilities. The purpose of this chapter is to draw from innovative techniques in translational research as it relates to health promotion for older adults that may be applicable for adults with intellectual disabilities. This chapter first summarizes the health promotion literature on adults with intellectual disabilities and the emerging translational strategies in this research. Following this, we examine the novel translational strategies employed in the gerontological literature to identify practices applicable to people with intellectual disabilities, and to draw recommendations for future research and practice.

Health interventions for people with intellectual disabilities

Health interventions for adults with intellectual disabilities address a variety of health topics through three main types of interventions:

- fitness/exercise only
- multi-component interventions
- healthcare and screening interventions.

Researchers have developed various curricula geared to people with intellectual disabilities to address health topics such as healthy eating, good self-care, physical activity and exercise maintenance, and screening adherence.

Interventions that provide opportunities to exercise may include balance, cardiovascular and endurance, resistance training, or sports activities. As summarized in a recent review (Heller et al. 2011), outcomes from interventions targeting physical activity for adults with intellectual disabilities have generally included improved balance, strength, and aerobic capacity, lower blood pressure, and weight loss, as well as some limited emotional and behavioural outcomes.

More comprehensive programmes incorporate physical activity and exercise, nutrition, and health education (which may cover such topics as nutrition and exercise, self-care, health advocacy, and stress reduction). Results of these studies have included improved fitness as well as changes in attitudes towards health promotion and positive psychosocial outcomes.

A third type of health promotion intervention features health screenings by health professionals (see Chapter 18). Generally, interventions to promote screening adherence among adults with intellectual disabilities have resulted in more subsequent clinical activities. Other benefits reported as a result of screenings have included less pain, fewer falls, fewer emergency room visits, and greater satisfaction (Robertson et al. 2011).

Moving health promotion for people with intellectual disabilities into the community

To set the stage for what we can learn from the gerontological health promotion literature, we first discuss innovative translational strategies being conducted by health promotion researchers among people with intellectual disabilities. These tactics are just starting to be recognized in disability research as those designing interventions look at ways to use evidence-based and promising practices in the community.

Translational research often relies upon methodological frameworks to ensure comprehensive considerations of disseminating and evaluating the impact of an intervention. The RE-AIM framework is utilized in ageing and is beginning to be used in disability research. This translational strategy operationalizes a method that researchers and community partners can use to appropriately implement and institutionalize a health promotion programme. Standing for Reach, Effectiveness, Adoption, Implementation, and Maintenance, this framework enhances the quality and impact of public health interventions (Glasgow et al. 1999). Next we discuss three examples of programmes for adults with intellectual disabilities that make use of this translational methodology:

1. The *Health Matters* programme (Marks et al. 2010b).
2. *Women Be Healthy* (Lunsky et al. 2003; Parish et al. 2012).
3. The Special Olympics community-based health promotion programmes (Heller et al. 2012).

Health Matters

Health Matters: The Exercise and Nutrition Health Education Curriculum for People with Developmental Disabilities (Marks et al. 2010b), originally titled *Exercise and Nutrition Health Education Curriculum for Adults with Developmental Disabilities* (Heller et al. 2001), is an intervention developed in the Rehabilitation Research and Training Center on Aging with Developmental Disabilities (RRTCADD) at the University of Illinois at Chicago (UIC). This comprehensive programme, initially tested in our university site, had participants with intellectual disabilities participate in exercise, nutrition and health education, and cooking classes. The curriculum is based on two theoretical frameworks: Bandura's Social Cognitive Theory of Social Learning (Bandura 1977) and the Trans-theoretical Model of Behaviour Change (Prochaska and Norcross 1979) (see Chapter 2). Its goals are to help the participants:

- understand the benefits of health-promoting behaviours (outcome expectations)
- increase their self-efficacy in performing exercise
- develop health promotion goals and action plans emanating from their personal preferences.

It is also based on person-centred planning, a theme that underlies much of the intellectual disability service framework. This programme was first evaluated using a randomized control trial, which found evidence that the programme had many psychological and attitudinal outcomes compared with the control group, such as improved fitness, increased exercise self-efficacy, more positive expected outcomes, fewer cognitive–emotional barriers, improved life satisfaction, and marginally lower depression (Heller et al. 2004; Rimmer et al. 2004).

Health Matters was originally held at our centre, and after developing the aforementioned evidence base we developed a Train-the-Trainer element. This generalized the programme to the community, enabling direct support providers at service agencies to teach the programme, which was found to be effective in increasing the health and exercise attitudes of the staff in addition to positive outcomes for the many participants with intellectual disabilities in the programmes that were implemented. Outcome for these participants included improved knowledge and self-efficacy, as well as fitness (Marks et al. 2010b). While Train-the-Trainer brought the programme to community settings, achieving sustainability required community academic partnerships aimed at building organizational capacity. HealthMatters™ Community Academic Partnerships (HM CAP) was created as a collaboration to enhance health status and optimize full community participation of people with intellectual disabilities. It introduces a new approach, in which two community-based organizations (NorthPointe Resources of Zion, Illinois and ARCA of Albuquerque, New Mexico) and an academic institution (University of Illinois at Chicago) work together to find practical solutions using evidence-based curricula and training to improve health. This collaboration is building an infrastructure to facilitate and sustain healthy choices and behaviours among people with intellectual disabilities to improve their health status (Marks et al. 2010a).

Women Be Healthy

The intervention *Women Be Healthy* (Lunsky et al. 2003; Parish et al. 2012) is also an example of translational research, moving from clinics to communities. This intervention promotes health screenings in adults with intellectual disabilities. Despite the health benefits of screening adherence, women with intellectual disabilities have strikingly low rates of cervical and breast cancer screening. Through psycho-educational sessions, this intervention improved breast cancer screening knowledge, but not knowledge of cervical screening. Currently, investigators are testing ways to revise the programme with *Women be Healthy Two*. They are developing training for family and paid caregivers who play a major role in women's access to care. They are also engaging stakeholders through workshops, health fairs, smart phone applications, website content, mailings, DVDs, and other social media outlets such as Facebook and YouTube. These translational efforts are underway using the RE-AIM framework (Parish et al. 2012).

Special Olympics

A health promotion programme funded by the Special Olympics in 2009 is an example of one dynamic way a health intervention for people with intellectual disabilities has been sustainably and meaningfully brought to communities. This one-year programme was disseminated in five sites and four countries (Kenya, Mauritius, Belgium, and the United States) and evaluated at the University of Illinois at Chicago (Heller et al. 2012). This programme led not only to benefits for the participating athletes, but also to increased community capacity and awareness of the importance of health promotion for individuals with intellectual disabilities. Partnerships formed with local universities, schools, businesses, and hospitals helped provide expertise and assistance for implementation. This programme proved to be sustainable, as several of the programmes continued to host the Special Olympics beyond the funding cycle. This inspired other programmes in these communities as well, such as development of social entrepreneurship initiatives of a newly formed parent group.

These examples demonstrate that translational strategies are emerging in health promotion for people with intellectual disabilities. However, this practice is still very new, with only a few studies (mostly not yet published in journals) implemented in communities. Hence, we look to gerontology to learn what new strategies are successfully bringing programmes to communities and integrating health promotion into naturally occurring settings.

Types of health interventions for older adults

Ageing health promotion interventions address diverse topics and approaches. Physical activity is the dominant topic or activity in most health promotion interventions, although many physical activity interventions are multi-faceted or only address exercise in an educational capacity. As with the interventions for intellectual disabilities, health promotion interventions for older adults can be categorized as:

- physical activity only
- multi-component interventions with physical activity and additional activities
- health screenings and assessments.

Other interventions include health education only or psychosocial only, and untraditional strategies, such as singing groups or volunteering. These types of interventions are expanded upon by their innovative elements in the following section.

Moving health promotion for older adults into the community

Gerontological health promotion is a broader and more vigorously researched field than health promotion for adults with intellectual disabilities. This field has many more health interventions, and now utilizes creative settings, innovative motivational strategies, and original activities. Programmes for older adults now are more often community-oriented and translational, moving away from clinics and towards more natural settings (Kolomer et al. 2010). This section explores what can be mined from these newer approaches for use with people with intellectual disabilities by looking at innovative target populations, theoretical orientations, settings, and strategies.

Target populations

Interventions for older adults are increasingly seeking to target more vulnerable populations. To address health disparities and deliver more culturally competent programming, many interventions are tailored for specific ethnic communities such as Native Americans (Klug et al. 2008) or African Americans (Ralston et al. 2007; Zoellner et al. 2009). These interventions employ strategies to appeal to these groups, often creating a community advisory board or using other community-based 'action research' approaches to best engage the target population.

Other interventions pursue hard-to-reach groups of older adults such as rural women (Folta et al. 2009), individuals who have difficulty leaving their house (Laforest et al. 2008), or men, who are typically under-represented in health promotion (Williamson 2011).

Advances in science and cultural changes manifest in evolving older adult needs and preferences over time, known as the 'cohort effect' (Ryder 1965). Health promotion uses new strategies to address these changing target populations, such as interventions targeting older workers (Hughes et al. 2011) and interventions for STI prevention in older women (Smith et al. 2010). The current cohort of older adults is growing more 'computer-savvy' than previous generations, providing a new channel for health promotion through Internet and computer interventions (Chu et al. 2009).

Settings

Leaving the clinics behind, health promotion is now more often taking place in locations where older adults naturally congregate, such as senior centres, libraries, senior housing, YMCAs, cultural centres, malls, and naturally occurring retirement communities (NORCs). Health promotion for older adults increasingly recognizes the impact of multiple levels of influence (Kolomer et al. 2010), that in order to be sustainable, healthy activities must take place within natural surroundings. Social ecological approaches have led to interventions in locations where participants might happen to be anyway. Older adults exist in a 'structural lag', a life phase lacking in the socially enforced structures of school and work (Riley et al. 1994), making ecological opportunities for intervention more complex and challenging. Gerontologists strive for new settings and novel ways to integrate health interventions into naturally occurring places.

Strategies

While health promotion in ageing is moving in innovative directions, many of the established health-promoting strategies are still employed, such as small group interventions, telephone counselling, and other motivational tactics. Instead of new strategies, the way these interventions are interpreted and used by those designing the interventions is new. Also, some health interventions for older adults employ unique and new ideas for interventions, such as storytelling to reduce blood pressure (Houston et al. 2011) and volunteering with children to increase neuro-cognitive plasticity (Carlson et al. 2009).

In keeping with the social ecological approach, intervention designers are dovetailing health promotion programmes with another activity. For example, a colorectal cancer screening education intervention was added to flu shots for older adults, significantly increasing screening adherence (Potter et al. 2011). In this way, health programmes are working within the confines of pre-existing structures to impact greater numbers of their target population.

As gerontologists seek new ways to incorporate health promotion into natural settings, they also look to move beyond simply encouraging older adults to make healthful changes and towards discovering what truly motivates older adults. Many interventions found innovative ways to incentivize health behaviour, whether directly through prizes (Finkelstein et al. 2008), friendly competition such as games (Studenski et al. 2010), or through more psychologically meaningful incentives such as volunteering (Reddy et al. 2007). As participation in health promotion is mostly voluntary, gerontologists continue to find creative ways to engage older adults in these activities.

To engage older adults in exercise, many health promotion researchers use creative approaches to physical activity. For example, Argentine Tango classes were used for a falls prevention workshop; this intervention increased balance and strength compared to the walking group control, and participants enjoyed it more (McKinley et al. 2008). Other interventions used singing to enhance lung capacity (Skingley and Bungay 2010). These innovative strategies remind participants that healthy activities are fun, and keep them engaged and excited to participate.

Many interventions utilize volunteering and civic engagement as a way to bestow health-promoting activities with greater meaning for participants, beyond merely their own health. Theoretical constructs that are used in this kind of intervention are social capital (de Souza and Grundy 2007) and 'generativity' (Fried et al. 2004). Other ways that civic engagement is present in ageing health promotion is through political organizations such as the 'Raging Grannies' (Hutchinson and Wexler 2007) and membership of a leisure group, the 'Red Hat Society' (Son et al. 2007). Group affiliation and civic commitment have meaning related to health behaviour within health promotion for older adults, endowing a layer of additional value and motivation to the intervention for the participant.

What disability researchers can learn from ageing: recommendations

Researchers designing interventions for adults with intellectual disabilities stand to learn much from health promotion programmes for older adults on ways to further integrate programming into communities and meaningfully engage target audiences. Through exploring what is new and interesting, this chapter recommends four ways that intellectual disability health promotion research can learn from ageing:

1. *Make use of natural settings*. In health promotion for older adults, research is consistently moving out of the clinics and into communities. To facilitate this same transition in disability research and further translate health promotion interventions in community settings, interventions need to address fully integrating health promotion in community settings for adults with intellectual disabilities.
2. *Use peer mentors, civic engagement, and volunteering*. Peer leaders are a popular means for delivering health promotion interventions in ageing. Social cognitive theory posits that health messages resonate more strongly when coming from a recognizable peer, a theory actualized in much of the ageing health promotion (Bandura 1977). Due to the unique lived experience of having an intellectual disability, peer leaders, such as those developed in the *Peer to Peer Health Messages* programme, could play a critical role in health promotion. Furthermore, use of health promotion strategies that incorporate civic engagement and volunteering could endow programmes with more meaning and could resonate for people with intellectual disabilities.
3. *Make health promotion fun*. Participation in health promotion is mostly voluntary. Thus, those designing interventions must ask themselves what truly excites their target audience and makes them want to be involved. The ageing literature reflects new ways that researchers can motivate participants to care about a programme and continue to practise the good health behaviours therein. Currently, there are health promotion programmes where older adults learn modern jazz dance, sing in a choir, wear costumes, go to protest marches, and read stories to children. These new ideas are essential for research to effectively translate to community settings. Adults with intellectual disabilities have interests as well, and this must be a factor in programme design.
4. *Make use of new modalities*. The novel use of technology has emerged in the ageing literature. Some studies have used the Internet to deliver otherwise traditional health promotion interventions (Lorig et al. 2008); others have helped older adults learn to use the Internet to retrieve health information (Shapira et al. 2007). This use of technology can also make interventions more fun by incorporating DVDs or video games. This may be of use for people with intellectual disabilities as well, as technology may compensate for some of the barriers people with disabilities often experience in traditional health promotion settings.

Limitations

There are some limitations to fully incorporating these recommendations into the intellectual disability health promotion field. One major limitation is the size of the population. While the population of adults with intellectual disabilities is growing, it is much smaller than the size of the general ageing population, thus limiting the target population and the researchers in the field.

Another major limitation is the workforce crisis within community organizations. Despite the increasing need for these services, in the USA the overall national annual Direct Service Provider (DSP) turnover rate ranges from 25 per cent to 75 per cent with an average of about 54 per cent (Hatton et al. 2001). This may be due to low wages, occupational risks and stress, which create difficulty for organizations to recruit, train, and retain DSPs. To effectively integrate health promotion into natural settings, new DSPs must receive effective healthcare education and efforts must be made to retain them (Marks et al. 2008).

Summary

- People with intellectual disabilities experience lower levels of healthy behaviours, as do older persons, making health promotion a key priority for these populations.
- Health promotion researchers increasingly focus on ways to incorporate interventions in communities by making them a part of everyday life instead of only in clinical settings, a strategy that is more established in ageing than in intellectual disability research.
- Some examples of community-based health promotion interventions for people with intellectual disabilities include *Health Matters, Women Be Healthy*, and Special Olympics programmes.
- Ageing health promotion utilizes many creative settings, innovative motivational strategies, and original activities to make programmes engaging and sustainable.
- Intellectual disability health promotion researchers can learn from ageing to make use of natural settings, peer mentors, and new modalities, and make health promotion fun.
- People with intellectual disabilities more commonly live longer; thus disability health promotion must look to ageing literature to learn from what is working to promote good health for older adults and bring health promotion to community settings.

Web resources

- Old age: http://www.easyhealth.org.uk/listing/old-age-(leaflets)
- Centers for Disease Control and Prevention – Healthy ageing for older adults: http://www.cdc.gov/aging/
- Centers for Disease Control and Prevention – Developmental disabilities: http://www.cdc.gov/ncbddd/developmentaldisabilities/index.html
- Rehabilitation Research and Training Center on Aging with Developmental Disabilities – Lifespan health and function: http://www.rrtcadd.org/
- Health Matters Program: http://healthmattersprogram.org/
- Experience Corps Program: http://www.experiencecorps.org/

Acknowledgement

This chapter was produced under grant number H133B080009 awarded by the US Department of Education's National Institute on Disability and Rehabilitation Research to the Rehabilitation Research and Training Center on Aging with Developmental Disabilities-Lifespan Health and Function at the University of Illinois at Chicago. The contents of this chapter do not necessarily represent the policy of the US Department of Education, and should not be assumed as being endorsed by the US Federal Government.

References

Bandura, A. (1977) *Social Learning Theory*. New York: General Learning Press.

Bittles, A., Petterson, B., Sullivan, S., Hussain, R., Glasson, E. and Montgomery, P. (2002) The influence of intellectual disability on life expectancy. *Journals of Gerontology A: Biological Sciences and Medical Sciences*, 57: M470–2.

Carlson, M.C., Erickson, K.I., Kramer, A.F., Voss, M.W., Bolea, N., Mielke, M. et al. (2009) Evidence for neurocognitive plasticity in at-risk older adults: the Experience Corps program. *Journals of Gerontology A: Biological Sciences and Medical Sciences*, 64: 1275–82.

Centers for Disease Control and Prevention (2010) *Behavioral Risk Factor Surveillance Survey*. Atlanta, GA: Centers for Disease Control and Prevention. Available at: http://www.cdc.gov/brfss/ [accessed 13 July 2012].

Chu, A., Huber, J., Mastel-Smith, B. and Cesario, S. (2009) 'Partnering with Seniors for Better Health': computer use and internet health information retrieval among older adults in a low socioeconomic community. *Journal of the Medical Library Association*, 97(1): 12–20.

De Souza, E.M. and Grundy, E. (2007) Intergenerational interaction, social capital and health: results from a randomised controlled trial in Brazil. *Social Science and Medicine*, 65: 1397–409.

Finkelstein, E.A., Brown, D.S., Brown, D.R. and Buchner, D.M. (2008) A randomized study of financial incentives to increase physical activity among sedentary older adults. *Preventive Medicine*, 47: 182–7.

Folta, S.C., Lichtenstein, A.H., Seguin, R.A., Goldberg, J.P., Kuder, J.F. and Nelson, M.E. (2009) The Strong Women–Healthy Hearts program: reducing cardiovascular disease risk factors in rural sedentary, overweight, and obese midlife and older women. *American Journal of Public Health*, 99: 1271–7.

Fried, L.P., Carlson, M.C., Freedman, M., Frick, K.D., Glass, T.A., Hill, J. et al. 2004. A social model for health promotion for an aging population: initial evidence on the Experience Corps model. *Journal of Urban Health*, 81: 64–78.

Glasgow, R.E., Vogt, T.M. and Boles, S.M. (1999) Evaluating the public health impact of health promotion interventions: the RE-AIM framework. *American Journal of Public Health*, 89: 1322–7.

Hatton, C., Rivers, M., Mason, H., Mason, L., Emerson, E., Kiernan, C. et al. 2001. Organizational culture and staff outcomes in services for people with intellectual disabilities. *Journal of Intellectual Disability Research*, 43: 206–18.

Heller, T., Marks, B. and Ailey, S.H. (2001) *Exercise and Nutrition Health Education Curriculum for Adults with Developmental Disabilities*. Chicago, IL: University of Illinois at Chicago, Rehabilitation Research and Training Center on Aging and Developmental Disabilities. Department of Disability and Human Development.

Heller, T., Hsieh, K. and Rimmer, J.H. (2004) Attitudinal and psychosocial outcomes of a fitness and health education program on adults with Down syndrome. *Journal Information*, 109(2): 175–85.

Heller, T., McCubbin, J.A., Drum, C. and Peterson, J. (2011) Physical activity and nutrition health promotion interventions: what is working for people with intellectual disabilities? *Intellectual and Developmental Disabilities*, 49: 26–36.

Heller, T., Hsieh, K., Badetti, L. and Parker, H. (2012) *The Special Olympics Community Based Health Promotion Programs: Program Evaluation Report*. Washington, DC: Special Olympics.

Houston, T.K., Allison, J.J., Sussman, M., Horn, W., Holt, C.L., Trobaugh, J. et al. (2011) Culturally appropriate storytelling to improve blood pressure: a randomized trial. *Annals of Internal Medicine*, 154: 77–84.

Hughes, S.L., Seymour, R.B., Campbell, R.T., Shaw, J.W., Fabiyi, C. and Sokas, R. (2011) Comparison of two health-promotion programs for older workers. *American Journal of Public Health*, 101: 883–90.

Hutchinson, S.L. and Wexler, B. (2007) Is 'raging' good for health? Older women's participation in the raging grannies. *Health Care for Women International*, 28: 88–118.

Klug, C., Toobert, D.J. and Fogerty, M. (2008) Healthy Changes™ for living with diabetes: an evidence-based community diabetes self-management program. *Diabetes Education*, 34: 1053–61.

Kolomer, S., Quinn, M.E. and Steele, K. (2010) Interdisciplinary health fairs for older adults and the value of interprofessional service learning. *Journal of Community Practice*, 18: 267–79.

Laforest, S., Nour, K., Gignac, M., Gauvin, L., Parisien, M. and Poirier, M.C. (2008) Short-term effects of a self-management intervention on health status of housebound older adults with arthritis. *Journal of Applied Gerontology*, 27: 539–67.

Lorig, K.R., Ritter, P.L., Dost, A., Plant, K., Laurent, D.D. and McNeil, I. (2008) The Expert Patients Programme online, a 1-year study of an Internet-based self-management programme for people with long-term conditions. *Chronic Illness*, 4: 247–56.

Lunsky, Y., Straiko, A. and Armstrong, S. (2003) Women be Healthy: evaluation of a women's health curriculum for women with intellectual disabilities. *Journal of Applied Research in Intellectual Disabilities*, 16: 247–53.

Marks, B., Sisirak, J. and Hsieh, K. (2008) Health services, health promotion, and health literacy: Report from the State of the Science in Aging with Developmental Disabilities Conference. *Disability and Health Journal*, 1: 136–42.

Marks, B., Sisirak, J. and Heller, T. (2010a) *Health Matters for People with Developmental Disabilities: Creating a Sustainable Health Promotion Program*. Baltimore, MD: Brookes Publishing.

Marks, B., Sisirak, J. and Heller, T. (2010b) *Health Matters: The Exercise, Nutrition and Health Education Curriculum for People with Developmental Disabilities*. Baltimore, MD: Brookes Publishing.

McKinley, P., Jacobson, A., Leroux, A., Bednarczyk, V., Rossignol, M. and Fung, J. (2008) Effect of a community-based Argentine tango dance program on functional balance and confidence in older adults. *Journal of Aging and Physical Activity*, 16: 435–53.

Parish, S.L., Rose, R.A., Luken, K., Swaine, J.G. and O'Hare, L. (2012) Cancer screening knowledge changes results from a randomized control trial of women with developmental disabilities. *Research on Social Work Practice*, 22: 43–53.

Potter, M.B., Somkin, C.P., Ackerson, L.M., Gomez, V., Dao, T., Horberg, M.A. et al. (2011) The FLU-FIT program: an effective colorectal cancer screening program for high volume flu shot clinics. *American Journal of Managed Care*, 17: 577–83.

Prochaska, J. and Norcross, J. (1979) *Systems of Psychotherapy: A Transtheoretical Perspective*. Homewood, IL: Dorsey Press.

Ralston, P.A., Furlow, J., Brickler-Hart, C., Baker, L., Austin, D., Ford, C.A. et al. (2007) The Community Wellness Program: an intergenerational seminar for African Americans. *Journal of Health Care for the Poor and Underserved*, 18: 21–7.

Reddy, D.M., Fried, L.P., Rand, C., McGill, S. and Simpson, C.F. (2007) Can older adult volunteers serve effectively to improve asthma management for children? Experience Corps Baltimore. *Journal of Asthma*, 44: 177–81.

Riley, M.W.E., Kahn, R.L.E., Foner, A.E. and Mack, K.A. (1994) *Age and Structural Lag: Society's Failure to Provide Meaningful Opportunities in Work, Family, and Leisure*. New York: Wiley.

Rimmer, J.H., Heller, T., Wang, E. and Valerio, I. (2004) Improvements in physical fitness in adults with Down syndrome. *American Journal of Mental Retardation*, 109(2): 165–74.

Robertson, J., Roberts, H., Emerson, E., Turner, S. and Greig, R. (2011) The impact of health checks for people with intellectual disabilities: a systematic review of evidence. *Journal of Intellectual Disability Research*, 55: 1009–19.

Ryder, N.B. (1965) The cohort as a concept in the study of social change. *American Sociological Review*, 30(6): 843–61.

Shapira, N., Barak, A. and Gal, I. (2007) Promoting older adults' well-being through Internet training and use. *Aging and Mental Health*, 11(5): 477–84.

Skingley, A. and Bungay, H. (2010) The Silver Song Club Project: singing to promote the health of older people. *British Journal of Community Nursing*, 15: 135–40.

Slevin, E., Taggart, L., McConkey, R., Cousins, W., Truesdale-Kennedy, M. and Dowling, S. (2011) *A Rapid Review of Literature Relating to Support for People with Intellectual Disabilities and their Family Carers when the Person has: Behaviours that Challenge and/or Mental Health Problems; or they are Advancing in Age*. Belfast: University of Ulster.

Smith, P., Cowell, J., McGarry, P. and Chandler, S. (2010) No sex please! We're over 50. *Working with Older People: Community Care Policy and Practice*, 14: 40–3.

Son, J.S., Kerstetter, D.L., Yarnal, C. and Baker, B.L. (2007) Promoting older women's health and well-being through social leisure environments: what we have learned from the Red Hat Society. *Journal of Women and Aging,* 19(3/4): 89–104.

Studenski, S., Perera, S., Hile, E., Keller, V., Spadola-Bogard, J. and Garcia, J. (2010) Interactive video dance games for healthy older adults. *Journal of Nutrition, Health and Aging*, 14: 850–2.

Williamson, T. (2011) Grouchy old men? Promoting older men's mental health and emotional well being. *Working with Older People: Community Care Policy and Practice*, 15: 164–76.

Zoellner, J., Powers, A., Avis-Williams, A., Ndirangu, M., Strickland, E. and Yadrick, K. (2009) Compliance and acceptability of maintaining a 6-month pedometer diary in a rural, African American community-based walking intervention. *Journal of Physical Activity and Health*, 6: 475–82.

Part 3

Health promotion in context

14 Health promotion within families

Malin Broberg and Beverley Temple

Introduction

Families with an individual with intellectual disabilities face ongoing challenges in their everyday life. For example, they are dependent on existing and functioning support services while interactions and changes within the family impact the individual with the disability and the family system as a whole. We sometimes call these families 'ordinary families under extraordinary circumstances' to point out that the families have the same needs, desires, and aspirations as other families but, because one or more of the children have special needs, the whole family must adapt to a special life situation involving other caregiving tasks that most families do not have to carry out, including continuously advocating for the child's right to support (see case study below for an example).

Being a primary caregiver to a family member with intellectual disabilities increases the risk for health problems, such as stress reactions and psychological and physical symptoms, and is associated with lower levels of involvement in paid work and more sick leave, both of which may lead to adverse economic consequences for the family. The primary focus of this chapter is on what could be done to promote health in families caring for an individual with intellectual disabilities. We present factors that influence the health of the individual with learning disability as well as his/her family by using the ecological model (Bronfenbrenner 1977; Algood et al. 2013).

Case study

The parents of Carissa, a 17-year-old with a moderate intellectual disability, are concerned about her health. She has been participating in sports at school and has been welcomed onto teams to play all types of sports. As the planning begins for her to transition out of the school system to the adult systems of support, they are concerned as to where they will find suitable activities for her. Previously the teams provided a social group as well as activities to keep her fit. Now it could prove difficult to find a place for her to interact with people of her own age without incurring a significant cost. Carissa has two older siblings who have recently gone to university, so they are not available to include Carissa in their activities. Carissa's parents are considering work programmes for her, but these do not address her physical activity and social belonging needs.

Understanding the ecological model

The ecological model recognizes that individuals and families exist within interconnected systems. There are four systems:

1. The first, the microsystem, includes the closest relationships between you and the persons you live with or people who act as your main support.
2. The second level of the ecological model, the mesosystem, includes interactions between people in the microsystem and other people you interact with on a daily basis such as day care, schools, and workplaces.
3. The third level, called the exosystem, affects the family indirectly and includes the effects of major institutions of society such as community support and health services.
4. The macrosystem, the outermost level of the ecological system, refers to our larger society and culture and includes cultural values, laws, societal regulations, and resources that have an indirect effect on you.

We place the factors that influence families' health within these system levels and propose and discuss support that can be offered at each level to promote family health (Dempsey and Keen 2008).

The microsystem

Parents of children with intellectual disabilities identify an increased risk for health problems attributed to the caregiving demands that increase stress and workload (Singer 2006; Singer et al. 2007). Parents' caregiving often interferes with their capacity to fulfil their other family, civic, and societal roles. A stressful situation in the family may have a negative impact on children with intellectual disabilities as well as on their siblings. Parents under stress, in general, interact less with their children, are more critical and, specifically, use more harsh discipline methods towards their children with intellectual disabilities compared with siblings. Raising a child with intellectual disabilities may in itself be more stressful then raising other children, since a child with intellectual disabilities is more likely to have behaviour problems compared with typically developing children. Communication difficulties, impaired social ability, difficult temperament, repetitive behaviour, demanding patterns of behaviour, and clinging are all child characteristics that are related to parental stress. Parenting stress and child behaviour are interconnected and have mutually escalating effects on each other (Baker et al. 2003).

Compared with typically developing children, children with intellectual disabilities show dramatically higher levels of psychological symptoms. The interactions that evolve over time between members in the immediate environment play a crucial role for the psychological development of individuals with intellectual disabilities. Negative interaction patterns can emerge slowly in the transactions between the parents' state of mind and the child's difficulties, for example, to respond to communication or signal their needs. Parents of these children are at increased risk of becoming less responsive and more directive in their parenting compared with their behaviour towards typically developing children (Pennington et al. 2004). Children with intellectual disabilities have also been found to experience greater risk of neglect and threat of violence compared with other children, and the risk is especially elevated in families where a parent also has a psychiatric or cognitive disability. Individuals with intellectual disabilities and mental health issues may create more difficulties for families, and it has been found that parental mental health issues also result in poorer mental health of children.

Health-promoting interventions in the microsystem

As described above, interactions in the microsystem are often impacted in several ways by the presence of a family member with intellectual disabilities, and all family members can benefit from interventions aimed at promoting healthy interactions within the microsystem. Health-promoting interventions for families of children with intellectual disabilities can roughly be categorized as follows: stress-reducing or parent-training or parent as trainers/therapists.

The point of departure in several interventions for parents of children with intellectual disabilities is that negative interactions and poor parental wellbeing and psychiatric symptoms are a consequence of stress. A variety of interventions have been designed to reduce the stress and/or increase the parents' resources to manage the stress. Parents usually appreciate and feel supported by different types of stress-reducing interventions, such as mindfulness and/ or acceptance therapy, relaxation and massage, and parent support groups. Practical support to facilitate family life, such as respite, can also decrease stress, anxiety, and insomnia and increase parental control/empowerment. Information and advice about services and the child's diagnosis and prognosis are important dimensions of support and are sometimes given in parent education programmes. Support may also come through the use of technology to connect parents across greater geographical areas with similar needs. Access for all should be a priority and there is a need to produce information in a format and language that is useful and available for all families.

Parent training programmes can be defined as interventions where parents actively acquire parenting skills to better manage difficult child behaviour or become more 'in tune' with the child. These programmes often focus on teaching more positive parenting techniques, such as being responsive to the child by letting the child lead the interaction, or using praise for positive behaviours while ignoring negative behaviours. Most studies on parent training programmes show positive effects on parent behaviour or child outcomes, or both.

Children with autism are often enrolled in more than 30 hours of intervention per week. When children with autism are offered different programmes, parents have to take on work and responsibilities beyond those expected of ordinary parents. To use parents as trainers for small children with autism is common practice; it increases the chance of skill generalization and gives the child possibilities of training over longer periods. When parents train their children, their knowledge of autism increases and the communication between parent and child increases. Parents of children in intensive training can, however, experience increased stress through the responsibility they assume for the training. Parents get less time for the other children in the family and experience a change in family life by having professionals in the home working with the child.

To summarize, it is clear from research that interventions and health promotion programmes that build on family strengths, support positive views of the child, increase positive parent–child interaction, and support parents' development of self-efficacy (instead of being problem- and deficiency-focused) are most effective.

The mesosystem

The second layer of the ecological model is called the mesosystem, and is made up of interactions between different microsystems. For example, the relationship between the child's school and his or her social activities are of importance for the child's and parents' sense of security. Continuity and the flexibility and willingness of the parents' workplace to accommodate the family's needs affect all family members indirectly. The factor described as most affected by caring for an individual with intellectual disabilities is time. Time restrictions and the disruption of daily life are more frequent in families of these children than in control families and are related to adjustment problems in parents. Families with children with intellectual disabilities devote more time to childcare and spend less time in social activities and enjoy less active free time than parents of typically developing children. As a result of the demands of caring, mothers of children with intellectual disabilities often report role restriction and limitations in pursuing a career. The more restricted the mother feels, the more likely she is to experience motherhood as frustrating, unhappy, and wearing. One major obstacle for mothers' employment is the difficulty in finding suitable day care for their child with intellectual disabilities and re-occurring ill-health and appointments with professionals for the child.

Receiving unsatisfactory social support is also strongly associated with difficulties in family functioning and parental mental health. Parents of children with intellectual disabilities have been found to have more limited numbers of social networks than parents of typically developing children. They have more contact with family members and less contact with friends than parents of typically developing children. Ongoing positive interactions with other support systems, such as parent support groups, assist healthy parenting as the child grows. Better collaboration between the school systems and healthcare systems would facilitate greater satisfaction for families and potentially more positive outcomes for these children. More positive perceptions of their child and their child's progress supports parents in a more positive view of their child and their interactions.

Health-promoting interventions in the mesosystem

Family members interact with each other and with other individuals and institutions in the surrounding society (schools, workplace, and so forth) and the reactions, behaviours, and support received in these interactions have consequences for the manoeuvres and choices made by the individual family members. Stress and coping by parents of children with disability have been found to be highly gender related, with women reporting both more stress and more constructive coping strategies such as problem solving. Fathers' reactions to the child's diagnosis seem to be somewhat delayed and fathers may initially avoid dealing with the impact of the disability on everyday life. By avoiding the impact of the disability, a certain distance to the child appears to follow.

Fathers, mothers, siblings, and the children themselves could benefit from interventions promoting the process of developing a close father–child relationship. When fathers take on more responsibility, the mother has the potential to engage in other important roles, for example at the workplace and socially, which can have a protective effect on her health. Fathers tend to report being less affected than mothers in terms of wellbeing in relation to the child with intellectual disabilities, and they are also commonly less engaged in childcare activities while focusing on problem solving outside the family system. Fathers are less likely to make use of psychological support or to participate in interventions related to children available through health services. This could be due to fathers not feeling the need for support, or that they do not expect to benefit from the support available. However, many fathers are motivated to participate in the care of children if, for instance, health services are willing to make appointments outside of office hours. Other fathers may need to be properly informed about how important they are for their child and partner. Father participation, engagement, and equal responsibility for the care of the individual with intellectual disabilities are related to better health and wellbeing of the mother.

One way to support families and facilitate their everyday life is for support systems to be better coordinated and interact more with each other and to have a clear family focus. Family-centred support is not a specific intervention but rather a comprehensive and multidisciplinary approach giving the family access to a variety of services, including specialized medical care, health maintenance, preventive services, coordination of care, family counselling, educational advice, and social support. A growing body of literature points to the importance of caring for children with special healthcare needs in the context of the family and including family members as equal partners in care. Family-centred care acknowledges the central role that families play in children's development, health, and wellbeing and encourages collaboration, information sharing, empowerment, and joint decision making between parents and professionals, all so as to give the child the best conditions for development. Family-centred services aim to support the choices made by families and endeavour to be flexible enough to ensure that services meet the needs of all individual family members. From the beginning of the child's life, the parents will have learned to advocate and coordinate the services and support for their child, yet parents sometimes meet attitudes that create barriers when they advocate for their family member since professionals do not always value the family's involvement, and this can lead to conflicts and a feeling of helplessness in parents.

Practically based family support using relational forms of support increases effects for parents, families, and children, and support is most effective when it is personalized and geared towards family needs such as increasing availability to social support, improving family functioning, and decreasing child behaviour problems. Research shows, however, that there are inequalities as to which families participate or are offered family-centred care; families of children with autism, parents with low socio-economic status, and parents from ethnic minorities are, for example, less likely to have access to family-centred care.

The exosystem

More distant relations that affect the child and the parent indirectly are found in the exosystem, which includes larger social institutions such as community support and health services. The movement of direct care of people with severe intellectual disabilities from institutional care to the community is usually positive for individuals with intellectual disabilities, but has placed families in new situations, where more is expected from them in terms of supporting their children at home. Parents indicate that the formal support they receive for themselves and their child is one of the most important factors for their coping with the situation. Families with children with disabilities are dependent on many different forms of support and one frequent problem is the lack of coordination between different support providers. Families often find it difficult to navigate the support system and usually they have to take responsibility as the coordinator of support. Families often have to be firm advocates for their children, for example to receive the supports that they need, or for their children to be included in schools and other places in society. Families who have a coordinator who can provide an overview and coordinate the family's different needs report better relationships with professionals and fewer unmet service needs.

The concept of quality of life assists in moving towards the importance of policy instead of focusing on personal responsibility within families. Even though it appears that government spending to support people with intellectual disabilities and their families has increased in many countries, numerous inequities remain and there is a need to improve the involvement of families and people with intellectual disabilities themselves in decisions about the delivery of service to facilitate better quality of life for families. Mothers of children with intellectual disabilities are less well integrated into society's workforce than other mothers and there is a need to focus on policies around adequate accessible child care, and family-friendly work and social environments. As people with intellectual disabilities age, their families want services that allow them to be able to 'age in place' where they will be integrated into formal housing, services to allow them continued independence but with ongoing supports. Using concepts such as family-based care and consumer-directed care will allow families to make choices about the needs that they have at that particular time, not as directed by policy makers for a general group of families. It is important to bear in mind that certain groups of families need extra support such as families with children with complex needs and families experiencing socio-economic hardship. Children with intellectual disabilities living in poverty are exposed to more adverse life events, thus increasing the risk for psychopathology. Greater economic hardships in families with children with intellectual disabilities have an impact on other family members' health as well, with parents demonstrating increased levels of psychological stress. To keep families with a child with intellectual disabilities out of poverty often requires that the social security system and the disability system collaborate and coordinate their services to ensure effective services and good quality of life for the whole family. Proper supports need to be put into place to allow parents to enter the employment world at the same time as good day care and respite services are made available to them (Emerson et al. 2010; Parish et al. 2010).

Health-promoting interventions in the exosystem

As described in relation to the mesosystem, families have varying needs, but on a community level there are also many common and re-occurring needs that can be taken care of if the community members and government are foresighted enough in the planning of services. Situations that are often perceived as difficult by families have to do with transitions due to normal development, for example from pre-school to school, from child to adult services, from living with the family to the move into community living; however, these are naturally and frequently occurring processes that the community should have overall plans for. As adolescents require more independence, appropriate employment or employment readiness programmes are required to enhance the sense of wellbeing and contribute to improved skills, knowledge, and ability of the adolescent to enter the workforce. Work experiences and being valued in society are important factors for healthy development for adolescents and adults with intellectual disabilities, and families play an important part in obtaining appropriate placements for their family members with intellectual disabilities since major gaps in services remain.

Eventually families need to care for their family members with intellectual disabilities who are dying; current palliative services have not met the needs of many of these families. Supports to ageing people may also need to consider services for people with intellectual disabilities and dementia. The beliefs and values held by families, staff, and policy makers will need to be considered, as these services become increasingly important to families and quality care for people with intellectual disabilities beyond the medical model of cure.

Long-term care, respite services, and support in future planning for ageing parents with adult children with intellectual disabilities will require greater service delivery forethought to appropriately assist families to have a good quality of life. Families remain active in advocating for inclusion and active living even as their adult children with intellectual disabilities age, but this needs to be supplemented by others to ensure continuing support and improved services when they are no longer able to advocate for their children themselves.

Overall, there is a need for better coordinated and high-quality services that promote the inclusion of individuals with a disability and their family members in general society, such as schools, after-school care, leisure activities, and general health promotion and support programmes. People with intellectual disabilities are known to have poorer health because of lack of access to quality health care appropriate for their needs, which creates increased stress on families as they attempt to advocate for, and get access to, these services. Liaison workers and family advocacy groups are types of services that may assist families to navigate systems and access appropriate services. These partnership models can assist families in making independent decisions and improve quality of life. Programmes will be enhanced by professionals who are educated and knowledgeable about disabilities, and this would improve professionals' confidence in working with people with intellectual disabilities.

The macrosystem

The macrosystem, the outermost layer of the ecological system, refers to institutional patterns or structures of a culture. For example, cultures vary in how much of the responsibility for children or adults with disabilities is placed upon the individual/family compared with society (for example, how individualistic or collectivistic the society is). Cultural values usually play a role in laws and societal policies for child care, disability pensions, supported employment, and independent living arrangements, all of which provide important support for individuals with disability and their family members. For instance, parents' allowance may enable parents to stay at home with the child during infancy and later access to child care and high-quality inclusive schooling outside the home may promote the child's social and language development and allow for parents to participate in working life.

How we view disability is also culturally based: in most societies disability is viewed as a tragedy and a challenging situation. When parents realize that their child has intellectual disabilities, most experience strong emotional reactions – a crisis. How this crisis develops, and what the consequences are, varies greatly depending on, for example, the circumstances and the personality of the parent but also the cultural beliefs and attitudes of society. Being a parent of a child with intellectual disabilities does not only include a loss – there is also the joy of becoming a parent. Parents may be able to find benefits in having a child with intellectual disabilities, and family, friends, and professionals who discourage them from doing so may impede the development of the positive aspects of caring. Even people who work professionally with parents of children with intellectual disabilities sometimes reduce, filter or change parents' narratives to be compatible with a 'tragedy discourse'. In this process, parents are reduced to being 'only sad' and the child's humanity is being reduced to his or her impairment. Families need to maintain their privacy and strengths in how they have chosen to provide support and care for their loved one. Society may also need to review the vision of caregiving provided by families of children and adults with intellectual disabilities as potential social capital.

Attitudes and perceptions of society also influence the support provided by society for people with intellectual disabilities and their families. There continues to be an effect on families of perceived stigmatization of disability in society. The importance of the support provided by professionals such as social workers needs to be highlighted and valued. Paid carers or family members often determine the types of activities that they consider to be valuable for people with intellectual disabilities, and this may interfere with the concept of inclusion as it was originally defined. As people with intellectual disabilities age, they develop more complex health needs but the system developed to support them is based on supporting well individuals. Social workers are increasingly responsible for the assessment and referral for health needs with which they are not familiar, which puts the health of people with intellectual disabilities at risk.

Spirituality and culture are important in the ways that families develop their understandings of their child and the ways that families develop coping strategies. There is a relation between belonging to an ethnic minority group and experiencing increased stress that most probably can be accounted for by a mix of economic and social structures as well as prejudices and discrimination in society. Countries enact policies based on their own culture and understandings of the developing needs of families with a child with intellectual disabilities. As the population of people with intellectual disabilities ages and they outlive their caregivers, a greater demand is placed on services to support this ageing group. The interface between societal changes, government policy, use of technology, and the workforce will all have an impact on the quality of life of many families with children with intellectual disabilities in the future.

Health-promoting interventions in the macrosystem

The WHO (2011) has emphasized that the degree or severity of a disability depends on the type and extent of impairment together with environmental factors. These factors interact to facilitate or limit activity and participation in daily life. This conceptual model to assess the degree of the disability could also translate to the experiences of family members. Family members explain that they are affected not just by the impairments in different cognitive or physical domains of the child, but also by the discourses and constraints of the environment. Increased awareness of the needs and rights of individuals with disabilities and their families to actively participate and be included in all areas of society is important for their wellbeing. According to the UN Convention on the Right of the Child (UNCRC 1990) and the UN Convention on the Rights of Persons with Disabilities (UNCRPD 2008), children and people with disabilities are to be perceived as active participants in their every-day life and participate in decision-making processes. Ratification of the conventions means that the signatories agree that inclusion and participation in everyday life are fundamental rights for all individuals. Legal documents and policies can be important tools in the work to improve support to individuals with disabilities and their families if they are used actively. Policy makers and support workers at all levels and in all areas need education on the UN conventions in order to take over some of the advocacy responsibility from family members. All citizens share the responsibility for creating a society where all individuals are equally valued and given the same rights to a good life; those who work to support individuals with disabilities and their families have a special responsibility to advocate for this population.

Summary

- Families of children with disabilities have the same needs, desires, and aspirations as other families but because one or more of the children have special needs the whole family must adapt to a special life situation, including continuously advocating for the child's right to support. This special life situation often leads to increased stress and negative health outcomes for family members.
- Interventions and health promotion programmes that build on family strengths, support positive views of the child, increase positive parent–child interaction, and support parents' development of self-efficacy, instead of being problem- and deficiency-focused, are most effective.
- Practically based family support increases effects for parents, families, and children. The support is most effective when it is personalized and geared towards family needs such as improving availability to social support, improving family functioning, and decreasing child behaviour problems.
- Increased awareness of the needs and rights of individuals with disabilities and their families to actively participate and be included in all areas of society is important for their wellbeing.

Useful resources

- Bali, K. and Childs, S. (2005) *The Art of Hiding Vegetables: Sneaky Ways to Feed Your Children Healthy Food*. Newton Abbott: White Ladder Press.
- Legge, B. (2002) *Can't Eat, Won't Eat: Dietary Difficulties and Autistic Spectrum Disorders*. London: Jessica Kingsley.
- Raising Children Network: http://raisingchildren.net.au/articles/screen_time.html/context/481
- A Review of Processes and Outcomes in Family-Centered Services for Children With a Disability: http://tec.sagepub.com/content/28/1/42.full.pdf
- Sleep: http://www.nas.org.uk
- UK National Autism Society fact sheet about autism and play: http://www.autism.org.uk/living-with-autism/communicating-and-interacting.aspx
- Wheeler, M. (2004) Mealtime and children on the Autism spectrum: beyond picky, fussy, and fads. *The Reporter*, 9(2): 13–19.
- Raising Children Network's web page on parentings a child with special needs: http://raisingchildren.net.au/special_needs/special_needs.html

Web resources

- Fact sheets about autism: http://www.med.monash.edu.au/spppm/research/devpsych/actnow/factsheet.html

General health information

- http://www.easyhealth.org.uk/
- www.intellectualdisability.info
- http://www.intellectualdisability.info/changing-values/i-have-downs-syndrome-but-dont-feel-sorry-for-me

References

Algood, C.L., Harris, C., & Hong, J.S. (2013). Parenting Success and Challenges for Families of Children with Disabilities: An Ecological Systems Analysis. *Journal of Human Behaviour in the Social Environment*, 23(2), 126–136.

Baker, B.L., McIntyre, L.L., Blacher, J., Crnic, K., Edlebrock, C. and Low, C (2003) Pre-school children with and without developmental delay: behaviour problems and parenting stress over time. *Journal of Intellectual Disability Research*, 47(4/5): 217–30.

Bronfenbrenner, U. (1977) Toward an experimental ecology of human development. *American Psychologist*, 32(7): 513–31.

Dempsey, I., & Keen, D. (2008). A review of processes and outcomes in family-centered services for children with a disability. *Topics in Early Childhood Special Education*, 28(1), 42–52. Available at: http://tec.sagepub.com/content/28/1/42.full.pdf

Emerson, E., Shahtahmasebi, S., Lancaster, G. and Berridge, D. (2010) Poverty transitions among families supporting a child with intellectual disability. *Journal of Intellectual and Developmental Disability*, 35(4): 224–34.

Olsson, M.B. (2008). Understanding Individual Differences in Adaptation in Parents of Children with Intellectual Disabilities: A Risk and Resilience Perspective. *International review of research in mental retardation*, 36, 281–315. http://www.pol.gu.se/digitalAssets/1328/1328180_int-review.pdf

Parish, S., Grinstein-Weiss, M., Yeong Hun, Y., Rose, R. and Rimmerman, A. (2010) Assets and income: disability-based disparities in the United States. *Social Work Research*, 34(2): 71–82.

Pennington, L., Goldbart, J. and Marshall, J. (2004) Interaction training for conversational partners of children with cerebral palsy: a systematic review. *International Journal of Language and Communication Disorders*, 39: 151–70.

Singer, G. (2006) Meta-analysis of comparative studies of depression in mothers of children with and without developmental disabilities. *American Journal on Mental Retardation*, 11(3): 155–69.

Singer, G.H., Ethridge, B.L., & Aldana, S.I. (2007). Primary and secondary effects of parenting and stress management interventions for parents of children with developmental disabilities: A meta-analysis. *Mental Retardation and Developmental Disabilities Research Reviews*, 13(4), 357–369.

United Nations High Commission for Human Rights (1990) *United Nations Convention on the Rights of the Child* (UNCRC). Available at: www.unicef.org/crc/ [accessed 22 June 2013].

United Nations Secretariat (2008) *United Nations Convention on the Rights of Persons with Disability* (UNCRPD). Available at: http://www.un.org/esa/socdev/enable/rights/convtexte.htm. [accessed 22 June 2013].

World Health Organization (WHO) (2011) *World Report on Disability*. Geneva: WHO.

Health promotion in schools

Laurence Taggart and David Stewart

Introduction

Over the last twenty years there has been an international growth in how educational facilities can promote the physical and mental health of children and young people. The 'Healthy School' approach incorporates the whole school, including teachers, support staff and cooks, as well as health professionals and the wider community. At the hub of this approach are the young person and their family: schools alone cannot change health.

This chapter illustrates how health promotion is integral to the overall learning of children and young people with intellectual disabilities in both mainstream and special school settings. It explores strategies by which teachers and support staff can ensure that health education is embedded as part of personal, social, and health education, and is cross-curricula in nature. Obesity, sexual health and personal relationships, smoking/alcohol and illicit drugs, and mental health (including suicide and bullying) are explored. The importance of working with parents and families and a range of other professionals is explored throughout this chapter.

Health-promoting schools

There is an important relationship between children and young people, teachers, families, the wider community, and the ability of any school to function at its best and achieve all that is expected from the process of formal school education. If young people in schools are happy and healthy they can learn, work, and play better (see Box 15.1 for the principles of a health-promoting school). A health-promoting school is one that works in a way that demonstrates a whole-school commitment to improving and protecting the health and wellbeing of the school community. More specifically, a health-promoting school is one that uses a *health-promoting schools* approach. A health-promoting school cannot be defined by the presence of special projects, educational activities or specific physical characteristics. Nor is it a programme with a beginning or an end.

A health-promoting schools approach is really a way of thinking and working that is adopted by the whole school to make the school the best possible place to learn, work, and play. The approach is defined by:

- People from across the school community working together to plan and deliver school activities; this includes pupils, parents, teachers, other staff, cooks, health professionals, and the wider community.
- An ongoing consideration of the broad range of factors that make up the school, to ensure that positive and comprehensive school systems, environments, and programmes and activities are provided. This means coordinated programmes through all the key stages with teachers sharing and planning their approaches and activities.

Box 15.1 Principles of health-promoting schools

- Promotes the physical and mental health of pupils
- Enhances the learning outcomes of pupils
- Upholds social justice and equity concepts
- Provides a safe and supportive environment
- Involves pupil participation and empowerment
- Links health and education issues and systems
- Addresses the health and wellbeing issues of all school staff
- Collaborates with parents and the local community
- Integrates health into the school's ongoing activities, curriculum, and assessment standards
- Sets realistic goals built on accurate data and sound scientific evidence
- Seeks continuous improvement through ongoing monitoring and evaluation

Taken from the International Union for Health Promotion and Education. Check out the website at: http://www.iuhpe.org/uploaded/Publications/Books_Reports/HPS_GuidelinesII_2009_English.pdf

Many schools that adopt such an approach find the health-promoting schools framework, as set out in Box 15.1, an extremely helpful instrument for ensuring their thinking and planning processes are comprehensive and consider all aspects that make up the school. According to the WHO (2011), a health-promoting school is one that constantly strengthens its capacity as a healthy setting for living, learning, and working.

The objectives of a health-promoting school are to:

- foster health and learning with all the measures at its disposal
- engage health and educational professionals, teachers, teachers' unions, students, parents, health providers, and community leaders in efforts to make the school a healthy place for its young people
- strive to provide a healthy environment along with school/community projects and out-reach, health promotion programmes for staff, nutrition and food safety programmes, opportunities for physical education and recreation, and programmes for counselling, social support, and mental health promotion
- implement policies and practices that respect an individual's wellbeing and dignity, provide multiple opportunities for success, and acknowledge good efforts and intentions as well as personal achievements
- strive to improve the health of school personnel, families, and community members as well as pupils; and work with community leaders to help them understand how the community contributes to, or undermines, health and education.

Health-promoting schools and four protective concepts

The health-promoting schools approach has the potential to integrate four key protective concepts that can positively empower the healthy development and wellbeing of children and young people with and without intellectual disabilities across schools:

- target obesity by promoting healthy eating and increasing physical activity
- prevent smoking, abuse of alcohol, and use of illicit drugs
- promote sexual health and relationship education
- develop emotional resilience and recognize mental health problems (including bullying and suicide risk).

Sipler (2006) has identified four types of strategies that have been shown to effectively support the health and wellbeing of young people in schools:

- decrease the risk factors that contribute to risky behaviour and poor health outcomes
- increase the protective factors that contribute to resiliency and healthy outcomes
- provide opportunities for young people to successfully meet the developmental needs of adolescence
- build healthy communities that support and nurture adolescents.

The role of personal development in achieving this is summarized in Figure 15.1.

Establishing health-promoting schools through a 'whole-school approach'

Schools can make a substantial contribution to a pupil's physical, mental, and social wellbeing. This has been recognized by many international initiatives, including those from the WHO, UNICEF, UNESCO, and the International Union for Health Promotion and Education (IUHPE). A range of strategies and programmes have evolved with diverse names, such as:

- Health-Promoting Schools
- Comprehensive School Health
- Child Friendly Schools
- FRESH initiative.

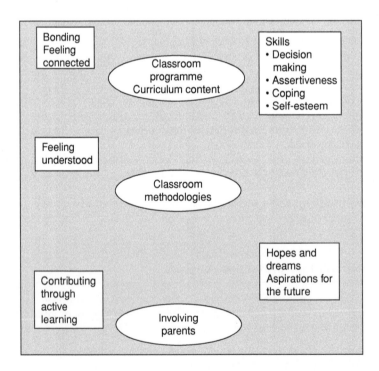

Figure 15.1 How personal development can reduce risk and enhance protective factors

Source: http://www.nicurriculum.org.uk/docs/key_stage_3/areas_of_learning/personal_development/ks3_pd_powerofteachers.pdf

Box 15.2 Establishing health promotion in schools: a whole-school approach

- Developing a supportive government/local authority policy for health-promoting schools
- Achieving administrative and senior management support
- Creating a small group that is actively engaged in leading and coordinating actions, including teachers, non-teaching staff, pupils, parents, healthcare professionals, and community members
- Conducting an audit of current health-promoting actions according to the six essential elements
- Establishing agreed goals and a strategy to achieve them
- Developing a health-promoting school charter
- Ensuring appropriate school staff and community partners undertake capacity-building programmes and that they have opportunities to put their skills into practice
- Celebrating milestones
- Allowing 3–4 years to complete specific goals

Taken from the International Union for Health Promotion and Education. Check out the website at: http://www.iuhpe.org/uploaded/Publications/Books_Reports/HPS_GuidelinesII_2009_English.pdf

However, these strategies share the connecting thread of a *whole-school approach* and recognition that all aspects of the life of the school are important in the promotion of the health of the young person. It has become clear in these approaches that it is necessary to do more than just offer health education classes in the curriculum if we wish schools to fulfil their potential in promoting the health of children and young people with and without intellectual disabilities. The IUHPE has provided guidelines for how schools could develop a whole-school approach for all children and young people (see Box 15.2 and Box 15.3).

Schools are at the front-line and together with a range of partners they must ensure effective health education, which is appropriate to need and open to scrutiny and assessment. This is about young people's rights.

There have been many strategies to support schools in delivering health education as part of a wider programme of Personal, Social, and Health Education (PSHE). Healthy Schools programmes have supported schools to develop not only their curriculums but encouraged a whole-school

Box 15.3 Essential elements of promoting health in schools

Healthy schools policy: such as healthy eating polices, promoting physical activity, drug awareness, respects policy

The school's physical environment: buildings, grounds, equipment, space

The school's social environment: quality of the relationships among and between teaching staff and pupils, parents and the wider community

Individual health skills and action competencies: including the formal and informal curriculum and associated activities, where pupils learn their age-related knowledge, understandings, skills, and experiences

Community links: including connections with families and wider community/groups as well as the school and pupil; appropriate consultations with relevant stakeholders are important

Health services: local healthcare services/professionals responsible for health care and promotion. They provide education, screening and assessment, and also mental health services/counselling to promote students' social and emotional development and address stress and anxiety

Taken from the International Union for Health Promotion and Education. Check out the website at: http://www.iuhpe.org/uploaded/Publications/Books_Reports/HPS_GuidelinesII_2009_English.pdf ethos for promoting health. Schools are encouraged to think of the emotional, physical, and learning environment provided. Useful guidance enjoins schools to consider involving the whole school community. The health of pupils, staff, families, and the immediate community are all-important. Some themes, as mentioned above, which are particularly relevant to young people with and without intellectual disabilities, include:

- targeting obesity by promoting healthy eating and increasing physical activity
- preventing smoking/alcohol/illicit drug use
- promoting sexual health and relationship education
- developing emotional resilience and recognizing mental health problems (including bullying and suicide risk).

All these themes are interrelated and interdependent. A good school would encourage participation and consultation with the school community. Ensuring that school improvements in health are evidence-based should have greater impact in embedding change.

Obesity

There is growing evidence that both young people and adults with intellectual disabilities are more likely to be obese compared with their non-disabled peers (see Chapter 5). Risk factors for obesity for this population include:

- genetic causes
- poverty
- physical disabilities
- the greater likelihood of a sedentary lifestyle
- low levels of exercise
- a high-fat diet
- long-term use of medications
- limited access to recreational activities.

Healthy eating

Young people with intellectual disabilities may have real issues with eating. They may be particularly fussy with food, and may have issues of not eating or eating too much. Unfortunately, food is often used as a control mechanism, particularly in relation to behaviour. Adults who may feel sorry for the young person may indulge them with less healthy items of food, which provide instant comfort. A child quickly learns how to manipulate an adult.

It is important for schools to reflect on the adult population with intellectual disabilities, and identify the issues affecting them, such as Type 2 diabetes (Taggart et al. 2012). As we know some of the health problems that afflict adults with intellectual disabilities, it would be prudent for schools to take steps to avoid the same fate befalling today's young people in the future. Ensuring that school meals are healthy and nutritious is a powerful way of introducing pupils to healthier options. Are there healthy choices? Is there always fruit? Do children have access to drinking water? Involving the young people in meal preparation and devising menus is helpful. Encouraging pupils to shop and choose healthier options promotes their understanding of healthier life choices (see Chapter 4).

Clearly, schools need to work with the young person but also with their family; encouraging healthy eating needs to be tackled sensitively, as some families will be struggling with budgets. Schemes such as 'Let's Get Cooking' are excellent, since they promote parents and their children cooking together, concentrating on healthy options. Discussions about packed lunches are important and school policies on the consumption of no fizzy drinks are helpful.

Physical activity

A reduction in physical activity levels in addition to high calorie intake can eventually lead to obesity. Thus to maintain a healthy weight, a combination of regular physical activity and a controlled diet is required (see Chapter 5). However, evidence suggests that the people with intellectual disabilities have lower levels of physical activity than their non-disabled peers. According to Emerson (2011), young people with intellectual disabilities are 3.7 times less likely to take part in exercise. This is an alarming statistic, as there is significant evidence that regular exercise can reduce the risk factors for many health problems (see Chapter 16).

It is clear that physical activity intervention programmes have beneficial effects immediately following the intervention and in the long term. However, barriers do exist to long-term adherence of physical activity for these young people. Shields et al. (2012) highlighted the most popular facilitators to physical activity in this population:

- the programme needs a social element to it (i.e. friends and/or family are included)
- the programme needs a variety of elements as opposed to one main theme in the intervention
- the programme could be tailor-made to fit individual ability and needs.

Substance abuse

Smoking

Generally, smoking among teenagers with severe intellectual disabilities is relatively rare, although the incidence is likely to be higher among those with more moderate disabilities. It is interesting to note that some take up smoking as adults. Could this be due to an inappropriate role model among the support staff? With many pupils having breathing problems, discussion needs to be had with adults about the issues of passive smoking. Although staff cannot smoke on the premises, some may still think that it is all right to work with someone when they still have a strong smell of smoke on their clothes.

Alcohol

As with other young people, people with intellectual disabilities need clear advice about sensible consumption of alcohol. Many pupils with intellectual disabilities will require medication that may have contraindications with alcohol, so they will need to be very clear about the consequences of drinking. Due to personal safety issues, advice will need to be given about the dangers of becoming intoxicated. They will also need to know that drinks can be spiked and therefore they need to be vigilant in social settings. Staff will need to be mindful that there may be students in the class who have foetal alcohol syndrome and are living with the consequence of alcohol consumption.

Drug education

Many of the students may be prescribed a range of medications that they take on a regular basis. Over time they may have become passive consumers of these medications. Do they know why they are taking the medication? Do they know the side-effects? Every effort must be taken to inform the student so that they can be empowered in their lives. Pupils need to be aware of the dangers of drugs and the risks. One needs to be sensitive, for there may be issues of drug abuse in their own home. Young women and men, perhaps with more mild intellectual disabilities, may through drug use be drawn into prostitution. They need clear education and advice to prevent these risks (see Chapter 12).

Sexual health and relationship education

The theme of PSHE is broad. One area that schools may have difficulty with implementing and teaching is that of sex and relationship education. In making the case for clear and supportive sex and relationship education for students with intellectual disabilities, it is often helpful to review the range of sources that have impacted on our knowledge, views, and attitudes (see Chapter 10). When one compares these to the experiences of many people with intellectual disabilities, it becomes very apparent when such education needs to be in place. We now consider some of the major influences.

Family

For many parents and families who may still be coming to terms with their child's disability, that they will need to consider sex education may be the last thing on their minds. They may feel at a loss, and clearly experience would tell us that they are looking to others for support. Siblings may feel inhibited or be jealous as parents direct considerable time to the sibling with the intellectual disability. They may wish to model themselves on siblings but may find that there are constraints, which then lead to frustrations. The school therefore needs to be confident in its own abilities and prepared to be supportive in what can be very embarrassing situations for parents. Training courses and support groups for parents are invaluable. It enables them to discuss issues in a safe and supportive environment. When working with parents, one must be sensitive to cultural and religious beliefs. Some communities may find this a difficult subject and may ask for different forums in which to meet.

Friends

Most non-disabled people cite their friends and peers as a great source of information while growing up, even if the information given and received is not always correct. Many young people with intellectual disabilities may not have a social network of friends. They may know children but they are not invited to parties or sleepovers – the sorts of occasions when the informal learning around relationships occurs. They may always have a support worker with them in a playground situation, hindering natural communication with peers. Regarding friendships and relationships, parents must realize the crucial part they will play in supporting and enabling these to be formed and sustained. There may need to be a great deal of engineering of social situations to enable this to happen. Many friendships end when students leave school and lose contact with their friends. Little wonder, then, that some will become depressed and isolated.

School

There appears to be very mixed picture in what is provided in sex and relationship education in mainstream and special schools. We cannot assume that a young person has had access to a full, rounded, and continuing education in this area of learning. A useful exercise in staff training is to ask staff to work in groups and decide what is allowed at any time, any place, certain times, certain places or never. There can often be a question of whose need is being met. Male and female staff may hold different views. Often what is clear is there has not been enough discussion and senior leadership has not provided enough guidance. If staff members are confused, then what hope for the students? Students have the right to a supportive and clear education.

Media

Pupils with intellectual disabilities may struggle to put in context much of what they see and hear in the media. Sexualized language in songs suddenly becomes part of vocabulary with little understanding. Television soaps may purport to be educational, but their storylines are more about getting audience figures. They can give out some very mixed messages in regard to relationships. For those who cannot read, a picture in a paper or magazine will be seen but not necessarily in the correct context.

While there are many other influences, those above help to illustrate the importance of students having a clear and informative education. With all these obvious gaps in their learning, it is essential that schools and children services step in.

Emotional resilience

A range of factors can affect students' emotional wellbeing and it is important that meaningful education and support is in place. Students arrive at school from a range of different family backgrounds; some may have experienced years of bullying, and consequently self-esteem may be very low. Having been bullied, some young people may have developed some bullying behaviours as a means of defence. Some may feel low or depressed, even feel a sense of loneliness and isolation.

Positive mental health or resilience

The Mental Health Foundation (2011) defines positive mental health as 'a state of well-being in which the individual realises his or her own abilities, he/she can cope with the normal stresses of life, can work productively and is able to make a contribution to his or her community': in other words, being resilient. Resilience is characterized by an individual who:

- develops emotionally, intellectually, and spiritually
- initiates, develops, and sustains mutually satisfying personal relationships
- faces problems, resolves them, and learns from them
- is confident and assertive
- is aware of others and empathizes with them
- enjoys solitude
- plays and has fun
- laughs both at him/herself and the world.

Resilience means having the ability to overcome daily challenges, facing everyday difficulties, and maintaining a sense of consistency in managing such struggles. Resilience is about promoting and maintaining positive mental health. There are a number of core components required that can enable a person to become resilient or versatile in light of the daily hassles and stresses involved in life:

Personal strengths or attributes

- using practical and emotional coping strategies
- having a range of problem-solving skills
- having clear and articulate communication skills
- having good social skills
- having high self-esteem
- having high self-efficacy
- having an internal locus of control
- having a positive self-identity and self-image
- having a sense of humour
- having a sense of control.

Ecological context/protective environments

- prior experience of challenges and how successful or not the young person was in overcoming these across their lifespan
- having support of consistent and loving relationships to aid the young person to overcome the adversity
- having external resources such as school, family, and community.

Perceived threat

- understanding the challenge (i.e. comprehensibility)
- having the internal and external resources to overcome the difficulty (i.e. manageability)
- having the motivation to want to challenge the difficulty (i.e. meaningfulness).

Resilient children and young people react to challenges in constructive ways, even in the face of seemingly overwhelming hardship and adversity. Resilient children survive risky environments because of their strong internal strengths and they are able to fight off or recover from their misfortune. They are also more likely to show sustained competence when under stress, or to rebound to previously healthy levels of competence following traumatic or stressful experiences. Resilience involves ongoing interactions between protective and vulnerability factors within the young person, between the young person and his or her surroundings, and among the various risk factors.

Mental ill-health

Mental ill-health and similar terms are used interchangeably to cover a wide range of negative feelings and behaviours from those that can be described as normal (such as feeling low or sad) to chronic and enduring feelings (e.g. thought disturbance, ideas of self-harm, feelings hopeless). These feelings and behaviours can last for a few hours or days through to more negative feelings and behaviours that last for weeks or even months and can lead to a diagnosis of a psychiatric condition. As part of personal, social, and health education, it is important to work with students on their emotions and their appreciation of the emotions of others. Students need to understand and manage their emotions.

Teachers and other staff can help children and young people develop emotional intelligence by encouraging them to identify their emotions and understand how these feelings are connected to their actions. In school settings, children can learn about their emotions through the stories they read. For example, a child in a story may experience some mixture of joy, sadness, anxiety or loss. One method used in classrooms includes circle time, which enables expression of emotions.

Circle time was developed by Jenny Mosley and is widely used in schools. Quality Circle Time (QCT) is a democratic and creative approach used to support teachers and other staff in managing a range of issues that affect the whole learning community. Quality Circle Time meetings for children involve carrying out activities, games and the practice of speaking and listening skills, often in a round. There are several key elements to the model, namely:

- improving the morale and self-esteem of staff
- listening systems for children and adults
- the Golden Rules: a system of behavioural rules for children
- incentives: a weekly celebration to congratulate the children for keeping the Golden Rules
- sanctions: the partial withdrawal of the Golden Time incentive
- lunchtime policy.

It is important that there are structures in place in schools not only to give young people a voice but also to ensure that voice is valued. The provision of counsellors in school who have skills in working with students with intellectual disabilities is invaluable. Over time they can build up good relationships with the students, encouraging them to be more confident.

Bullying

Young people with intellectual disabilities may be at particular risk of bullying from their peers without disabilities as they are easily identified as a marginalized group. The National Autistic Society (2006) examined bullying and found that two out of five children with autism have been bullied, and three out of five of those with Asperger's syndrome and high-functioning autism have been bullied. A Mencap Report (2007) revealed that eight out of ten children with an intellectual disability were bullied, and six out of ten had been physically hurt. As a result, Mencap launched an anti-bullying campaign to stop the bullying of children and young people with an intellectual disability.

Given the associations between school bullying and victimization and poor mental health, schools should prioritize the implementation of anti-bullying policies and interventions. Many interventions have been found to directly reduce bullying. For example, Vreeman and Carroll (2007) pointed out the value of multi-disciplinary whole-school approaches, including a combination of school-wide sanctions, teacher training, classroom curriculum, conflict resolution training, and individual counselling. This contrasted with curriculum interventions (video-tapes, lectures, and written curriculum), which were less successful. Social skills training and individual, group, and family interventions have been found to help young people with intellectual disabilities who have been bullied to increase social competence and peer relations (Mishna 2003). Individual, familial, peer, and school factors have been identified that can place a young person at risk for participating in bullying behaviour (see Box 15.4).

Suicide

There are few reports of deliberate self-harm in children and young people with intellectual disabilities. It is recognized that behaviour such as cutting oneself, running into vehicles, and jumping from heights do occur in this population. There is also recognition that self-injury, aggression, and screaming might be behavioural equivalents of depression, especially in people with severe or profound disabilities (Marston et al. 1997). Despite this, the majority of attention is directed to self-injurious behaviour. Self-harm refers to any self-inflicted behaviour that can cause tissue damage to the child's own body. Lunsky (2004) studied 98 adults with intellectual disabilities and 33 of this sample reported suicidal thoughts. Twenty-three people said that they thought about killing themselves and 11 said how they would carry out the act (3 with an overdose of medication, 3 slashing their wrists, 4 jumping, 1 with a knife, and 1 by shooting). Eleven people with intellectual disabilities in this study had also reported previous suicide attempts.

Giannini et al. (2010) argued that rates of suicide risk factors are higher in those with intellectual disabilities than in the general population, although suicide rates may be lower. They reviewed the literature and identified the following risk factors associated with suicide in people with intellectual disabilities:

- psychiatric disorders
- depressive disorders
- post-traumatic stress disorder
- psychotic disorders
- sleep and eating disturbances
- sadness

Box 15.4 Risk factors for bullying peers

Individual risk factors
- impulsive, hot-headed, dominant personality lacking empathy
- difficulty conforming to rules and low frustration tolerance
- positive attitudes towards violence
- physically aggressive
- gradually decreasing interest in school (achievement).

Family risk factors
- lack of parental warmth and involvement
- overly permissive or excessively harsh discipline/physical punishment by parents
- lack of parental supervision.

Peer risk factors
- friends/peers with positive attitudes towards violence
- exposure to models of bullying.

School risk factors
- lack of supervision during breaks (e.g. lunchrooms, playgrounds, hallways, locker rooms, and bathrooms)
- unsupervised interactions between different grades during breaks
- indifferent or accepting teacher attitudes towards bullying
- indifferent or accepting student attitudes towards bullying
- inconsistent enforcement of the rules

- psychomotor retardation
- somatization
- family discord
- bereavement
- history of physical or sexual abuse
- certain medications
- conduct disorders
- self-injury
- behavioural issues.

The majority of self-harmers do not come to the attention of health services, thus schools need to raise awareness about positive mental health and help-seeking. Children and adolescents may present to a hospital after self-harm. However, specialist assessment and psychosocial support may not be available. Hawton et al. (2003) outlined the need for school-based mental health initiatives aimed at education and promotion of mental health, targeting anxiety, depression, poor self-esteem, and impulsivity. They suggested screening pupils and helping teachers recognize such pupils. They recommended:

- the use of help lines
- self-referral agencies
- school counselling services.

Warning signs of suicide in young people include:

- change in eating and sleeping habits
- withdrawal from friends, family, and regular activities
- violent or rebellious behaviour, or running away

- drug or alcohol abuse
- unusual neglect of personal appearance
- radical personality change
- persistent boredom, difficulty concentrating, or a decline in the quality of school work
- frequent complaints about physical symptoms often related to emotions, such as stomach ache or headache, fatigue
- loss of interest in pleasurable activities
- not tolerating praise or rewards
- complaining of being 'rotten inside'
- putting affairs in order, giving away favourite possessions, cleaning room, throwing things away
- becoming suddenly cheerful after a period of depression
- giving verbal hints with statements such as: 'I won't be a problem for you much longer'; 'Nothing matters'; 'It's no use', and 'I won't see you again'.

(adapted from: http://www.familymentalhealth.com/suicide.htm)

Summary

- A 'Healthy School' approach should be employed across the whole school with a focus on obesity, sexual health and personal relationships, smoking/alcohol and illicit drug use, and mental health (including suicide and bullying).
- Teachers, classroom support assistants, cooks, health professionals, communities, and families must work together to make the school a healthy place for its young people.
- Given the high rates of mental ill-health reported in young people with intellectual disabilities, schools should provide initiatives aimed at education and promotion of resilience targeting depression/anxiety, low self-esteem, disempowerment, and bullying.

Useful resources

Obesity

- *The 3 Fives*: WHO Advice document available at: http://www.who.int/foodsafety/consumer/3x5_SA_en.pdf

Sexual health and personal relationships

- *Living Your Life*: The sex education and personal development resource for people with intellectual difficulties and disabilities: www.brook.org.uk
- *All About Us*: Family Planning Association CD-ROM: www.fpa.org.uk
- *Let's Plan It*: A planning guide to creating programmes of sex and relationship education for people with intellectual disabilities across a wide range of ages and abilities. Image in Action: www.imageinaction.org

Substance abuse

- http://www.easyhealth.org.uk/listing/smoking-(leaflets)
- http://www.ldhealthnetwork.org.uk/docs/trigg.pub

Resilience

- Watch and listen to how this school promotes emotional resilience within its young people: http://www.teachersmedia.co.uk/videos/helping-children-stay-mentally-strong
- Promoting resilience: https://www.naeyc.org/files/yc/file/201103/PromotingResilience_Pizzolongo0311.pdf
- Jenny Mosley's website: http://www.circle-time.co.uk/

Web resources

Bullying

- http://ec.europa.eu/justice_home/daphnetoolkit/files/others/europe_violence/2.1.pdf
- http://www.youtube.com/watch?v=t1bcbtz2eJE
- http://www.niabf.org.uk/cms/images/stories/documents/resources/All%20About%20Me%20KS2.pdf

Suicide

- http://www.selfinjurysupport.org.uk/files/docs/hidden-pain/hidden-pain-full-report.pdf
- http://www.selfinjurysupport.org.uk/hidden-pain-self-injury-and-people-learning-disabilities
- http://www.wellatschool.org/index.php?option=com_content&view=article&id=126&Itemid=381

References

Emerson, E. (2011) Health status and health risks of the 'hidden majority' of adults with intellectual disability. *Intellectual and Developmental Disabilities*, 49: 155–65.

Giannini, M.J., Bergmark, B., Kreshover, S., Elias, E., Plummer, C. and O'Keefe, C. (2010) Understanding suicide and disability through three major disabling conditions: intellectual disability, spinal cord injury and multiple sclerosis. *Disability and Health Journal*, 3: 74–8.

Hawton, K., Rodham, K., Evans, E. and Wetherall, E. (2003) Deliberate self-harm in adolescents: self report survey in schools in England. *British Medical Journal*, 325: 1207–11.

Lunsky, Y. (2004) Suicidality in a clinical and community sample of adults with mental retardation. *Research in Developmental Disabilities*, 25: 231–43.

Marston, G.M., Perry, D.W. and Roy, A. (1997) Manifestations of depression in people with intellectual disability. *Journal of Intellectual Disability Research*, 41: 476–80.

Mencap (2007) *Bullying Wrecks Lives: The Experiences of Children and Young People with a Learning Disability.* Available at: http://www.mencap.org.uk/sites/default/files/documents/2008-03/Bullying%20wrecks%20lives.pdf [accessed 18 May 2013].

Mental Health Foundation (2011) http://www.mentalhealth.org.uk/help-information/mental-health-a-z/?letter=P [accessed 12 December 2012].

Mishna, F. (2003) Learning disabilities and bullying: double jeopardy. *Journal of Learning Disabilities*, 36(4): 336–47.

National Autistic Society (NAS) (2006) *B is for Bullied.* London: NAS.

Shields, N., Synnot, A.J. and Barr, M. (2012) Perceived barriers and facilitators to physical activity for children with disability: a systematic review. *British Journal of Sports Medicine*, 46(14): 989–97.

Sipler, E. (2006) *The Power of Teachers in a Young Person's World: The Rationale for Teaching Personal Development in Post Primary Schools in Northern Ireland.* Belfast: CCEA.

Taggart, L., Truesdale-Kennedy, M. and Coates, V. (2012) Management and quality indicators of diabetes mellitus in people with intellectual disabilities. *Journal of Intellectual Disability Research* (DOI: 10.1111/j.1365-2788.2012.01633.x).

Vreeman, R.C. and Carroll, A.E. (2007) A systematic review of school-based interventions to prevent bullying. *Archives of Pediatric and Adolescent Medicine*, 161: 78–88.

World Health Organization (WHO) (2011) *Health Promoting Schools.* Geneva: WHO. Available at: http://www.who.int/school_youth_health/gshi/hps/en/index.html [accessed 12 October 2012].

16 Physical activity, exercise, and sport

Karen Nankervis, Wendy Cousins, Hana Válková,
and Tadhg Macintyre

Introduction

Substantial empirical evidence confirms that regular participation in physical activity contributes to health in individuals of all ages, gender, and ability. Yet numerous studies have found that people with disabilities are less likely to engage in physical activity, are more sedentary, and tend to be less fit than their peers (Temple et al. 2006). This chapter provides an overview of the evidence that sets out the value of exercise and sport participation by people with an intellectual disability and, where available, the cascading benefits for families and workers. Strategies to promote involvement in exercise and sport are addressed, with a focus on evidence-based strategies that can be incorporated into practice and undertaken in environments that promote community inclusion and experiences. Recommendations for promoting exercise and sport participation for people with intellectual disabilities are also provided.

Physical activity and exercise

The term *physical activity* is generally defined as any bodily movement produced by the skeletal muscles that results in energy expenditure (measured in kilocalories or kilojoules). Physical activity in daily life can be categorized into occupational, sports, conditioning, household, or other activities. While the terms exercise and physical activity are sometimes used interchangeably, exercise is considered a subset of physical activity defined by the fact that is planned, structured, and repetitive and has, as a final or an intermediate objective, the improvement or maintenance of physical fitness (Caspersen et al. 1985). Being physically fit has been defined as the ability to carry out daily tasks with vigour and alertness, without undue fatigue and with ample energy to enjoy leisure-time pursuits and to meet unforeseen emergencies. There are three primary components of physical fitness: cardiovascular endurance, muscular strength and endurance, and flexibility (Rimmer 2009).

Sport

Sport is physical activity that involves competition, scorekeeping, rules, and an outcome that cannot be predetermined. Sports are usually divided into several categories: individual sports, such as gymnastics; dual sports, such as tennis; and team sports, such as football. The European Sports Charter (Council of Europe 1992: Article 2) defines sport as 'all forms of physical activity, which through casual or organized participation, aim at expressing or improving physical fitness and mental well being, forming social relationships or obtaining results in competition at all levels'. This definition highlights sport as one of the domains through which people can be physically active but also points to the role of sport in promoting psychological wellbeing and increasing social capital. There is no reason to suggest that the benefits of sport are in any way less applicable to people with intellectual disabilities (Robertson and Emerson 2010). Sport for people with disabilities is not a new concept, but its full potential as a powerful means to foster greater inclusion and wellbeing is only beginning to be realized (Sport for Development and Peace International Working Group 2008).

Benefits of participation

For people with intellectual disabilities, physical activity, exercise, and sport offer opportunities to engage in experiences that provide physical, psychological, and social benefits. Regular exercise can also help prevent many health conditions prevalent in this population, including cardiovascular disease, high blood pressure, obesity, Type 2 diabetes, and mental health difficulties (Johnson 2009). Engaging in a moderate amount of physical activity will result in improved mood and emotional states. Exercise can promote psychological wellbeing as well as improve quality of life (Association for Applied Sport Psychology 2012). Participation in sports by people with disabilities can increase their sense of wellbeing by changing how they think and feel about themselves. Furthermore, it can foster inclusion by changing how communities think and feel about people with intellectual disabilities (Sport for Development and Peace International Working Group 2008). Positive effects are not limited to the individual, as benefits may also extend to families and communities by reducing isolation and increasing parental involvement (Harada et al. 2011). However, our current knowledge is mainly relevant to people with mild-to-moderate levels of intellectual disability; less is known about the benefits of physical activity for people with severe-to-profound intellectual disability, as little research has been undertaken with this cohort.

It is known that people with intellectual disabilities tend to be less active than people without disabilities and lead sedentary lifestyles that can further compromise their health. There is a large body of research that demonstrates that people with an intellectual disability do not meet guidelines for physical activity and that their levels of engagement in exercise and sport are lower than those of non-disabled people. A variety of reasons are thought to contribute to this, including lack of access, lack of information on appropriate physical activity, lack of support in the community, and the nature of their disabilities (Johnson 2009); low levels of participation have been reported where people had high to very high support needs (Darcy and Dowse 2012). Other evidence suggests that people with a disability are more likely to be excluded from sport when their disability is combined with a low income and wider social disadvantage (Sport England 2002).

The right to participate

The right to participate in exercise and sport is enshrined in the UN Convention on the Rights of People with Disabilities (2007), Article 30.5 (see Box 16.1). This is the first legally binding international instrument to address the rights of people with disabilities with regard to sport. In particular, it requires that children with disabilities be included in physical education within the school system 'to the fullest extent possible' and enjoy equal access

---

Box 16.1 The UN Convention on the Rights of Persons with Disabilities, Article 30.5

With a view to enabling persons with disabilities to participate on an equal basis with others in recreational, leisure and sporting activities, States Parties shall take appropriate measures:

(a) To encourage and promote the participation, to the fullest extent possible, of persons with disabilities in mainstream sporting activities at all levels;

(b) To ensure that persons with disabilities have an opportunity to organize, develop and participate in disability-specific sporting and recreational activities and, to this end, encourage the provision, on an equal basis with others, of appropriate instruction, training and resources;

(c) To ensure that persons with disabilities have access to sporting, recreational and tourism venues;

(d) To ensure that children with disabilities have equal access with other children to participation in play, recreation and leisure and sporting activities, including those activities in the school system;

(e) To ensure that persons with disabilities have access to services from those involved in the organization of recreational, tourism, leisure and sporting activities.

(UN 2007)

---

to play. This legislation marks another step away from the historical framing of disability as a medically defined social welfare issue and towards a rights-based approach in support of inclusion.

World Health Organization guidelines on physical activity

Physical inactivity has been identified as a leading risk factor for global mortality. The rise in levels of inactivity in many countries has major implications for the prevalence of non-communicable diseases (NCDs) and for general health across the world. To address this issue, the WHO (2010) developed global recommendations for frequency, duration, intensity, type, and total amount of physical activity needed for the maintenance of health and the prevention of NCDs. These recommendations can also be applied to people with disabilities (see Table 16.1). However, it is recognized that they may need to be adjusted for each individual based on their exercise capacity and specific health risks or limitations.

Developing exercise programmes

People with intellectual disabilities have the same essential needs as the general population in terms of improving their health and fitness. Good foundations need to be laid early in the life course and it should be assumed that children with an intellectual disability will be active participants in sports and exercise. This will help contribute to the development of positive attitudes towards physical activity throughout life (Hannon 2005).

An exercise programme should include the three common elements of cardiovascular endurance, strength, and flexibility (see Box 16.2). A physician should always approve an individual's structured fitness programme. The more strenuous the exercise programme, the greater the importance in having appropriate medical evaluation before commencing it. When developing an exercise programme for people with intellectual disabilities, it is important

Table 16.1 World Health Organization (WHO) recommendations for physical activity

Age 5–17 years	Age 18–64 years	Age 65 years and over
For children and young people of this age group, physical activity includes play, games, sports, transportation, recreation, physical education, or planned exercise, in the context of family, school, and community activities. To improve cardiorespiratory and muscular fitness, bone health, cardiovascular and metabolic health biomarkers, and reduce symptoms of anxiety and depression, the following activities are also recommended:	For adults of this age group, physical activity includes recreational or leisure-time physical activity, transportation (e.g. walking or cycling), occupational (i.e. work), household chores, play, games, sports or planned exercise, in the context of daily, family, and community activities. To improve cardiorespiratory and muscular fitness, bone health, and reduce the risk of NCDs and depression, the following are recommended:	For adults of this age group, physical activity includes recreational or leisure-time physical activity, transportation (e.g. walking or cycling), occupational (if the person is still engaged in work), household chores, play, games, sports or planned exercise, in the context of daily, family, and community activities. To improve cardiorespiratory and muscular fitness, bone and functional health, and reduce the risk of NCDs, depression, and cognitive decline, the following are recommended:
At least 60 minutes of moderate- to vigorous-intensity physical activity daily	Adults aged 18–64 years should do at least 150 minutes of moderate-intensity aerobic physical activity throughout the week, or do at least 75 minutes of vigorous-intensity aerobic physical activity throughout the week, or an equivalent combination of moderate- and vigorous-intensity activity	Adults aged 65 years and above should do at least 150 minutes of moderate-intensity aerobic physical activity throughout the week, or do at least 75 minutes of vigorous-intensity aerobic physical activity throughout the week, or an equivalent combination of moderate- and vigorous-intensity activity
Physical activity of amounts greater than 60 minutes daily will provide additional health benefits	Aerobic activity should be performed in bouts of at least 10 minutes duration	Aerobic activity should be performed in bouts of at least 10 minutes duration
Most daily physical activity should be aerobic. Vigorous-intensity activities should be incorporated, including those that strengthen muscle and bone, at least three times per week	For additional health benefits, adults should increase their moderate-intensity aerobic physical activity to 300 minutes per week, or engage in 150 minutes of vigorous-intensity aerobic physical activity per week, or an equivalent combination of moderate- and vigorous-intensity activity	For additional health benefits, adults aged 65 years and above should increase their moderate intensity aerobic physical activity to 300 minutes per week, or engage in 150 minutes of vigorous-intensity aerobic physical activity per week, or an equivalent combination of moderate- and vigorous-intensity activity. Adults of this age group with poor mobility should perform physical activity to enhance balance and prevent falls on three or more days per week
	Muscle-strengthening activities should be done involving major muscle groups on two or more days a week	Muscle-strengthening activities should be done involving major muscle groups on two or more days a week
		When Individuals cannot do the recommended amounts of physical activity due to health conditions, they should be as physically active as their abilities and conditions allow

NCDs, non-communicable diseases.

Source: Adapted from World Health Organization (WHO 2010).

Box 16.2 Stages in the development of an exercise programme

1   The intensity of the exercise should be built up gradually.
2   Various reinforcing events should be employed to increase the person's motivation to exercise.
3   The person's opinion about the exercise should be assessed by allowing them to choose between various exercise options.

(Lancioni and O'Reilly 1998)

---

to ensure that a range of physical activities are available so that the personal interests of each person can be identified and addressed in terms of that individual's support needs. There are many activities that can be used to improve fitness, including swimming, cycling, equestrian sports, dancing, and skating. Participating in competitive sports tournaments at weekends can be an enjoyable change of pace from the usual fitness routine and can be highly motivating for some individuals (Rimmer 2009).

Special Olympics

The Special Olympics has been at the forefront of developing physical activity programmes for individuals with intellectual disabilities since 1968, when the movement was formally established as an international non-profit organization, with the First International Summer Games at Soldier Field in Chicago, Illinois (see Box 16.3). Through weekly training and regular events and competitions, the Special Olympics aims to engage people with intellectual disabilities, and their families and communities, using sport as a means to transform lives. The movement provides year-round training and competitions for more than four million athletes around the world.

Sport has the capacity to change a person with a disability in a profound way. For some, participation marks their first experience of human agency, in that it enables them to make choices and to take risks on their own. For others, the acquisition of skills and accomplishments can help build the self-confidence needed to take on other life challenges such as pursuing education or employment (Sport for Development and Peace International Working Group 2008). Research studies have shown that the benefits of participating in Special Olympics include reductions in maladaptive behaviours (Weiss 2008), the development of a sense of success, skills acquisition, and increases in social competence for athletes. In addition, a longer time spent participating in the programme was also associated with more activities, hobbies, jobs, chores, clubs, and friends (Dykens and Cohen 1996). The Special Olympics has also been found to have positive benefits for the families of participants (Glidden et al. 2011) and in particular has been found to function as valued support for the mothers of competitors (Weiss 2008). On

---

Box 16.3 Special Olympics Mission Statement

The mission of Special Olympics is to provide year-round sports training and athletic competition in a variety of Olympic-type sports for children and adults with intellectual disabilities, giving them continuing opportunities to develop physical fitness, demonstrate courage, experience joy and participate in a sharing of gifts, skills and friendship with their families, other Special Olympics athletes and the community.

(Special Olympics 2010: para. 1)

a wider stage, the Special Olympics serves as an engine of change to provide opportunities for individuals with intellectual disabilities to become more visible in society (Harada et al. 2011). The Unified Sports® initiative combines players with intellectual disabilities with non-disabled partners in the same sports teams for training and competition. Alongside the development of sporting skills, this programme promotes social inclusion by offering athletes a platform to socialize with peers and to take part in the life of their community (McConkey et al. 2012).

However, despite the well-documented benefits of participation in Special Olympics, the frequency, duration, and intensity of the programme does not, itself, provide enough physical activity to affect physical fitness levels (Marks et al. 2005). To address this issue, a wider set of programmes needs to be developed for this population that involve exercise and physical activity; targeted interventions to increase levels of sports participation by people with intellectual disabilities are required (Robertson and Emerson 2010).

Strategies for promoting physical activity and participation in exercise and sport

The importance of sport and physical activity needs to be recognized, and their importance underlined by strategic action at national, regional, and local level (Hannon 2005). Policy development is critical. As a minimum standard, equitable access to facilities is essential. However, for people with an intellectual disability, physical access alone may not be enough for them to engage in activities. They will require support from professional staff and carers, who should be informed and aware of the importance of physical activity for this population.

The staff of health clubs and sporting organizations in the wider community need to know that people with an intellectual disability have the right and need to actively participate in sports and exercise. Access to facilities should be socially enabled and trainers should have patience with those who take longer to learn, as well as the skills to modify and adapt programmes to suit the personal needs of people with intellectual disabilities. A qualitative study found that parents who sought inclusive sport involvement for their children soon gave up their effort if they felt rejected by staff and other participants; however, staff with positive inclusion attitudes and abilities could lead to more successful outcomes (Tsai and Fung 2009). The successful inclusion of people with intellectual disabilities in community-based physical activities should be a planned, regular activity along with targeted strategies to address the skills and attitudes of the community members in that environment. The attitude of carers has been found to be a significant predictor of intention to support physical activity, highlighting the need for carer interventions that emphasize the benefits of physical activity for people with intellectual disabilities (Martin et al. 2011). It will be difficult to change the physical activity patterns of people with intellectual disabilities if staff or family members are not proactive in encouraging participation. A strong need exists to provide education about the process of engaging people with intellectual disability in physical activity (Temple and Walkley 2007). Finding creative ways to keep people exercising beyond a few weeks or months can be challenging, although there are many ways to encourage lifestyle changes in people with developmental disabilities using behavioural strategies. Examples of some potentially useful strategies are outlined in Box 16.4.

Box 16.4 Some strategies for encouraging people with intellectual disabilities to exercise

- Develop a reward system that reinforces small accomplishments in the exercise programme. Completing one month of exercise without missing a session, or trying a new activity, should be rewarded.
- Offer a 'buddy' system that will allow the person to exercise with a friend or another person they enjoy being around.

- Keep records of performance. It is critical to know how much and how often the person is exercising. Plan a reward when a targeted goal is achieved.
- In group homes or other congregate care settings, keep wall charts to record progress. Many people with intellectual disabilities will enjoy seeing their names on the board and following their progress as they increase their physical activity levels. A wall chart may show a photo of the person exercising with blank boxes next to his or her name. Upon completion of the exercise session, the person places a checkmark √ in the box. Some people may enjoy keeping track of how many boxes are filled with checkmarks.
- When developing a reinforcement system, try to stay away from high fat food items. For example, substitute a Friday night pizza outing with bowling or a trip to see a movie.

(Adapted from Rimmer 2009)

Conclusion

Participation in sport and physical activity leads to improved levels of physical health and psychological wellbeing, and is therefore a key aspect of health promotion for everyone. People with intellectual disabilities have lower rates of participation than the general population and face barriers to becoming more involved. A key challenge for policy makers, professionals, and carers is to encourage and promote their participation to the fullest extent possible through the development of public policy, the creation of supportive environments, and the growth of personal skills.

Summary

- Active participation in sport, exercise, and other physical activities is critical to the health and wellbeing of people with intellectual disabilities as well as providing benefits to their carers. As such, physical activity needs to be a routine part of each individual's daily life.
- The right to participate in exercise and sport is enshrined in the UN Convention on the Rights of People with Disabilities (2007).
- The WHO (2010) has developed global recommendations on physical activity necessary for the maintenance of health. These recommendations can also be applied to people with disabilities and adjusted for each individual based on their exercise capacity and specific health risks or limitations.
- An exercise programme should include elements of cardiovascular endurance, strength, and flexibility, and should be approved by the person's physician. Making a range of physical activities available allows for the development and encouragement of personal interests.
- Professional staff and carers should be informed and aware of the importance of physical activity for people with intellectual disabilities and use behavioural strategies to encourage and reinforce participation.

Web resources

- International Federation of Adapted Physical Activity: http://www.ifapa.biz/
- National Center on Health, Physical Activity, and Disability (NCHPAD): http://www.ncpad.org/Aboutus

- P.E. Central – Adapted physical activity: http://www.pecentral.org/adapted/adaptedmenu. html
- Special Olympics resources: http://resources.specialolympics.org/ResourcesDefault.aspx
- UK Sports Association for people with learning disability: http://www.uksportsassociation. org/

References

Association for Applied Sport Psychology (2012) *Psychological Benefits of Exercise.* Available at: https://www. appliedsportpsych.org/Resource-Center/health-and-fitness/articles/psych-benefits-of-exercise [accessed 20 January 2013].

Caspersen, C.J., Powell, K.E. and Christenson, G.M. (1985) Physical activity, exercise and physical fitness: definitions and distinctions for health-related research. *Public Health Reports*, 100(2): 126–31.

Council of Europe (1992) *The European Sports Charter.* Available at: http://www.coe.int/t/dg4/epas/resources/ charter_en.asp [accessed 20 January 2013].

Darcy, S. and Dowse, L. (2012) In search of a level playing field? The constraints and benefits of sport participation for people with intellectual disability. *Disability and Society*, 28(3): 393–407.

Dykens, E.M. and Cohen, D.J. (1996) Effects of Special Olympics International on social competence in persons with mental retardation. *Journal of the American Academy of Child and Adolescent Psychiatry*, 35: 223–9.

Glidden, L.M., Bamberger, K.T., Draheim, R. and Kersh, J. (2011) Parent and athlete perceptions of Special Olympics participation: utility and danger of proxy responding. *Intellectual and Developmental Disabilities*, 49(1): 37–45.

Hannon, F. (2005) *Promoting the Participation of People with Disabilities in Physical Activity and Sport in Ireland.* Dublin: National Disability Authority.

Harada, C.M., Siperstein, G.N., Parker, R.C. and Lenox, D (2011) Promoting social inclusion for people with intellectual disabilities through sport: Special Olympics International, global sport initiatives and strategies. *Sport in Society*, 14(9): 1131–49.

Johnson, C. (2009) The benefits of physical activity for youth with developmental disabilities: a systematic review. *American Journal of Health Promotion*, 23(3): 157–67.

Lancioni, G.E. and O'Reilly, M.F. (1998) A review of research on physical exercise with people with severe and profound developmental disabilities. *Research in Developmental Disabilities*, 19: 477–92.

Marks, B., Heller, T., Sisirak, J., Hsieh, K. and Pastorfield, C. (2005) *Health Promotion Pilot Programmes Evaluation: Improving Athletes' Health*, Final Report. Washington, DC: Special Olympics International.

Martin, E., McKenzie, K., Newman, E., Bowden, K. and Morris, P.G. (2011) Care staff intentions to support adults with an intellectual disability to engage in physical activity: an application of the Theory of Planned Behavior. *Research in Developmental Disabilities*, 32(2): 2535–41.

McConkey, R., Dowling, S., Hassan, D. and Menke, S. (2012) Promoting social inclusion through Unified Sports for youth with intellectual disabilities: a five-nation study. *Journal of Intellectual Disability Research* (DOI: 10.1111/j.1365-2788.2012.01587.x).

Rimmer, J.H. (2009) *Developmental Disability and Fitness.* Available at: http://www.ncpad.org/104/795/Devel opmental~Disability~and~Fitness [accessed 20 January 2013].

Robertson, J. and Emerson, E. (2010) Participation in sports by people with intellectual disabilities in England. *Journal of Applied Research in Intellectual Disabilities*, 23: 616–22.

Special Olympics (2010) *Mission Statement.* Available at: http://www.specialolympics.org/mission.aspx [accessed 19 May 2013].

Sport England (2002) *Adults with a Disability and Sport National Survey 2000–2001: Headline Findings.* London: Sport England.

Sport for Development and Peace International Working Group (2008) *Harnessing the Power of Sport for Development and Peace: Recommendations to Governments.* Toronto: Right to Play. Available at: http:// www.righttoplay.com/uk/news-and-media/Pages/HarnessingthePowerofSports.aspx [accessed 22 June 2013].

Temple, V.A. and Walkley, J.W. (2007) Perspectives of constraining and enabling factors for health-promoting physical activity by adults with intellectual disability. *Journal of Intellectual and Developmental Disability*, 32(1): 28–38.

Temple, V.A., Frey, G.C. and Stanish, H.I. (2006) Physical activity of adults with mental retardation: review and research needs. *American Journal of Health Promotion*, 21: 2–12.

Tsai, E.H.L. and Fung, L. (2009) Parents' experiences and decisions on inclusive sport participation of their children with intellectual disabilities. *Adapted Physical Activity Quarterly*, 26(2): 151–71.

United Nations (2007) *The United Nations Convention on the Rights of Persons with Disabilities.* Available at: http://www.un.org/disabilities/default.asp?id=150 [accessed 20 January 2013].

Weiss, J.A. (2008) The role of Special Olympics for mothers of adult athletes with intellectual disability. *American Journal on Mental Retardation*, 113(4): 241–53.

World Health Organization (WHO) (2010) *Global Recommendations on Physical Activity for Health*. Geneva: WHO. Available at: http://whqlibdoc.who.int/publications/2010/9789241599979_eng.pdf [accessed 20 January 2013].

The role of healthcare professionals

Robert Davis and Nick Lennox

Introduction

Health promotional activities are not dependent on contact with healthcare professionals; nevertheless, we need to consider the role of these professionals. While much of the health promotional activity directed at the person with intellectual disability is initiated through the social supports around them (their family and support staff), health professionals have key roles within this process. This role may vary depending on the setting of the interaction and on the particular responsibilities of the individual health professional. The health professional may act as an educator, an advocate, a facilitator, a monitor, a behavioural re-enforcer and coordinator. Effective health services require a collaborative approach between healthcare professionals and those that support people with intellectual disabilities throughout their lifespan. It is important that the person with intellectual disabilities remains central to the process.

International context of healthcare delivery

The delivery of health care for the non-disabled population will vary from country to country and even state to state. Healthcare outcomes do not necessarily improve with the amount of money spent on health services. Access to health care varies from predominantly private health services, where the user pays, through to services where there is universal access to health services. There is a varying emphasis on delivery of acute healthcare services, primary health services, preventative health care, and health promotion. Factors that impact on this emphasis within these constituencies include health legislation, cultural expectations, socio-economic status, and political philosophies. Within these health services, healthcare delivery may vary for the intellectually disabled population, with some countries having specialized services, others relying on access through the generic services and some with a mix of both approaches. In most situations, it has been expected that the generic services would pick up the skill set and provide services for this population. However, there has often been very little exposure to intellectual disabilities within undergraduate programmes and health professionals have indicated a need for training and specialized supports.

Services within the UK evolved from pre-existing services that supported people with intellectual disabilities living within institutions. Policy makers decided that with the devolution of the institutions during the 1980s, they would maintain the existing health support infrastructure. This included psychiatrists with a special interest in the health of people with intellectual disabilities and a range of supports including nurses with specific training in intellectual disabilities, psychologists, and allied health professionals. People with intellectual disabilities continue to have access to community-based nurses with specialized skills in intellectual disability. The

2001 White Paper *Valuing People* in the UK (Department of Health 2001) indicated a range of unmet needs and advocated the need to deliver flexible quality services with additional support when necessary. The regional health authorities across the UK are funded to provide health services for people with intellectual disabilities in their region and have the flexibility to respond to identified health needs.

In the Netherlands, at the time of de-institutionalization in the 1990s, physicians working within the institutions had already developed specialized skills and had a training programme in place with over 130 doctors with specialized skills. This group went on to develop a formalized specialty training programme and continued to support primary healthcare physicians with specialized care supported by nurses and allied health professionals with specialized skills. There is a specific tax in the Netherlands that supports funding for health and other services for people with disabilities.

In the USA, services vary from state to state. Some services are closely integrated with university centres and research institutes that provide high-quality integrated healthcare management. In other states, services have evolved from institution-based care with a mix of more specialized service providers and support from local generic services. The Developmental Disability Nurses Association has developed a postgraduate qualification entitled 'The Certificate of Developmental Disability'. There is a wide variation in access and in the quality of care varying from 'state of the art' to minimal access to services.

Within Canada and Australia, the bulk of health care is community based within the generic services with some states having access to more specialized referral centres to support GPs and psychiatrists. In Australia, there used to be undergraduate nursing programmes that specialized in intellectual disabilities; however, these were devolved years ago. The numbers of nurses familiar with the health issues of people with intellectual disabilities are diminishing. Some nurses with specialized skills have remained in the field and there are limited numbers coming through a few postgraduate programmes. Currently, there is limited access to skilled nurses who mainly support individuals with complex physical health problems. Services in New Zealand are similar to those in Australia but also have some of the features of those in the UK, with regional health authorities directing local health services. In all these countries, direct support staff have little or no training in health issues for people with intellectual disabilities.

The role of health promotion in mainstream health promotion

While individual healthcare providers, health professionals, and organizations indicate that they have roles and even a stakehold in improving public health through health promotion, outcomes are dependent on how effective they are at working together. Health promotion within the non-disabled population draws on a wide range of professionals that includes doctors, nurses, teachers, dieticians, psychotherapists, health visitors, dental health workers, dentists, exercise physiologists and fitness trainers, social workers, and mental health professionals. Health promotion involves developing a socio-economic environment that best supports good health outcomes for the population, and as such is not the sole responsibility of any one professional group or even the health sector.

Effective health promotion requires a comprehensive team approach by different healthcare professionals. Health professionals as health promoters have to work within many other disciplines: 'No single profession has a monopoly of health promotion wisdom or is equipped to perform all the necessary tasks' (Kemm and Close 1995: 15). The differing skill sets and perspectives help inform each health professional as well as those who are the target of the health promotional activity. Successful collaboration requires a mutual respect for other members of the team, an understanding of each other's roles, values, responsibilities, and ways of working.

Within the non-disabled population, the major areas targeted by health promotion activities include:

- tobacco consumption
- healthy diets
- obesity
- physical activity and exercise
- domestic violence
- alcohol avoidance
- sun exposure
- cancer screening and prevention
- road safety
- safe sex.

In all these areas, health professionals working in clinical settings have roles in identifying those at risk, informing individuals of their risk and the implications of continuing exposure to that risk, advising on risk reduction programmes, and ongoing monitoring and support. This may involve obtaining further information, including their family history, and extending the examination to include further tests. This actively engages the patient in the process and provides greater incentive for adjustment in their behaviour. The health professional is often in a position of trust and can be an effective agent for change. For instance, smoking cessation is far more successful when counselling and medication is followed up with a planned review. These follow-up reviews provide a means to acknowledge achievements of the individual and encourage continued participation.

In a number of these areas there is a need for a multi-disciplinary approach. Obesity may involve a dietician, physician, and perhaps a diabetes educator. In this situation, it is important that the health promotional message is consistent and that communication between the professionals and between the patient and professional is maintained. Changes in physical activity may involve options that do not include healthcare professionals but the person's health might impact on their ability to participate. Changes in packaging laws for cigarettes, bans on advertising, and the introduction of bans on smoking in shared spaces have come about by determined campaigns initiated by health professionals.

Healthcare professionals have advocacy roles within the community at large. It is important that research provides an evidence base for advice on health promotion. This research should not only inform the form and content of the particular recommendation or health promotional activity but should also investigate the response to advice: whether there was a change in behaviour or the level of health promotional activity and the eventual health outcome for the person and the population.

Translating mainstream health promotion for people with intellectual disabilities

Although, to a large extent, health professionals have similar roles and responsibilities, in the field of health promotion for people with intellectual disabilities there are some fundamental differences in the way these areas are translated. People with intellectual disabilities may have problems understanding and accessing the range of health promotional literacy and messages directed at the non-disabled population through the media. This might be due to language difficulties or difficulties in understanding what appears an abstract concept. For example, people with intellectual disabilities who see people smoking around them find it hard to understand that smoking is a health hazard. The message may need to be more direct or linked to a desired health outcome, such as helping with a cough or doing better at a sport. Group activities directed at day programmes may be another way of improving the understanding of the risk.

A range of health promotional materials have been developed for people with intellectual disabilities on a number of topics including depression, breast examination, diet, exercise, cervical smears, safe sex, and healthy diets (see www.easyhealth.org.uk). These are available to people with intellectual disabilities and their carers through the Internet. Some have been reviewed by healthcare professionals and provide a valuable resource to support people with intellectual disabilities.

Health promotion over a lifetime

Health promotion is important throughout life, particularly at times of transition. While the type of health professionals may vary with the particular transition, they will often play key roles at these times. Initially, there is a need for the paediatrician and nursing staff to counsel and support parents at the diagnosis of the intellectual disability. At that stage, parents want to know of any immediate health concerns including preventative health measures. They will also want access to information and other resources throughout this early phase. Support will be needed through the early intervention programme from allied health professionals, including speech pathologists, physiotherapists, and psychologists. Health issues through childhood may include the need for specific immunization, diet and exercise, management and identification of mobility issues, epilepsy, vision and hearing problems.

Transition into adulthood brings with it a new set of issues including the need for education on human relations, pregnancy, and sexually transmitted disease as well as education on smoking, and regular cervical smears and mammograms. Transition into old age brings about another set of health issues. There is a need to identify cardiac risk factors, for example cholesterol, high blood sugars, and obesity. Carers and people with intellectual disabilities need to be aware of issues such as dementia, and the higher risks of stomach and gall bladder cancers.

Healthcare professionals' knowledge of the health of people with intellectual disabilities

The knowledge of professionals about the health of people with intellectual disabilities will vary across constituencies. As previously stated, the UK and the Netherlands have dedicated specialized health services that have direct contact with people with intellectual disabilities, which can provide support to health professionals supporting people with intellectual disabilities. However, most people with intellectual disabilities will access services through the primary healthcare system. It is therefore important that our knowledge of the common problems faced by people with intellectual disabilities in general (van Schrojenstein Lantman-de Valk et al. 1997; Ouellette-Kuntz et al. 2005; van Schrojenstein Lantman-de Valk and Walsh 2008), and those specific to the more common aetiologies, are incorporated into undergraduate training of health professionals who are likely to come in contact with them.

Surveys of GPs in Australia showed that, while GPs were willing to provide care for this group, they recognized that there was a lack in their undergraduate training (Phillips et al. 2004). Research in Australia, Scotland, and Wales has shown that regular health checks or assessments have been able to identify important health problems in this population (Jones and Kerr 1997; Cooper et al. 2006; Lennox et al. 2006). Many of these would best be dealt with by systematic health promotion that targets people with disability and their family and formal carers. Some health promotional activities will target problems that are specific to this population. Health problems identified within the IASSID Health targets (see Web Resources) that warrant attention through health promotion activity include constipation, epilepsy, vision and hearing problems, safe use of medications, mental health, obesity, under-nutrition, swallowing difficulties, respiratory disease, and dental problems. The health professionals involved in health promotion will vary depending on a range of factors.

Constipation

Constipation is an important and often life-long health problem for people with intellectual disabilities that can impact on continence, behaviour, and indeed the level of independence of an individual. This problem is best identified in childhood with the support of parents in diet management and the development of good toileting habits. This awareness and support will need to continue through adult life with paid carers and accommodation services supporting the diet and reinforcing good bowel habits. Health professionals that may have contact with the person and their carers over this time include a paediatrician, practice nurse, dietician, GP, continence nurse, occupational therapist, and gastroenterologist.

Epilepsy

Epilepsy may involve a neurologist, an occupational therapist, a specialized nurse counsellor, a GP, and a pharmacist in its management. Managing the epilepsy is not just about the right medication and treatment, but involves education of the patient and carers in recognizing the need to avoid situations that might unnecessarily put the person at risk. For example, avoiding behaviours such as missing sleep or watching television for too long that might trigger a seizure, recognizing the prodromal features of a seizure, keeping a record of seizures, and ensuring that those supporting the person with a seizure are aware of the immediate management for seizures. This education needs to target not only the person with direct responsibility for the epileptic individual, but those involved with services that support this population.

Respiratory disease

Respiratory disease in people with intellectual disabilities significantly contributes to their higher mortality under the age of 45 years (Haveman 2004). It is therefore important that they and their carers ensure that their vaccinations for influenza and pneumococcus are current. This may be the responsibility of the primary healthcare physician or the practice nurse. Those particularly at risk are the frailer individuals with cerebral palsy and patients with Down syndrome. While living in supported settings, people with intellectual disabilities may be required to have regular health checks. However, those living with their parents or living in the community may need to be proactively encouraged to ensure their immunization status is up to date. A particular group at risk are those with a history of aspiration and past chest infections. Staff members who support people with intellectual disabilities need to be aware that those who have any problems with coughing and spluttering during meals need to be reviewed and that this might involve a speech therapist and a dietician.

Dental problems

People with intellectual disabilities are at particular risk of dental disease. They will also tend to present late for these problems. Health promotion and preventive health care play an important role in managing dental problems in the wider community. People with intellectual disabilities may have problems in cooperating for simple dental examinations and in organizing themselves for regular reviews. Familiarity with a dentist and dental therapist makes this a lot easier for all concerned. An active promotion of dental health throughout the person's life starting in childhood and continuing on through adulthood is important. People with intellectual disabilities and their carers need to be aware of the need for good dental hygiene. Regular brushing, appropriate diet, and regular dental health checks are a part of this management. This needs to be integrated into their support programme.

Visual impairment

There is a high prevalence of visual impairment in people with intellectual disabilities (Evenhuis et al. 2001), which increases with age. Visual impairment is often undiagnosed, as it is difficult to carry out the standard tests of visual acuity in this population. However, significant visual impairment can impact on the person's quality of life. While the use of spectacles may not be tolerated, the awareness of the problem may make it necessary to adjust the person's physical environment. This may involve the removal of clutter in the person's living space or better defining doorways with darker or contrasting colours. Again health promotion needs to make those around people with intellectual disabilities aware that this is a potential problem and encourage regular review. Health professionals involved in this process may include the GP, the optometrist, the ophthalmologist, and the occupational therapist.

Hearing problems

Hearing problems are more prevalent in people with intellectual disabilities, which again increase with age. Regular audiometry and examination of the ears is recommended. This can be incorporated into a regular health check up but those patients who are not regularly checked, and their carers, need to be made aware of the potential problem and advised as to the most appropriate review. Health professionals involved include audiologists, GPs, and ear, nose and throat (ENT) specialists.

Under-nutrition and swallowing difficulties

Under-nutrition and swallowing difficulties can be major health issues for a small but significant number of people with intellectual disabilities, and may become of particular concern when the individual who is already compromised loses more weight. Regular weighing and close scrutiny of the diet are therefore important components of these people's management plan. Those supporting them need to be aware of their vulnerability and the need to keep a close eye on their weight. Regular weight assessment of all people with intellectual disabilities in supported accommodation and review of those where there is significant weight loss have been used as preventative health measures in some jurisdictions. Should there be a significant weight reduction, health practitioners may be required to intervene. Health professionals involved may be the GP, dietician, speech pathologist, gastroenterologist, and ENT surgeon.

Safe use of medication

Due to high rates of psychiatric disorders, epilepsy, and difficulties with behaviour management, many people with intellectual disabilities are prescribed psychoactive medications that have significant side-effect profiles. The cognitive and communication problems in this group mean that, without a proactive review, side-effects may not be picked up until relatively late. Carers and people with intellectual disabilities therefore need to be aware of potential problems and the need for regular review. This can include access to information on the medication the person is taking. People involved may include the GP, the pharmacist, the neurologist, and psychiatrist.

Obesity

Obesity and the range of health problems associated with it, such as diabetes, has become a major problem in the general population. People with intellectual disabilities have been shown to have higher rates of obesity. Within Australia, this seems be a problem among those in the mild range of intellectual disabilities who live independently or with their parents. The other group of people at risk of obesity are those taking psychotropic medications that are associated with weight gain. This underscores the need to set up health promotion activities that are accessible to this group. Access to cheap high calorie food sources and lack of affordable health alternatives has been part of the problem. Regular review of weight combined with information on healthy diet alternatives is one means of making this population, and those that support them, aware of the most appropriate management. Health professionals that might contribute to this process include dieticians, GPs, diabetes educators, exercise physiologists, and pharmacists.

Aetiologically specific risks

Some of the underlying aetiologies for intellectual disability carry with them increased risks of a range of health problems. Table 17.1 documents some of these problems. Knowledge of the increase in risk allows for preventative strategies to be put in place and for earlier diagnosis and treatment. While the increase in risk in more common conditions is well documented, it is good practice to anticipate the aetiologically specific health problems and provide people with intellectual disabilities, parents, staff, and carers with background information. The classic example of how the aetiology of a disability has an impact on important preventive health and health promotional issues is Prader-Willi syndrome. Lifestyle factors are extremely important in Prader-Willi syndrome where the food-seeking behaviour associated with this condition can lead to gross obesity and a range of complications, including diabetes and sleep apnoea. It is therefore extremely important that parents and carers actively encourage a healthy diet, restrict and monitor access to food, and regularly review weight. It is also important that other people within the person's life are aware that access to food may need to be restricted. Parents will often need support and regular reviews with health professionals, including the paediatrician, dietician, and community nurse.

Table 17.1 Health promotion and aetiological groups

Aetiology	Health issues	Health promotional activity
Down syndrome	Dementia	Awareness of onset with ageing
	Hypothyroidism	Need for yearly blood test
	Atlanto-axial instability	Need to review if at risk (gymnastics)
	Respiratory infections	Pneumococcal and influenza vaccine
Cornelia de Lange syndrome	Oesophageal reflux	Common problem, need for endoscopy, may result in escalation of self-injury
Tuberous sclerosis	Malignant tumours	Need for regular health check; review if change in epilepsy or behaviour
Cerebral palsy	Osteoporosis	Encourage exercise, sun exposure, vitamin D supplements
	Oesophagitis	Monitor and look for symptoms, pain at night, night-time waking
	Respiratory infections	Posture, monitor aspiration, pneumococcal and influenza vaccine
Fragile X syndrome	Attention-deficit hyperactivity disorder	Identify and support with medication and behavioural strategies
Rett sydrome	Scollosis	Review by orthopaedic surgeon
	Osteopenia/osteoporosis	Maintain mobility, promote exercise

Health checks in people with intellectual disability

There is growing evidence to show that regular health checks or assessments, or screening based on the health vulnerabilities of people with intellectual disabilities are effective in identifying health problems (Jones and Kerr 1997; Cooper et al. 2006; Lennox et al. 2006). It has been shown that annual checks on average reveal one previously unidentified health problem per patient. The health screen is also a way of ensuring that regular health promotional activity takes place. Review of weight, diet, and exercise with carers is an opportunity to review the individual's current health status and to promote and facilitate activities that bring about a healthier lifestyle. The individual's immunization record needs to be reviewed and updated. Health checks can include a number of pathology tests such as blood lipids, cholesterol, fasting glucose, thyroid screens, *Helicobacter* antibodies, vitamin D, folate, and vitamin B12. It is also important to screen for vision and hearing impairment and mental health disorders. Table 17.2 links the health issues identified at a health check with the type of health professional involved in managing that problem.

Table 17.2 Health screens and health promotional activity

Health check: frequency	Health professionals involved	Health promotional activity
Blood pressure and dyslipidaemia: yearly	GP, practice nurse	Healthy diet, regular checks, target those with family history of cardiac disease and obesity
Oral health: 6 monthly	Dentist, dental nurse, dental hygienist, general practitioner (GP)	Training in brushing techniques, regular brushing, diet
Hearing/audiology: 3–5 yearly	GP, audiologist, ear, nose and throat (ENT) specialist	Awareness of people with intellectual disabilities, staff, and carers
Vision/acuity: 3–5 yearly	GP, optometrist, ophthalmologist	Awareness of people with intellectual disabilities, staff, and carers
Medication review: 6 monthly	GP, psychiatrist, neurologist, pharmacist	Awareness efficacy and side-effects
Thyroid screen: yearly	GP, practice nurse	Promote awareness, particularly in Down syndrome
Diabetes: yearly fasting blood glucose	GP, practice nurse, endocrinologist, diabetes educator, dietician	Need for health check, diet and weight monitoring, education about diabetes
Lifestyle factors: yearly review including weight	GP, community nurse, dietician, exercise physiologist, occupational therapist	Status of smoking and nutrition; promotion of exercise and healthy diet
Women's health: breast exam and mammogram	GP, radiographer, radiologist, community nurse, breast surgeon	Breast exam (frequency), teach self-examination and awareness, follow up if family history, examination by carers, educate about mammography
Men's health Prostate: PSA of questionable value Testicular exam: yearly	GP, practice nurse, community nurse, urologist	Awareness of high frequency in older men, symptoms, promote importance of lumps in testicles, follow up if family history
Epilepsy	GP, neurologist, community nurse, occupational therapist, epilepsy educator	Risks of epilepsy, environmental management, adverse effects of medication, monitoring
Mental health: yearly	GP, psychiatrist, mental health nurse, psychologist, behaviourist	Awareness of staff, behaviour change or secondary sign, manage stress within environment

PSA, prostate-specific antigen.

Table 17.3 Example of person-centred care plan that includes health promotion activities: person with intellectual disability and Lennox Gastaux syndrome (epilepsy)

Goals – changes to be achieved	Required treatments and services, including patient actions	Person/services responsible: who and when*
Patient and carers have clear understanding of epilepsy risks and person's role in management	Personnel education Ensure understands need for regular sleep and avoidance of potential triggers to epilepsy, such as TV	GP and practice nurse: 3 monthly Neurologist: 6-monthly Counsellor, epilepsy support organization: as required
Optimal medication management	Ensure person understands correct use of medications Home medicine review, education on adverse effects Organize medication packaging	GP: 3-monthly Pharmacist: monthly
Have epilepsy management plan in place to respond to seizures	Draw up epilepsy management plan, ensure staff aware and trained in necessary procedures e.g. rolling over, use of intra-nasal midazolam for seizures	GP initiate and review: yearly Neurologist review: yearly Service coordinator review: yearly
Safety from falls and accidents	Ensure a safe physical environment and that activities do not put person at risk	GP: initiate and yearly review Occupational therapist: initiate and yearly review
Maintain healthy diet and optimum weight range	Maintain healthy nutrition and weight control	GP and dietician: 3 monthly Health educator for support services
Maintain optimal physical activity and access to community	Development of exercise programme suitable to needs of patient; may need to adjust to gait or to the risk of falls	GP: initiate and review yearly Exercise physiologist: ongoing Occupational therapist; social worker; counsellor, epilepsy support organization: as required

*Contact details could be included. GP, general practitioner.

Integrating health promotion into each person's person-centred plan

This population is more reliant than the general population on those around them to have access to health promotional material and to respond to this. As such, it is important to have a framework that establishes: the important goals to maintain good health outcomes; the required treatment and services, including the patient's actions; who is responsible; and how and when outcomes are reviewed. This healthcare plan incorporates team care arrangements and can be initiated by the primary care health practitioner or be a part of the support services for the individual, for example incorporated into an individual's person-centred plan by the service provider. Table 17.3 is an example of a person-centred plan that has within it a number of health promotional activities directed at the person with intellectual disability.

Summary

- Health professionals play a number of key roles in health promotion. Their roles will vary depending on their specific profession, the health system in which they work, and the timing of, and the reason for, the interaction with the person with intellectual disabilities and their carers.

- Most of the high-priority health problems requiring health promotional activities are the same as those for the general population; however, the health promotional activity may need to be modified in its content for its target audience if it is to impact people with intellectual disabilities.
- Health professionals are in a position to identify individuals who need access to this activity, the timing and type of health promotional activity they need, and where they will find the resources.
- Advances have been made in the screening of people with intellectual disabilities and identifying specific health problems. When this is linked to a person-centred plan, there is scope to include health promotion as part of that plan.
- There are a range of appropriate resources available to people with intellectual disabilities and their carers, which are detailed throughout this book, that focus upon health education/literacy, health promotion initiatives, and health screening opportunities.

Web resources

- *Health Guidelines for Adults with an Intellectual Disability*, IASSID: www.iassid.org/pdf/healthguidelines-2002.pdf

- Going to the doctor: http://www.easyhealth.org.uk/listing/doctors-(leaflets)

- Information for supporting a person with intellectual disabilities to go into hospital: http://www.easyhealth.org.uk/listing/hospital-(leaflets)

- Accessing physiotherapy: http://www.easyhealth.org.uk/sites/default/files/physiotherapy.pdf

- Accessing an occupational therapist: http://www.easyhealth.org.uk/sites/default/files/occupational_therapy.pdf

- What to do in an emergency: http://www.easyhealth.org.uk/listing/what-to-do-in-an-emergency-(leaflets)

- Going for an X-ray or scan: http://www.easyhealth.org.uk/categories/x-rays-and-scans-(leaflets)

References

Cooper, S.A., Morrison, J., Melville, C., Finlayson, J., Allan, L., Martin, G. et al. (2006) Improving the health of people with intellectual disabilities: outcomes of a health screening programme after 1 year. *Journal of Intellectual Disability Research*, 50(9): 667–77.

Department of Health (2001) *Valuing People: A New Strategy for Learning Disability for the 21st Century – A White Paper*. London: The Stationery Office.

Evenhuis, H., Theunissen, M., Denkers, I., Verschuure, H. and Kemme, H. (2001) Prevalence of visual and hearing impairment in a Dutch institutionalized population with intellectual disability. *Journal of Intellectual Disability Research*, 45(5): 457–64.

Haveman, M. (2004) Disease epidemiology and aging people with intellectual disabilities. *Journal of Policy and Practice in Intellectual Disabilities*, 1(1): 16–23.

Jones, R.G. and Kerr, M.P. (1997) A randomized control trial of an opportunistic health screening tool in primary care for people with intellectual disability. *Journal of Intellectual Disability Research*, 41(5): 409–15.

Kemm, J. and Close, A. (1995) *Health Promotion: Theory and Practice*. Basingstoke: Macmillan.

Lennox, N., Rey-Conde, T. and Cooling, N. (2006) Comprehensive health assessments during de-institutionalization: an observational study. *Journal of Intellectual Disability Research*, 50(10): 719–24.

Ouellette-Kuntz, H., Garcin, N., Lewis, M.E., Minnes, P., Martin, C. and Holden, J.J. (2005) Addressing health disparities through promoting equity for individuals with intellectual disability. *Canadian Journal of Public Health*, 96(suppl. 2): S8–S22.

Phillips, A., Morrison, J. and Davis, R.W. (2004) General practitioners' educational needs in intellectual disability health. *Journal of Intellectual Disability Research*, 48(2): 142–9.

Van Schrojenstein Lantman-de Valk, H. and Walsh, P.N. (2008) Managing health problems in persons with intellectual disabilities. *British Medical Journal*, 337: a2507.

Van Schrojenstein Lantman-de Valk, H.M.J., van den Akker, M., Maaskant, M.A., Haveman, M.J., Urlings, H.F.J., Kessels, A.G.H. et al. (1997) Prevalence and incidence of health problems in people with intellectual disability. *Journal of Intellectual Disability Research*, 41(1): 42–51.

18 Health checks

Nick Lennox and Janet Robertson

Introduction

The poor health of people with intellectual disability has been well documented across the developed world. People with intellectual disability have poorer health than their non-disabled peers and their health inequities are, to a significant extent, avoidable (Ouellette-Kuntz et al. 2005; Krahn et al. 2006; Emerson et al. 2009; Emerson and Baines 2010). The poorer health of people with intellectual disabilities is partly due to barriers to identifying the need for health care and accessing timely services (Mencap 2007; Michael and Richardson 2008). When medical clinicians review people with intellectual disability, they often find unrecognized or poorly managed medical conditions and uptake of health screening that is substantially less than that among the non-disabled population (Beange et al. 1995; Khan et al. 2012). The urgent need for effective action to identify and better manage health conditions is best exemplified by the early mortality among this population. Australian record linkage data have demonstrated that people with severe intellectual disability die up to 20 years younger than the non-disabled population (Bittles et al. 2002). Data from England for 2004 to 2008 found that people with intellectual disability died 15 years younger than people without intellectual disability (Glover and Ayub 2010). When mortality is examined in detail, it is common for previously unrecognized conditions to explain the preventable death of the person (New South Wales Community Services Commission 2001). The implementation of health checks has been recommended internationally as a key component of health policy responses needed to improve the health of people with intellectual disability (Santos et al. 2002).

History of health checks

Health checks or assessments originated in the early twentieth century in the USA, when Dr. E.L. Fisk convinced life insurance companies that the screening of yearly insurance applications would prolong life and increase actuarial savings (Reith 1989). The 'annual check-up' became common practice in North America; however, by the 1990s it was established that there was little evidence to support their implementation and they were not recommended (Katz 1996).

In the UK, interest in geriatric health screening began in the 1950s with numerous surveys of hospital and general practice populations that identified undisclosed morbidity (van Haastregt et al. 2000). In 1990, the UK NHS introduced contracts for GPs that required all patients aged over 75 years to be offered a general assessment and home visit at least once a year. Most meta-analyses and systematic reviews suggest benefits arise from this process (van Haastregt et al. 2000; Elkan et al. 2001; Stuck et al. 2002). Emerging from geriatric health screening were the first studies involving elderly people with intellectual disability (Gunsett et al. 1989; Carlsen et al. 1994). These early descriptive studies suggested benefits for elderly people with intellectual disability and resulted in further and more rigorous examination of the process in people with intellectual disability of all ages, as described below.

Why perform a health check?

Health checks may:

- prompt primary care services to be more proactive because people with intellectual disability may not raise problems themselves, making a reactive approach ineffective (Martin et al. 1997)
- make people with intellectual disability more aware of the medical implications of the symptoms they experience and improve communication of these symptoms to their carers and healthcare providers (Beange et al. 1995; Martin et al. 2004)
- increase the likelihood that carers will see behaviour or complaints made by people with intellectual disability as manifestations of illness (Wilson and Haire 1990); and
- as a result provides a way to detect, treat, and prevent new health conditions in this population (Wilson and Haire 1990; Jones et al. 2010).

Health checks also provide a record of the person's health history and a measure of their current health status. This documentation can be useful for on-going health care, especially as paid carers frequently change, and long-term recall of health status by the person with an intellectual disability or their carers can be difficult and inaccurate (Martin 2003; Jones et al. 2010). Furthermore, health checks may be cost-effective, as early detection of new or underlying medical conditions may reduce the health costs associated with managing more severe physical and mental illness, or secondary challenging behaviour (Gunsett et al. 1989).

What is a health check?

A health check can be variously understood to mean:

- a tool-directed evaluation by a generic health service provider (usually a GP or a practice nurse) (Cooper et al. 2006; Lennox 2007; Lennox et al. 2010, 2011)
- a systematic evaluation performed by a specialist health service provider (Wilson and Haire 1990; Beange et al. 1995; Khan et al. 2012).

These processes vary substantially in how they are delivered, which process is undertaken, the setting of delivery, and the expertise of those delivering the intervention. The intervention may involve a physician with a special interest in this population actively recruiting motivated individuals and performing a one-on-one assessment with the clear purpose of finding unmet health needs and actively influencing on-going health care. However, although a clinician with specialist knowledge of intellectual disability is likely to provide the optimal health benefit when performing a health assessment, such individuals are not universally available in the UK and are almost completely inaccessible in countries such as Australia, New Zealand, and Canada, where specialist medical or allied health training programmes in the health of adults with intellectual disability do not exist. Such clinicians do, however, exist in Holland (see Chapter 17).

The lack of specialist and experienced clinicians has resulted in the pragmatic decision to develop assessment tools or health checks that can be widely implemented by generic primary healthcare providers (i.e. the GP and practice nurse). Of note is that the health systems of these implementing countries are centred on a primary care model, making the primary care setting the ideal context for health checks, unlike in the USA where patients can directly access specialist services. In the USA, a nurse-driven health assessment process independent of primary care has been trialled by Hahn and Aronow (2005).

We suggest the following definition for health checks in people with intellectual disability: 'the systematic gathering of a comprehensive health history that includes the person's current and past health information, and their psycho-social context'. This history is reviewed by a primary care health professional, considered and clarified where necessary, and leads to a directed, systematic physical and mental health examination which results in identification of any unmet health needs that are documented and optimally acted upon. The process optimally includes specific information about commonly missed and syndrome-specific health conditions to inform the person with intellectual disability, their caregivers, and the health professional.

Differences regarding terminology

The preferred term for this process in the UK is 'health check', while in other countries such as Australia the term 'health assessment' is commonly used. Both processes involve the systematic collation of the person's health and wellbeing history, which is taken to the healthcare provider who performs a healthcare review, communicates their findings, and recommends action, such as immunization, treatment and management of disease.

A number of approaches and tools have been developed to deliver health checks in the UK, New Zealand, and Australia. These include:

- the Cardiff Health Check
- the OK Health Check
- the 21st Century Health Check
- the Comprehensive Health Assessment Program (CHAP).

In the UK, the Royal College of General Practitioners (RCGP) has produced a step-by-step guide to assist GPs to deliver annual health checks for patients with intellectual disability (Hoghton and RCGP Learning Disabilities Group 2010). This guide focuses on the Cardiff Health Check, and the guide includes a template for this health check along with health checklists for specific syndromes such as Down syndrome and Rett syndrome. The Australian CHAP has been licensed by most state governments for use by disability departments and, in July 2006, the federal government introduced a payment to reimburse GPs to perform the assessment. A case study of the use of the CHAP is given below.

Case study

Tony is a 37-year-old man who lived at 'Conflux', a 24-hour supported accommodation, with two other men and attended 'Out There' community access programme during weekdays. He was 'a bit grumpy and slowing down a bit' according to his residential support staff, 'but what do you expect at his age?' commented a support worker who had known Tony for two years. He was otherwise thought to be well. His parents had died nine years previously and he had occasional contact with three older siblings. His family's doctor, who had known him from childhood, had retired, and Tony now attended a new practice around the corner from his current residence. The staff completed a CHAP and had to contact Tony's family for some details of his past history, which had been archived by Conflux. They organized with the practice nurse to come to the practice on a Wednesday and she performed much of the assessment in collaboration with Tony's GP. Tony said he had felt unwell for some time and he appeared unhappy. On examination he was found to have enlarged lymph nodes, a 5-kg unexplained weight loss, and no clear history of tetanus/diphtheria immunization, or vision or hearing testing since childhood. Consulting with his previous GP's notes found that he had been appropriately immunized. Further investigation was required of the other findings, which revealed hearing loss that was only partly due to the impacted wax in his right ear, and the discovery of a lymphoma. He was referred to the local tertiary hospital and, over time, received chemotherapy that resulted in remission and resolution of his symptoms.

Key elements of health checks

It remains unclear which elements of the health check process are essential to improve health outcomes among people with intellectual disability. Indeed, even in the extensive literature on health assessment in the elderly general population, the issue of the essential characteristics of the process have not been clarified (Stuck et al. 2002).

The key elements of the health check in people with intellectual disability appear to be that it should be:

1. *Credible*: increasing the authority of the process in the eyes of all who use it.
2. *Usable*: ensuring it is understood and as easy, as possible, to complete.
3. *Accessible*: gathering a health story in an accessible form.
4. *Empowering*: educating people with intellectual disability, parents, carers, and primary health care provider.
5. *Instructive*: directing an examination by a healthcare provider to address unmet health needs.
6. *Evidence-based*.
7. *Comprehensive*: covering all the important areas of health care, especially those where unmet needs are common.
8. *Action oriented*: attempting to ensure health needs are addressed once identified.

Evidence for the impact of health checks for people with intellectual disability

A systematic review of the impact of health checks on the health and wellbeing of people with intellectual disability identified 38 relevant studies (Robertson et al. 2011). The majority of studies were from the UK and Ireland, but there were also studies from Australia, USA, and New Zealand. In total, over 5000 people with intellectual disability received health checks in the course of the studies included in the review.

Health checks consistently led to detection of unmet health needs. The proportion of those who had previously undetected health conditions identified ranged from 51 per cent to 94 per cent (Cassidy et al. 2002; Baxter et al. 2006; Chauhan et al. 2012). The number of previously undetected or unmanaged health needs identified per participant ranged from 2.2 additional diagnoses (Carlsen et al. 1994) to 5.2 health problems requiring intervention (Aronow and Hahn 2005). The health conditions identified included serious and life-threatening conditions such as:

- testicular cancer
- dementia
- breast cancer
- Type 2 diabetes.

Some of the most frequently identified conditions were what might be considered 'less serious' health conditions, such as:

- obesity
- ear wax
- skin conditions
- dental problems
- constipation.

Studies consistently provide evidence of health checks leading to targeted actions to address identified health needs (McConkey et al. 2002; Martin et al. 2004; Aronow and Hahn 2005; Baxter et al. 2006; Lennox et al. 2006, 2010, 2011; Lennox 2007). Targeted actions identified were consistent with the notion that health checks facilitate the identification of previously undiagnosed health needs. Actions included relatively routine procedures such as ear wax removal and referral for skin conditions, as well as a number of life-saving actions including provision of a pacemaker and surgery for cancer.

When subjected to the rigour of a pooled analysis of two randomized controlled trials (RCTs) (Lennox 2007; Lennox et al. 2010) and a non-randomized matched control group study (Cooper et al. 2006) ($N = 795$), these descriptive findings were confirmed. Health checks resulted in a clear overall trend for identification of unmet health needs and highly statistically significant improvements in vision testing, hearing testing, hearing loss identified, hepatitis B immunization, and tetanus/diphtheria immunization (Lennox et al. 2011).

The experience of people with intellectual disability, caregivers, and GPs

The experience of health checks has been explored in people with intellectual disability, their caregivers, and GPs. When interviewed after the health check, most people with intellectual disability were unable to distinguish the consultation from their usual GP visit (Lennox 2008; Lennox et al. 2012); however, some people with intellectual disability were reluctant to participate in invasive tests (Martin et al. 2004).

An Australian telephone survey of GPs and residential support staff, before and after they were involved in a health check, indicated overall support for the process and the objectives of improving healthcare delivery to their patients (Lennox 2008). This support was underlined by the vast majority of GPs (92 per cent), who agreed to participate in the RCT of the CHAP. Usually in RCTs, only 10 per cent of potential study participants agree to participate (Lennox 2007). After completing the health check, many GPs identified better health care and ultimately better health outcomes for people with intellectual disability, especially the detection of previously unidentified health problems. The GPs reported concerns about the additional time needed to complete the consultation process and the disability service providers' organizational capacity to coordinate all parties to attend annual health checks. The GPs were also concerned about the ability of support staff to communicate with people with intellectual disability and their patient's ability to comply, as some had a fear of doctors (Lennox et al. 2012). Others have found a reluctance on the part of GPs to undertake health checks (Kerr et al. 1996; McConkey et al. 2002; Perry et al. 2010); however, enhanced training for specific practices has resulted in an increase in uptake (Perry et al. 2010).

A further potential barrier is low uptake of health screening. For example, 29 per cent of those scheduled to have health checks do not have them (Felce et al. 2008) and only 33 per cent of offered health checks are translated into actual checks (Perry et al. 2010). A telephone call by a community nurse to confirm attendance and answer queries has been found to increase uptake (Jones et al. 2010). Once health checks have been conducted, there may be barriers that prevent identified health needs from being translated into action to address these needs. In a study in Northern Ireland, health screens were conducted by a specialist health screening service and outcomes forwarded to the patient's own GP with a referral letter if necessary (McConkey et al. 2002). However, as many as half of GPs took no further action on the referrals, with 49 per cent not recalling having received a referral letter for the patient. The authors suggest that the most central reason for involving GPs more closely with health screening is that they are in a position to ensure that problems detected are attended to.

Limitations of the evidence

The systematic review by Robertson et al. (2011) demonstrated several limitations of the evidence relating to health checks for people with intellectual disability. First, only two RCTs in one country, Australia, have been conducted, involving relatively small populations (albeit the largest RCTs involving people with intellectual disability) (Lennox 2007; Lennox et al. 2010). In contrast, the elderly health assessment process has been extensively tested by many RCTs, four meta-analyses, and systematic reviews. Second, socio-cultural influences, including socio-economic position, cultural background or ethnicity, gender, and severity of the disability have not been examined in the context of the effects of health checks. Third, benefits from the health check have only been demonstrated in the short term; to date, no studies involving measures of health outcomes beyond one year have been published. Longitudinal studies provide significant challenges, including funding, resource issues, and participant attrition, but these studies are essential to determine whether the process confers longer-term health benefits.

The future of health checks

Health checks have been widely implemented in the UK and Australia but with limited implementation in New Zealand. Current interest in examining the evidence for, or implementation of, health checks has been shown in the USA, Canada, the Philippines, and Thailand.

Given the on-going implementation of health checks and increased and widespread interest in this process, further, rigorous evaluation of health checks is needed. These evaluations would preferably examine quantitative outcomes using gold-standard methodology (i.e. RCTs) and investigate the experience of all those involved in the health check, using more detailed, qualitative interviews of participants. Ideally, further research in different countries that considers their unique health and social support systems needs to be undertaken to confirm the otherwise limited evidence base for health assessments in people with intellectual disability.

Optimal frequency of health checks and cost–benefit analyses

Although it is common for health checks to be performed annually, and one study has concluded that annual checks seem appropriate (Felce et al. 2008), the optimal periodicity of the process remains unknown. Only two studies have examined the cost of health checks and found that health checks are relatively inexpensive and are not associated with higher health care costs when compared with treatment received by a matched control group (Romeo et al. 2009; Gordon et al. 2012).

Development of health checks for people with different syndromes

A potential refinement to the health check process would be a redesign making it more specific for people with different syndromes. This specificity would allow a more focused assessment of the often unique and unmet health needs of specific groups. A more specific process would support each of the participants to tailor care, especially where the person has a rarely encountered syndrome with specific needs including the identification of known associated conditions, such as the high risk of renal tumours in people with tuberous sclerosis. Specificity has already been addressed by the inclusion of syndrome-specific morbidity in the CHAP and of syndrome-specific checklists in the RCGP health checks guide (Hoghton and RCGP Learning Disabilities Group 2010) (see Web Resources).

Information technology systems and fidelity with emerging evidence

Many disability services and primary care services have computerized records and many countries are moving to electronic health records. These technological advances are likely to decrease the time and organizational burden of performing health checks and integration of the process into electronic systems. Legitimate privacy concerns are associated with any electronic record-sharing process, especially when the person involved may have difficulties with consent. These concerns need to be addressed, but must not be allowed to be used as an excuse for the exclusion of people with impaired capacity. The benefits of accurate and up-to-date health records are potentially enormous in a population that experiences fragmentation of services, loss of important health information and, in particular, the use of multiple medications.

Finally, it is important that the fidelity of the health check process remains consistent with emerging evidence and that the assessment tools keep pace with changing recommendations. For example, since the CHAP was developed in the late 1990s, constant changes to recommendations for immunizations, health screening, and new technologies, such as the use of comparative genomic hybridization (CGH) microarray technology to identify the cause of the person's disability, have arisen.

Summary

- Health checks provide a way to detect, treat, manage, and prevent new health conditions.
- The uptake of health screening for people with intellectual disability is substantially lower than that among the non-disabled population, despite the poorer health experienced by those with intellectual disability.
- Approaches and tools developed to deliver health checks include the Cardiff Health Check, the OK Health Check, the 21st Century Health Check, and the Comprehensive Health Assessment Program (CHAP).
- Health checks should be credible, usable, accessible, empowering, instructive, evidence-based, comprehensive, and action-oriented.
- Evidence suggests that health checks consistently lead to the detection of unmet health needs and to targeted actions to address identified health needs, and that they are acceptable to GPs, carers, and people with intellectual disabilities.
- Given the on-going implementation of health checks, and increased and widespread interest in this process, further rigorous evaluation of health checks is needed.
- The fidelity of the health check process must remain consistent with emerging evidence and the assessment tools must keep pace with changing recommendations.
- The benefits of accurate and up-to-date health records are potentially enormous in a population that experiences fragmentation of services, loss of important health information and, in particular, the use of multiple medications.

Web resources

- The RCGP health checks guide is available from the RCGP website: http://www.rcgp.org.uk/clinical-and-research/clinical-resources/learning-disabilities.aspx

- A training package to help support clinicians deliver annual health checks is available at: http://www.gptom.com/

- General Medical Council website designed to help doctors provide better care for people with learning disabilities is available at: http://www.gmc-uk.org/learningdisabilities/default.aspx

- Health checks and specific assessments, including the Cardiff Health Check and the OK Health Check: http://www.easyhealth.org.uk/listing/health-checks-and-assessments-(leaflets)

- Improving Health and Lives: Learning Disability Observatory: http://www.improving healthandlives.org.uk/

References

Aronow, H.U. and Hahn, J.E. (2005) Stay Well and Healthy! Pilot study findings from an inhome preventive healthcare programme for persons ageing with intellectual and/or developmental disabilities. *Journal of Applied Research in Intellectual Disabilities*, 18: 163–73.

Baxter, H., Lowe, K., Houston, H., Jones, G., Felce, D. and Kerr, M. (2006) Previously unidentified morbidity in patients with intellectual disability. *British Journal of General Practice*, 56: 93–8.

Beange, H., McElduff, A. and Baker, W. (1995) Medical disorders of adults with mental retardation: a population study. *American Journal of Mental Retardation*, 99: 595–604.

Bittles, A.H., Petterson, B.A., Sullivan, S.G., Hussain, R., Glasson, E. and Montgomery, P. (2002) The influence of intellectual disability on life expectancy. *Journals of Gerontology Series A: Biological Sciences and Medical Sciences*, 57: M470–2.

Carlsen, W.R., Galluzzi, K.E., Forman, L.F. and Cavalieri, T.A. (1994) Comprehensive geriatric assessment – applications for community-residing, elderly people with mental-retardation developmental-disabilities. *Mental Retardation*, 32: 334–40.

Cassidy, G., Martin, D.M., Martin, G.H.B. and Roy, A. (2002) Health checks for people with learning disabilities. *Journal of Intellectual Disabilities*, 6: 123–36.

Chauhan, U., Reeve, J., Kontopantelis, E., Hinder, S., Nelson, P. and Doran, T. (2012) *Impact of the English Directly Enhanced Service (DES) for Learning Disability*. Manchester: Health Sciences Research Group, University of Manchester.

Cooper, S.A., Morrison, J., Melville, C., Finlayson, J., Allan, L., Martin, G. et al. (2006) Improving the health of people with intellectual disabilities: outcomes of a health screening programme after 1 year. *Journal of Intellectual Disability Research*, 50: 667–77.

Elkan, R., Kendrick, D., Dewey, M., Hewitt, M., Robinson, J., Blair, M. et al. (2001) Effectiveness of home based support for older people: systematic review and meta-analysis. *British Medical Journal*, 323: 719–25.

Emerson, E. and Baines, S. (2010) *The Estimated Prevalence of Austism among Adults with Learning Disabilities in England*. London: Department of Health.

Emerson, E., Madden, R., Robertson, J., Graham, H., Hatton, C. and Llewellyn, G. (2009) *Intellectual and Physical Disability, Social Mobility, Social Inclusion and Health*. CeDR Research Report. Lancaster: Lancaster University, Centre for Disability Research.

Felce, D., Baxter, H., Lowe, K., Dunstan, F., Houston, H., Jones, G. et al. (2008) The impact of repeated health checks for adults with intellectual disabilities. *Journal of Applied Research in Intellectual Disabilities*, 21: 585–96.

Glover, G. and Ayub, M. (2010) *How People with Learning Disabilites Die*. Improving Health and Lives: Learning Disabilities Observatory. London: Public Health England.

Gordon, L., Holden, E., Ware, R., Taylor, M. and Lennox, N. (2012) Comprehensive health assessments for adults with intellectual disability living in the community – weighing up the costs and benefits. *Australian Family Physician*, 41(12): 969–72.

Gunsett, R.P., Mulick, J.A., Fernald, W.B. and Martin, J.L. (1989) Brief report: indications for medical screening prior to behavioral programming for severely and profoundly mentally retarded clients. *Journal of Autism and Developmental Disorders*, 19: 167–72.

Hahn, J.E. and Aronow, H.U. (2005) A pilot of a gerontological advanced practice nurse preventive intervention. *Journal of Applied Research in Intellectual Disabilities*, 18: 131–42.

Hoghton, M. and RCGP Learning Disabilities Group (2010) *A Step by Step Guide for GP Practices: Annual Health Checks for People with a Learning Disability*. London: The Royal College of General Practitioners.

Jones, J., Hathaway, D., Gilhooley, M., Leech, A. and Macleod, S. (2010) Down syndrome health screening – the Fife model. *British Journal of Learning Disabilities*, 38: 5–9.

Katz, A. (1996) Canadian Task Force on the periodic health examination – annual checkup revisited. *Canadian Family Physician*, 42: 1637–8.

Kerr, M.P., Richards, D. and Glover, G. (1996) Primary care for people with an intellectual disability – a group practice survey. *Journal of Applied Research in Intellectual Disabilities*, 9: 347–52.

Khan, N.Z., Gallo, L.A., Arghir, A., Budisteanu, B., Budisteanu, M., Dobrescu, I. et al. (2012) Autism and the grand challenges in global mental health. *Autism Research*, 5: 156–9.

Krahn, G.L., Hammond, L. and Turner, A. (2006) A cascade of disparities: health and health care access for people with intellectual disabilities. *Mental Retardation and Developmental Disabilities Research Reviews,* 12: 70–82.

Lennox, N. (2007) *A randomized cluster study of an intervention aimed at improving the health outcomes of adults with an intellectual disability.* Unpublished PhD thesis, University of Queensland, Brisbane, QLD.

Lennox, N. (2008) *Views of health assessments from intellectually disabled people, carers and general practitioners.* Paper presented at the 13th World Congress of the International Association for the Scientific Study of Intellectual Disabilities. *Journal of Intellectual Disability Research,* 52: 742.

Lennox, N., Rey-Conde, T. and Cooling, N. (2006) Comprehensive health assessments during de-institutionalization: an observational study. *Journal of Intellectual Disability Research,* 50: 719–24.

Lennox, N., Bain, C., Rey-Conde, T., Taylor, M., Boyle, F., Purdie, D., and Ware, R. (2010) Cluster randomized-controlled trial of interventions to improve health for adults with intellectual disability who live in private dwellings. *Journal of Applied Research in Intellectual Disabilities,* 23: 303-11.

Lennox, N.G., Ware, R.S., Bain, C., Taylor Gomez, M. and Cooper, S.A. (2011) Effects of health screening for adults with intellectual disability: a pooled analysis. *British Journal of General Practice,* 61: 193–6.

Lennox, N.G., Brolan, C.E., Dean, J., Ware, R.S., Boyle, F.M., Taylor Gomez, M. et al. (2012) General practitioners' views on perceived and actual gains, benefits, and barriers associated with the implementation of an Australian health assessment for people with intellectual disability. *Journal of Intellectual Disability Research* (DOI: 10.1111/j.1365-2788.2012.01586.x).

Martin, D., Roy, A. and Wells, M. (1997) Health gain through health checks: improving access to primary health care for people with intellectual disability. *Journal of Intellectual Disability Research,* 41: 401–8.

Martin, G. (2003) Annual health reviews for patients with severe learning disabilities. *Journal of Intellectual Disabilities,* 7: 9–21.

Martin, G., Philip, L., Bates, L. and Warwick, J. (2004) Evaluation of a nurse led annual review of patients with severe intellectual disabilities, needs identified and needs met, in a large group practice. *Journal of Learning Disabilities,* 8: 235–46.

McConkey, R., Moore, G. and Marshall, D. (2002) Changes in the attitudes of GPs to the health screening of patients with learning disabilities. *Journal of Intellectual Disabilities,* 6: 373–84.

Mencap (2007) *Death by Indifference.* London: Mencap.

Michael, J. and Richardson, A. (2008) Healthcare for all: the independent inquiry into access to healthcare for people with learning disabilities. *Tizard Learning Disability Review,* 13: 28–34.

New South Wales Community Services Commission (2001) *Disability, Death and the Responsibility of Care: A review of the Characteristics and Circumstances of 211 People with Disabilities who Died in Care between 1991–1998 in NSW.* Sydney, NSW: NSWCSC.

Ouellette-Kuntz, H., Garcin, N., Lewis, M.E., Minnes, P., Martin, C. and Holden, J. (2005) Addressing health disparities through promoting equity for individuals with intellectual disability. *Canadian Journal of Public Health: Revue Canadienne de Sante Publique,* 96(suppl. 2): S8–S22.

Perry, J., Kerr, M., Felce, D., Bartley, S. and Tomlinson, J. (2010) *Monitoring the Public Health Impact of Health Checks for Adults with a Learning Disability in Wales.* Cardiff: NHS Wales, Public Health Wales/WCLD.

Reith, P. (1989) Adapting the selective periodic health exam to a college-aged population. *Journal of the American College of Health,* 38: 109–13.

Robertson, J., Roberts, H., Emerson, E., Turner, S. and Greig, R. (2011) The impact of health checks for people with intellectual disabilities: a systematic review of evidence. *Journal of Intellectual Disability Research,* 55: 1009–19.

Romeo, R., Knapp, M., Morrison, J., Melville, C., Allan, L., Finlayson, J. et al. (2009) Cost estimation of a health-check intervention for adults with intellectual disabilities in the UK. *Journal of Intellectual Disability Research,* 53: 426–39.

Santos, R., Evenhuis, H., Stewart, L., Kerr, M., McElduff, A., Fraser, W. et al. (2002) *Health Guidelines for Adults with an Intellectual Disability.* An IASSID Publication. Available at: http://www.intellectualdisability. info/how-to../health-guidelines-for-adults-with-an-intellectual-disability#top [accessed 16 November 2012].

Stuck, A.E., Egger, M., Hammer, A., Minder, C.E. and Beck, J.C. (2002) Home visits to prevent nursing home admission and functional decline in elderly people – systematic review and meta-regression analysis. *Journal of the American Medical Association,* 287: 1022–8.

Van Haastregt, J.C.M., Diederiks, J.P.M., Van Rossum, E., De Witte, L.P. and Crebolder, H.F.J.M. (2000) Effects of preventive home visits to elderly people living in the community: systematic review. *British Medical Journal,* 320: 754–8.

Wilson, D. and Haire, A. (1990) Health care screening for people with mental handicap living in the community. *British Medical Journal,* 301: 1379–81.

19

Ethics

William F. Sullivan and John Heng

Introduction

James is a friendly man with Down syndrome who works with many people. Although highly susceptible to influenza and severely affected by it, he also has an acute fear of needles and refuses to be vaccinated. Jane has Prader-Willi syndrome. She finds it difficult to manage her weight and snacks frequently. At home, her parents allow her to eat whatever and whenever she wants. Mary has intellectual disabilities in the borderline range. Her few 'friends' supply her with amphetamines in return for sexual favours. Mark has intellectual disabilities of unknown aetiology, poor communication, and serious behavioural issues, such as self-injury. Staff members at the group home where he lives find it a challenge to bring him to his family physician and do so, reluctantly, only when he is in a crisis. Each of these persons could benefit from interventions for illness prevention and health promotion, but there are ethical issues involved.

The right to preventive care and health promotion

The UN Universal Declaration on Human Rights (1948) asserts that every human being has the right to health care. The UN International Covenant on Economic, Social, and Cultural Rights (1966) describes this right as an entitlement to 'the highest standard of mental and physical health that a society can provide' (art. 12). The WHO Charters, Ottawa (1986) and Bangkok (2005) clarify that this right includes health promotion.

In 2006, the UN used these documents to develop the Convention on the Rights of Persons with Disabilities, which numerous countries have ratified. This Convention outlines the right to health care of persons with disabilities in three ways:

- Persons with disabilities have the 'right to enjoyment of the highest attainable standard of health without discrimination on the basis of disability'.
- They have a right to services 'specifically because of their disability'.
- Healthcare professionals are urged to provide 'care of the same quality to persons with disabilities as to others, including the basis of free and informed consent, by . . . training and the promulgation of ethical standards' (art. 25).

These developments supply the legal basis for preventing illness and promoting health in people with intellectual disabilities. Crucially, they highlight the importance of ethical attitudes and conduct in healthcare professionals who provide services to these individuals. While this is an excellent starting point, the task of developing standards of illness prevention and health promotion for this population 'specifically because of their disability', and of elaborating the ethical principles that ought to inform and guide these standards, remains.

A number of comprehensive clinical guidelines for preventive care and health promotion covering people with intellectual disabilities have been or are being formulated (Lennox and

Diggens 1999; Sullivan et al. 2011b). Guidelines applicable to the general population are not always transferable to these persons. Many have health issues that present different manifestations and diverge in prevalence, age of onset, rate of progression, and degree of severity. They may also interact in complex ways (Haverman et al. 2009). Life-cycle transitions, changes in surroundings, decreases in level of support, disruption or loss of relationships can have a much greater negative effect on people with intellectual disabilities than on others.

Equally important are ethical guidelines covering illness prevention and health promotion for people with intellectual disabilities. Developing clinical and ethical standards should proceed in tandem. Specifying good outcomes for this population through sound clinical standards cannot be achieved without some understanding of why these outcomes are good, worthwhile or valuable. This chapter contributes to reflection and discussion of some ethical principles that should guide those caring for people with intellectual disabilities.

The good of relationships

The bio-psycho-social-spiritual model of health care has been the theoretical basis for providing holistic care in family medicine, nursing, and other health disciplines involved in primary care. Sulmasy (2002) explicated this model in terms of a series of human and other relationships. For people with intellectual disabilities, the influence and impact of these relationships are especially significant (Sullivan et al. 2006). Quite often, poor health, distressed behaviour, and premature death of people with intellectual disabilities can result from disruption of their relationships and the cascading effects that these disruptions have (Krahn et al. 2006). For example, biological, environmental, psycho-affective or social factors, or some combination of these, might contribute to distressed behaviours in a person with intellectual disabilities. Recognizing the good of relationships to persons with intellectual disabilities has implications for preventing illness and promoting their health. There is an ethical duty to promote healthy relationships as much as possible.

One cautionary note is important regarding the application of the bio-psycho-social-spiritual model. Some healthcare providers might treat each of the domains as separate for assessment and intervention and begin sequentially with the biological. When applied to people with intellectual disabilities, however, interactions among these domains often occur. These interactions should be recognized and appropriate targets for illness prevention and health promotion selected on the basis of them. For instance, a programme to promote good nutrition or physical fitness might be difficult to implement without enhancing the person's environment and social support, such as in the situation of Jane, as described above. In other situations, such as that of Mark, described above, preventing problem behaviours, such as self-injury, is hard to achieve until communication problems that might have precipitated it are addressed. Weaning a person with intellectual disabilities from harmful addictions and risky behaviours, such as those of Mary, described above, might be challenging without helping the person to receive the environmental, social, and spiritual resources and supports necessary for self-restraint and resilience.

Since the relationships of family members and other regular carers are important to this population, their perspectives regarding illness prevention and health promotion should be solicited, and they should be involved as much as possible as partners in care (Sullivan et al. 2006). Many people with intellectual disabilities, such as Jane, as described above, live with family members or in residences that do not promote healthy lifestyles for various reasons. This could be due to their carers' lack of knowledge, resources or support. Sadly, some people with intellectual disabilities, such as the case of Mary above, also live in environments where they suffer from neglect or abuse by those with whom they live and associate. In these situations, primary care providers should be vigilant about these factors and willing to take on the role of advocate as much as possible.

The ethical relationship between the person with intellectual disabilities and the primary care provider

Health care entails the participation of at least two persons, the patient who is in need and the healthcare professional possessing the requisite knowledge and skills. People with intellectual disabilities are particularly vulnerable owing to their impaired intellectual and adaptive functioning, diminished decision-making capacity, and other disadvantages related to personal, environmental, and social factors (Krahn et al. 2006). Given such vulnerability, Pellegrino and Thomasma (1988) emphasize the role of ethics in the relationship between patient and healthcare provider. The provider must always be trustworthy, putting aside self-interest to promote the person's wellbeing. They call this 'beneficence in trust', which is the first and foremost ethical principle founded on the very nature of health care. This entails that the provider's judgement always be informed both by his or her medical expertise and experience, and by knowledge of the person's need and situation. This knowledge can only be acquired if the care provider is attentive to the person's situation, willing to spend time understanding the person's needs and perspectives.

Primary care providers need to be aware of unconscious negative attitudes and mistaken beliefs regarding people with intellectual disabilities that arise from their lack of knowledge and infrequent contact with this group. These could impede the care provider's ability to recognize certain physical and mental health issues that should be addressed (Marks and Heller 2003). For example, there might be lower expectations that a person with intellectual disabilities can maintain an active lifestyle and healthy nutrition compared with non-disabled persons. Or a primary care provider might assume that it is not worthwhile discussing with a person, such as James, described above, his anxiety about flu vaccinations. There might also be 'diagnostic overshadowing', a failure to deal with behavioural issues wrongly attributed to the person's disabilities. This could lead to ignoring signs of physical or psycho-affective distresses or mental health issues that would normally concern primary care providers of persons without these disabilities (Holland 2000). It could result in overlooking the need to be *pro-active* in anticipating factors likely to cause distress, such as the loss of a relationship or a new situation. The person's mental health should be monitored in order to prevent the occurrence or escalation of problem behaviours.

People with intellectual disabilities often have difficulty recognizing and communicating health issues and experience distress in doing so. They might communicate some bits of information but fail to volunteer relevant information regarding the 'big picture'. Health and lifestyle advice and instructions, educational material, and even the office environment should be modified to take into account these persons' level of understanding and needs. Such adaptations can have a significant influence on the patient's ability to follow through with a plan of care.

People with intellectual disabilities typically have various and complex health issues. Given the busy primary care setting, finding the time and resources to deal with illness prevention and health promotion is not easy. In many practices, visits by people with intellectual disabilities might be irregular and undertaken out of necessity so that care providers tend to focus their time and attention on assessing and treating the complex and most urgent health conditions that are present, leaving aside issues of preventive care and health promotion. Also, people with intellectual disabilities often receive care and support from multiple healthcare professionals and agencies in a variety of programmes. An overall picture of what targets of illness prevention and health promotion need to be addressed might require coordinating the multiple sources of information that result from fragmented education, healthcare, and social support systems. For example, in Ontario, Canada, it has only recently been possible to combine health and social services data to track access to healthcare services among the roughly 65,000 adults with intellectual disabilities in that province. Preliminary analyses indicate that only about 20 per cent of these adults had a preventive care assessment during a two-year period, and very few of these assessments were specifically adapted for primary care of adults with intellectual disabilities.

Tools such as the Comprehensive Health Assessment Program (CHAP) developed in Queensland, Australia (Lennox et al. 2007) and the Preventive Care Checklist and Health Watch Tables for specific syndromes developed by the Developmental Disabilities Primary Care Initiative in Canada (Sullivan et al. 2011a) can assist primary care providers in assembling better information for health promotion and undertaking appropriate assessments. A key recommendation is for primary care providers to offer at least a regular (perhaps annual) preventive care assessment to all people with intellectual disabilities, using assessments that include considering their specific health issues. Primary care providers should also be willing to take on the role of case coordinator or assist the person in finding someone appropriate for that role. More clinics specializing in the care of people with intellectual disabilities organized around interdisciplinary teams are needed.

Respect for human dignity

The ethical right of persons with intellectual and developmental disabilities to the benefits of health promotion is based upon respect for their intrinsic or inherent dignity as human beings. This dignity does not diminish because of absent or impaired intellectual or adaptive functioning.

Respecting this dignity entails *optimizing* the extent to which persons can flourish with holistic care in a supportive environment that includes inter-personal relationships, even if they live with severe disabling limitations, while *minimizing* the burdens and distresses arising from screening, monitoring, and other preventive and health-promoting measures. Decisions about the type and frequency of screening or surveillance measures, as well as any health promotion programmes, should take into account not only the medical benefits and risks to the patient, but also how they could be less intrusive and burdensome. Often this requires adaptations of standard procedures, such as cervical smears, dental examinations, and others that are likely to elicit confusion, fear or anxiety in people with intellectual disabilities, or are perceived as burdensome and intrusive. The perspectives of people with intellectual disabilities and those of their family and other regular carers regarding tolerability and impact should always be considered, and more acceptable alternatives should be offered whenever possible.

Justice in illness prevention and health promotion should be understood as bridging the gap in health disparities by ensuring *equality of opportunity and access* to available public health promotion programmes, but also *equitable* access to those programmes designed specifically for them (Ouellette-Kuntz et al. 2005).

Autonomy and informed consent

Respect for autonomy is often the only ethical principle that is appealed to in preventive care and health promotion, but other ethical considerations are relevant. Autonomy is understood by ethicists both in terms of freedom from external constraints and freedom to decide and act on decisions. These present two ways of thinking about patient consent: a right to refuse what healthcare professionals propose and a right to be supported in the person's self-determined decisions. The first presupposes that the person understands and appreciates the significance of the proposed intervention; the second that the person is in a position to know what he or she needs and can ask for it. Neither of these capacities should be assumed to be present in all patients and in all circumstances.

Like everyone else, the capacity of people with intellectual disabilities to make free, informed, and value-based decisions varies according to the type and complexity of decision and personal and situational factors that might influence understanding and judgement.

Generally, persons with *mild* intellectual disabilities do not differ significantly from those without such disabilities in their capacity to make free and informed decisions in health care and research (Gunn et al. 2000). Persons with *moderate* intellectual disabilities might not have all the skills for a full range of complex decisions. Here, support from family members and other carers might enable them to participate in the decision-making process. It is unlikely that a person whose intellectual and functional abilities are in the *severe to profound* range of intellectual disabilities (for example, a person with an IQ score below 40 who needs significant supports in the areas of self-care, health, and safety) is capable of providing informed consent for most health care (Dinerstein et al. 1999). Nevertheless, the healthcare professional should always conduct a thorough assessment of the person's decision-making capacities. This is important not only for persons with moderate intellectual disabilities, in whom such capacities are uncertain, but also for those with mild and borderline intellectual disabilities, in whom such capacities might routinely (but sometimes mistakenly) be assumed.

Factors that mitigate capacity for free and informed consent in people with intellectual disabilities include living in residential care settings, lack of decision-making opportunities, lack of previous healthcare experiences, and a tendency to ready acquiescence (Goldsmith et al. 2008). Witnessing something traumatic in health care might influence the person with intellectual disabilities to refuse to consent to a test or intervention that he or she associates with that negative experience, even if it has a low risk of harm. People with intellectual disabilities might be unable to communicate well verbally or at all. Healthcare professionals should then use alternative modes of communication. The involvement of interpreters who know the person well can be very helpful here. Finally, a considerable number of people with intellectual disabilities may also have some form of affective disorder or psychiatric illness, which, if severe, could affect decision-making capacity.

In most jurisdictions, the law and healthcare policies stipulate that individuals are presumed to have the capacity to make free and informed decisions regarding their care unless it can be demonstrated otherwise. This capacity should be re-assessed, at least informally, each time there are grounds to question it and, if absent, a substitute decision maker should be authorized.

The stated legal and healthcare policies, however, treat the capacity of people to make free and informed decisions in health care as an all-or-none attribute. In practice, many different types of capacities are involved. They include the ability to form goals of care, to understand information, to judge the accuracy of the information provided and the trustworthiness of the persons providing it, to weigh the likely benefits and risks of harm of possible alternatives based on values and commitments, and to communicate the decision. People with intellectual disabilities might be capable of some but not all of these capacities (Heng and Sullivan 2007). The ethical principle of beneficence in trust entails that they should be given the opportunity to participate as much as possible in decision making, even if they fail to meet the legal or healthcare policy standard.

In illness prevention and health promotion, among the various capacities involved in decision making, that of weighing different options in light of the person's values and commitments is particularly important. It reflects a person's affirmation that a test or intervention is good or worthwhile because it contributes to his or her overall wellbeing and the commitments that he or she has, even if what is required is disagreeable in the short term. Such interventions include dental or eye examinations, screening for cancer, and participating in programmes to improve nutrition or physical fitness, or to reduce harmful addictions. People with intellectual disabilities might be capable of such value-based and commitment-based affirmations, or they might not. For instance, James, Jane, and Mark, as described at the beginning of this chapter, cannot simply be presumed to have this capacity.

Perhaps the most ethically troubling situations relate to instances when a person with intellectual and developmental disabilities is assessed to be capable of withholding consent according to legal standards and refuses a relatively non-intrusive preventive screen or test or a necessary intervention that is likely to avert significant future harm. For instance, many adults, like James, who live or work in environments in which the risk of transmission of infections such as influenza or hepatitis B is high, might value their life and work, but be assessed by the legal standard for capacity to consent to be capable of refusing vaccination. An individual with Prader-Willi syndrome, such as Jane, might meet the legal standard for the capacity to withhold consent from programming to curb food-seeking behaviours. A person who is assessed to be capable of a *healthcare* decision, such as refusing to participate in counselling to address a drug addiction or avoid risky sexual behaviours might be incapable of making an informed decision in *another area of life,* which could exacerbate their addiction. For instance, they might be vulnerable, like Mary, to exploitation from persons who provide the attention that they seek and enjoy.

The ethical principle of beneficence in trust entails that health professionals should take the time to discern the broader picture behind refusals to consent in people with intellectual disabilities and to discuss concerns with them. In some cases, they may need support, in particular from family members and others whom the patient trusts, to realize that a refusal is incompatible with their own deeply held values and cherished commitments. In talking things over, a creative solution to overcoming the impasse that is acceptable to the person can sometimes be found. In other cases, a pervasive incapacity to understand or judge the significance of overall or long-term benefit of interventions could be grounds for involving a substitute decision maker. This is ethically different from the situation in which the person has such a capacity but the healthcare professional or carer disagrees with the person's decision. In this situation, the person's decision should be respected.

Summary

- Both clinical and ethical guidelines for illness prevention and health promotion are important.
- Ethical care entails promoting health in the relationships of people with intellectual disabilities as much as possible.
- The relationship between the healthcare professional and the person with intellectual disabilities should be based on the principle of beneficence in trust – this entails that the healthcare professional should get to know the person well.
- Respecting the dignity of people with intellectual disabilities entails minimizing the burdens and distresses arising from tests, monitoring, and other preventive and health-promoting measures.
- Justice entails not only providing equal access to generic illness prevention and health promotion programmes and services, but also ensuring that they are adapted specifically for people with intellectual disabilities.
- Respect for autonomy entails a case-by-case assessment of the various capacities involved in decision making in people with intellectual disabilities as well as their specific vulnerabilities. In some cases, support from carers whom these persons trust can help them make decisions that are based on their values and commitments.

Web resources

- Developmental Disabilities Primary Care Initiative: http://www.surreyplace.on.ca/Primary-Care/Pages/Home.aspx
- Understanding intellectual disability and health: http://www.intellectualdisability.info/

References

Dinerstein, R.D., Herr, S.S. and O'Sullivan, J.L. (1999) *A Guide to Consent*. Washington, DC: American Association on Mental Retardation.

Goldsmith, L., Skirton, H. and Webb, C. (2008) Informed consent to healthcare interventions in people with learning disabilities: an integrative review. *Journal of Advanced Nursing*, 64(6): 549–63.

Gunn, M.J., Wong, J.G., Clare, I.C. and Holland, A.J. (2000) Medical research and incompetent adults. *Journal of Mental Health Law*, 2: 60–72.

Haverman, M.J., Heller, T., Lee, L.A., Maaskant, M.A., Shoostari, S. and Stydom, A. (2009) *Report of the State of Science on Health Risks and Ageing in People with Intellectual Disabilities*. Dortmund, Germany: IASSID Special Interest Research Group on Ageing and Intellectual Disabilities.

Heng, J. and Sullivan, W.F. (2007) Ethics of consent in people with intellectual and developmental disabilities, in I. Brown and M. Percy (eds.) *A Comprehensive Guide to Intellectual and Developmental Disabilities*. Boston, MA: Paul H. Brookes.

Holland, A.J. (2000) Ageing and learning disability. *British Journal of Psychiatry*, 176(1): 26–31.

Krahn, G.L., Hammond, L. and Turner, A. (2006) A cascade of disparities: health and health care access for people with intellectual disabilities. *Mental Retardation and Developmental Disabilities Research Review*, 12(1): 70–82.

Lennox, N. and Diggens, J. (eds.) (1999) *Management Guidelines: People with Developmental and Intellectual Disabilities*. Melbourne, VIC: Therapeutic Guidelines Ltd.

Lennox, N., Bain, C., Rey-Conde, T., Purdie, D., Bush, R. and Pandeya N. (2007) Effects of a comprehensive health assessment programme for Australian adults with intellectual disability: a cluster randomized trial. *International Journal of Epidemiology*, 36(1): 139–46.

Marks, B.A. and Heller, T. (2003) Bridging the equity gap: health promotion for adults with intellectual and developmental disabilities. *Nursing Clinics of North America*, 38(2): 205–28.

Ouellette-Kuntz, H., Garcin, N., Lewis, M.E., Minnes, P., Martin, C. and Holden, J.J. (2005) Addressing health disparities through promoting equity for individuals with intellectual disability. *Canadian Journal of Public Health*, 96(suppl. 2): 8–22.

Pellegrino, E.D. and Thomasma, D.C. (1988) *For the Patient's Good: The Restoration of Beneficence in Health Care*. Oxford: Oxford University Press.

Sullivan, W.F., Heng, J., Cameron, D., Lunsky, Y., Cheetham, T. and Hennen, B. (2006) Consensus Guidelines for Primary Health Care of Adults with Developmental Disabilities. *Canadian Family Physician*, 52(11): 1410–18.

Sullivan, W.F., Berg, J.M., Bradley, E., Cheetham, T. and Denton, R. (2011a) Primary care of adults with developmental disabilities: Canadian consensus guidelines. *Canadian Family Physician*, 57(5): 541–53.

Sullivan, W.F., Berg, J.M., Bradley, E., Cheetham, T. and Foster-Gibson C. (2011b) *Tools for the Primary Care of People with Developmental Disabilities*. Toronto: MUMS Guideline Clearinghouse.

Sulmasy, D.P. (2002) A bio-psycho-social-spiritual model for the care of patients at the end of life. *Gerontologist*, 42(spec no. 3): 24–33.

United Nations (1948) *The Universal Declaration on Human Rights*. Available from: http://www.un.org/en/documents/udhr/index.shtml [accessed 23 June 2013].

United Nations (1966) *The Covenant on Economic, Social, and Cultural Rights* (ICESCR). Available from: http://www.ohchr.org/EN/ProfessionalInterest/Pages/CESCR.asp [accessed 23 June 2013].

United Nations (2006) *The Convention on the Rights of Persons with Disabilities*. Available from: http://www.un.org/esa/socdev/enable/rights/convtexte.htm [accessed 23 June 2013].

World Health Organization (WHO) (1986) *The Ottawa Charter of Health Promotion*. Available from: http://www.who.int/healthpromotion/conferences/previous/ottawa/en/ [accessed 23 June 2013].

World Health Organization (WHO) (2005) *The Bangkok Charter of Health Promotion in a Globalized World*. Available from: http://www.who.int/healthpromotion/conferences/6gchp/bangkok_charter/en/ [accessed 23 June 2013].

20

Evaluating health promotion programmes

Paul Fleming and Wendy Cousins

Introduction

Health promotion has developed significantly since its inception with the Lalonde Report (Lalonde 1974) and its formal promulgation by the WHO through the Ottawa Charter in 1986 (WHO 1986). However, there is often a gap between policy intention and its implementation: 'Governments mediate, through their architecture of machinery and policy, access to rights and, by extension, to services' (Lawson et al. 2008: 3). There is a need for people with intellectual disabilities and their carers to break through this architecture to obtain the services they require. One possible bridging mechanism is the evidence and insights provided by programme evaluation. Elsewhere in this book, health promotion strategies for key health topic areas have been explored and ethical issues considered. It should be noted, however, that no matter how well developed the theoretical and practice-based elements of health promotion programmes are, we inevitably come to the key question: 'How do we know that health promotion interventions improve the health status of people with intellectual disabilities at all levels from individual to population?'

This chapter seeks to define the concept of evaluation and identify its integral role within health promotion practice. It explores the key elements of evaluation planning and implementation in health promotion programmes, particularly as they affect people with intellectual disabilities. We also recognize that the engagement with health promotion by people with intellectual disabilities and their caregivers will have collateral effects on their significant others, those who commission and deliver health promotion programmes, and the wider community. Those who advocate for the rights of people with intellectual disabilities, as they monitor the effects of health promotion interventions on this population, will also have an interest in the nature and outcomes of evaluation (Brolan et al. 2012; Feldman et al. 2012).

Good practice: know why you are evaluating

In developing good practice in health promotion programme planning, it is essential that we not only deliver well-planned interventions, but that we also build in the means to assure ourselves that the interventions have been efficacious for the target group/population and, for this purpose, evaluation strategies are employed. By doing this we hold ourselves accountable and seek to improve programme design and delivery (Wright 1999). Evaluation, however, is a term that is widely used but not always fully understood. Many of us will be familiar with the 'evaluation form' at the end of a training course or conference. These forms, sometimes dubbed 'happy sheets', tend to canvass a subjective opinion related to perceived performance of facilitators, perceived learning and opinions on the organizational aspects of the event. There is usually no indication as to how learning has been measured or how it is to be carried back to the 'real world'. These forms are used as a measure of customer satisfaction and a proxy for success or failure. Another approach often taken, particularly in the realm of health promotion interventions, is to belatedly think of undertaking some form of evaluation close to the end of the implementation phase of an intervention. At this late stage, the programme providers will begin to seek out some way of ascertaining whether or not the intervention has 'worked' in terms of both its process and the expected outcomes. Often this approach has been seen in the context of either using surplus funds in a project or as a way of using unexpended funds in a budget before the end of a financial year. It is worthy of note that this type of practice is common when programmes are commissioned, planned, and delivered by those with little formal education in health promotion. In both of these examples, the links with properly planned and implemented evaluation strategies is, to say the least, tenuous. Nevertheless, it should be remembered that programme evaluation, which moves beyond the merely superficial, is a cornerstone of evidence-based practice.

Defining evaluation

It is therefore vital that we move beyond these somewhat superficial approaches to evaluation. An obvious starting point when asking 'why evaluate?' is to explore a range of definitions; a large number of definitions of evaluation have been generated over time, particularly since the 1990s. In its Glossary of Health Promotion (WHO 1998a: 12), WHO defines health promotion evaluation as simply 'an assessment of the extent to which health promotion actions achieve a "valued" outcome'. This mirrors Tones' definition, which states that 'evaluation is essentially about determining the extent to which certain valued goals have been achieved' (Tones 1998: 52). This, of course, leads to the questions of how value is defined, agreed, and measured. It could lead to the situation where, for example, the health promotion practitioner may wish to facilitate the reduction of obesity in an intellectually disabled client group through healthy-eating strategies as a valued goal. The client group themselves, however, may place less value on this goal than on the empowerment derived from getting together with friends to eat and to make eating choices that are not necessarily dictated by health considerations, thus receiving both individual and collective gratification from the experience. In this scenario there is, or may possibly be, disagreement as to the value of the outcome, which can only be resolved by a participatory, negotiated agreement on what is actually valued.

Interestingly, in the same year in which WHO defined health promotion evaluation, in its now widely accepted document *Health Promotion Evaluation: Recommendations to Policy Makers* (WHO 1998b), evaluation was defined as 'the systematic examination and assessment of the features of an initiative and its effects, in order to produce information that can be used by those who have an interest in its improvement or effectiveness' (p. 12). This definition emphasizes that evaluation is a deliberate endeavour, which, therefore, must be approached systematically through coherent planning. It is also reckoned to be comprehensive in nature in that it focuses on both 'features' – principles, characteristics, and processes – and also outcomes (effects). The final element worthy of note is that the overall purpose of evaluation is to improve effectiveness. This is also a key emphasis in Springett's definition when she states that 'the aim of evaluation is to contribute towards solving practical problems, in terms of what works and why. It is about collecting information to inform action. Most of all, it is about learning from experience' (Springett 2001: 144). This definition focuses more on the use to which evaluation is put – to the solving of real-life problems through assessment of acceptability, effectiveness, and efficiency – and to the fact that learning from experience is an important element in driving the evaluation agenda in order to improve our practice and thus improve health promotion processes and health outcomes for the client group (Springett 1998).

However, this is not always quite as simple as it appears. Other underlying questions may have an influence on the nature and outcomes of evaluation. The first of these is 'for whom is the evaluation being undertaken?' This somewhat innocuous question may actually have ethical implications for what can be evaluated and how the findings of an evaluation can be used and disseminated. At its root is the issue of whether the evaluation could be open to inappropriate influence from any of the key players. Given that evaluation is in itself a form of research, it is useful to take on board Whitehead's (1993) indication that there are issues relating to ownership and dissemination rights between funders, practitioners (researchers), the community, and the wider public. Ownership can determine those elements of an evaluation that will/will not be disseminated to key interests and/or placed in the public domain. Beyond ownership, however, there may also be pressures from funders and commissioners to demonstrate that their funding is being appropriately targeted and successfully used. Health promotion practitioners may, in some cases, come under pressure to present evaluation results that demonstrate this in spite of the evidence. There may also be pressure from client groups to show success for a strategic direction for which they have strongly advocated even when the available evidence for its efficacy is weak.

In both of these examples, there is pressure for the evaluation to support the agenda of an entity with vested interests as opposed to making unbiased observations of the programme process and outcomes. Such pressure must be resisted if an ethical approach to evaluation is to be maintained, as pressure for evaluation to demonstrate success often does not take into account the multi-factorial nature of health promotion. The effects of factors such as inappropriate/inadequate funding levels for programmes, unrealistic methodological expectations, and/or the use of inappropriately qualified staff can lead to unrealistic expectations of the programme provider. This desire for a 'good news story' may also see pressure brought to bear on the practitioners to ensure that positive outcomes can be demonstrated and negative outcomes downplayed or suppressed. It is therefore imperative that any evaluation is underpinned by a sound ethical framework such as that suggested by the United Nations Evaluation Group (UNEG) in their Ethical Guidelines for Evaluation (UNEG 2012), which encourage responsible use of power, ensuring credibility and the responsible use of resources.

These principles are demonstrated in the UN's approach to evaluation of human rights and gender equity (UNEG 2011). So in basing evaluation on a sound ethical footing, it must always be uppermost in the health promotion practitioner's mind that improvement of programme delivery is paramount. The pressures to use evaluation to serve other agendas of key players such as policy makers, funders, and various pressure groups must be resisted. A further perspective drawing on a number of themes in these definitions is given by Øvretveit (1998: 9) when he indicates that, in the wider context of health interventions, evaluation is 'attributing value to an intervention by gathering reliable and valid information about it in a systematic way, and by making comparisons, for the purposes of making more informed decisions or understanding casual mechanisms or general principles'. Here Øvretveit seeks to place value on an intervention by comparing it with other programmes or initiatives that seek the same outcome or choose to use the same strategies. Evidence for comparison from other programmes can be obtained from systematic reviews (Sweet and Moynihan 2007) where large numbers of studies are examined under strict criteria to ascertain if they meet specific research standards and thus make effective contributions to the body of knowledge; meta-analyses take systematic reviews further and combine the data statistically (Lyman and Kuderer 2005). Øvretveit also makes clear that the veracity of the information on which such comparisons are made is of importance in enabling a sound judgement to be made of the components that are used to construct an effective, efficient, and acceptable intervention.

In considering these definitions of evaluation, however, it should also be noted that several major initiatives over the last 20 years have attempted to bring insight, coherence, and agreement to the wider topic of evaluation in health promotion. A seminal initiative in 2001 was undertaken for WHO Europe by a Working Group that was a collaboration between WHO Europe, Health Canada, the Centers for Disease Control (CDC) in the United States, and the then Health Development Authority in England (Rootman et al. 2001). This work, interestingly, concluded that evaluation in health promotion was 'the systematic examination and assessment of features of a programme or other intervention in order to produce knowledge that different stakeholders can use for a variety of purposes' (Rootman et al. 2001: 26). They also indicated that the scope of health promotion interventions should be empowering, participatory, holistic, intersectoral, equitable, sustainable, and multi-agency.

To ensure that clients in the field of intellectual disabilities are equitably encouraged to develop control over their own health by actively encouraging their participation in a sustainable, multi-agency evaluation strategy can be a particular challenge, especially where issues such as low health literacy affect the target population (Parker 2000). This WHO document remains, however, one of the most comprehensive and thought-provoking contributions to the field of evaluation in health promotion and in particular makes a strong contribution to the development of large programmes which source major funding and are aimed at larger populations. It should be noted, however, that its use for small, local programmes may be more limited. For instance, its generic logic model for planning and evaluating health promotion contains a level of detail and complexity that make it less accessible to practitioners seeking to implement evaluation on smaller scale programmes that are common in the field of intellectual disability. These programmes might be better served by a logic model such as Ewles and Simnett's Health Promotion Planning Model (Scriven 2010).

A slightly earlier, but equally important initiative that is still ongoing, is the Global Programme on Health Promotion Effectiveness (GPHPE). This is a multi-partner collaboration between the WHO and the International Union for Health Promotion and Education (IUHPE), which originated from action sparked by a publication by the IUPHE: *The Evidence of Health Promotion Effectiveness: Shaping Public Health in a New Europe* (IUHPE/EC 1997). The aim of the GPHPE has been to review and build evidence in health promotion, debating what counts as evidence of effectiveness, reviewing such evidence, and then translating evidence to users such as policy makers, health promotion practitioners, and researchers (WHO 2012). In a significant monograph published in 2007, GPHPE established a global context for the evaluation of effectiveness in health promotion (IUHPE 2007). This document went far beyond the traditional evaluation targets of increases in knowledge on a limited agenda of health topics and individual lifestyle behaviour and sought to examine evidence of effectiveness through such lenses as globalization, urbanization, governance, and conceptual frameworks such as the social determinants of health (Marmot and Wilkinson 2006).

When considering such a multi-faceted approach to evaluation, it should be noted that when evaluating real-life health promotion programmes with real people who have intellectual disabilities, the principles of evaluation are essentially no different to those of any other client group. It is, however, important to keep in mind that, when working with people with intellectual disabilities, empowerment of this vulnerable group needs careful planning and facilitation. Creative strategies may need to be adopted. For example, it has been demonstrated that young people with intellectual disabilities and communication impairments can express their ideas and feelings with the aid of non-verbal communication techniques such as Talking Mats™ (Mitchell 2010). This concept of empowerment sits at the very centre of the health promotion paradigm as a core issue in enabling all individuals to optimize their autonomy in health and other choices (WHO 2010).

The Ottawa Charter stated that the aim of health promotion is to enable all people and communities to 'increase control over, and improve their health' (WHO 1986). Empowerment is the primary benchmark against which interventions have been measured ever since Ottawa to validate their veracity as health promotion interventions. In the context of intellectual disability, we do need to keep in mind when undertaking evaluation the fact that there is wide variation in the characteristics of people in the intellectually disabled population. Intellectually disabled people occupy a spectrum from those who live independent lives to living in residential care; those who engage in significant employment and generally order their own lives with minimal input from others, to those who are unable to make any independent decisions. The issue of co-morbidities and/or multiple disabilities is also a factor in creating independence or minimizing the assistance and support required from others. In addition to acknowledging diversity of need, it should also be recognized that ethnicity, culture, and life-stage are also factors for consideration. It is therefore vital that at the service delivery and monitoring levels of evaluation, the principles and delivery elements of any health promotion intervention are viewed in the context of their contribution to the autonomy of the target audience.

Good practice: know what you are evaluating and how

In evaluating any health promotion intervention, Green and Kreuter's PRECEDE–PROCEED model of health promotion programme planning and evaluation indicates a sequence of evaluation that begins with process evaluation and then moves through impact evaluation to outcome evaluation (Green and Kreuter 2005). This approach immediately generates two key questions:

- Can we learn anything about *process*: the manner in which we planned and delivered the programme and the effects that were experienced by any or all of the key players involved?
- Did we achieve the *outcomes* that were planned for the health promotion programme?

These two questions immediately highlight the fact that there are two key areas of focus for evaluation: process and outcome (in which we will include impact).

Process evaluation

The first of these questions focuses, essentially, on the issue of the actions that were involved in planning and delivering a health promotion intervention. Process may be viewed from a number of perspectives, but it has been helpfully identified by Nutbeam (1998: 39-40) as addressing three key aspects of health promotion:

- Programme reach – did the programme reach all of the target population?
- Programme acceptability – was the programme acceptable to the target population?
- Programme integrity – is the programme implemented as planned?

It should be noted that each of these elements of process evaluation can make use of formative evaluation techniques that are descriptive in character (Green and South 2006). Here, information is gathered throughout the implementation of the programme and is used contemporaneously to make changes that will facilitate achievement of optimal outcomes (Tones and Green 2004).

Each of these elements has, as Nutbeam notes, specific challenges. In terms of *programme reach,* the smaller the population, the easier it is to monitor the coverage of the target population by the intervention. In the case of people with intellectual disabilities, client groups in education, care, residential or social settings can be relatively easily monitored. Sources of evidence can be simple observation noted appropriately in a written record (e.g. weight loss/gain, food diaries, exercise engaged in). When it comes to larger target populations such as the intellectually disabled population at municipal, regional or national level, gathering appropriate evidence is a much more difficult proposition. Variability in service delivery across different localities may mean evaluation is difficult (Slevin et al. 2011), and there is always the danger that those who have less access through geographical isolation, lack of strong advocates or limited financial resources may not be reached by a health promotion intervention. Monitoring for larger populations may require a more sophisticated approach involving population sampling or surveillance to detect involvement with a programme or to use proxies such as reporting from, for example, selected schools, day centres, and residential facilities to ascertain coverage.

Programme acceptability is the second element of process evaluation and focuses primarily on the responses of the target group to the intervention. Hearing the voices of people with intellectual disabilities is crucial.

It is now widely recognized that people with disabilities want to have a say about what happens in the services they attend, to help shape policy and influence how services are run (Health Service Executive 2012). Evaluation processes can also be targeted at their circle of significant others and day-to-day service providers, and also those involved in commissioning and delivering the intervention. Here we need to ascertain how the target group has responded to their experience during the health promotion process. Again, a range of methods of soliciting responses will be required. It is desirable, where possible, to ascertain clients' subjective views on issues such as appropriateness of aims and objectives in the context of their opinions/reactions; perceptions of appropriate participation in planning the intervention; the extent to which clients felt that they remained in control during the intervention; comfort with key actions in the intervention including perceptions of issues such as embarrassment, inconvenience or even pain. In other words, was the intervention enjoyed or endured? Sources of evidence here would include surveys based on semi-structured interview schedules delivered through individual interviews (Barriball and While 1994) or focus groups (Lane et al. 2001), or the use of rapid appraisal methods (Harvey et al. 2001), all of which are possible and appropriate for intellectually disabled populations with, where necessary, appropriate support.

Box 20.1 An educational support project in which people with intellectual disabilities, their families, and care staff were taught how to collaborate in the improvement of services

In 2010, the School of Nursing and Human Sciences at Dublin City University, Ireland created an education module, developed in partnership with local service providers to train teams of people with intellectual disabilities, their family members, and staff in ways to improve services. Called Improving Service with Co-operative Learning, the module is intended to create a 'legacy effect' for both students and services and to promote the ideal of inclusive, tertiary-level education and lifelong learning for people with intellectual disabilities. Early indications suggest that this form of educational support has the potential to assist with the translation of policies on service-user involvement into practice and empower participants.

(Corby et al. 2013)

The third element of process evaluation focuses on programme integrity, which seeks to ascertain whether or not the planned elements of a programme were delivered as envisaged and, if not, what were the factors that either detracted or enhanced the delivery. Programme integrity therefore describes whether or not each objective of the programme was successfully implemented and, if not, why not. Did specific methods of engagement with the client group work as envisaged? Was the way in which the programme was implemented seen to be professional and skilled, and if not, why not? This element requires honest and acute observation by either the health promotion practitioner or an independent observer/evaluator to detail the factors that would have contributed to the success or failure of the various facets of the programme. Honest answers to these and other evaluation questions can provide a rich learning experience from which health promotion practitioners can both learn from their mistakes and also identify what works well.

Impact and outcome evaluation

The second question posed above relates to the issue of *outcome*, which, in its widest sense, refers to the range of consequences from the implementation of a health promotion programme. When considering this aspect of evaluation, the terms 'result', 'impact', and 'outcome' are used extensively in the health promotion evaluation literature with some breadth of interpretation over their exact meanings (Green and South 2006). Indeed, to bring clarity to the use of the terms 'impact' and 'outcome', Green and South have suggested that it is helpful to simply use the term 'outcome' and 'to distinguish between immediate-, short- and longer-term outcomes'. In general, their view reflects the widely held view that, while it is not possible to make absolute distinctions between these terms, the key difference lies in the time period over which they are measured. 'Impact' is defined as 'the immediate effect that health promotion programmes have on people, stakeholders and settings to influence the determinants of health, i.e. the outcomes of individual objectives within a health promotion intervention.

Health promotion programmes may have a range of immediate effects on individuals and on social and physical settings' (Department of Human Services, Victoria, Australia 2008). Tones and Tilford (2001) advocate in this context the use of 'intermediate indicators' to measure the outcomes of individual health promotion interventions that will contribute to the ultimate health improvement outcomes. The key area of enquiry here is to ascertain if the programme has made a difference for the client group. Exemplars of impact evaluation could be drawn from many areas of work in intellectual disability such as obesity (Slevin et al. 2010) and sexual health (Cambridge 1998). In the case of a long-term health promotion programme that seeks to achieve a high rate of adoption of safer sexual practice in those who are sexually active with two or more partners, a range of intermediate indicators will relate to immediate and short-term *impact*. This would include changes in belief relating to condom use (cost, ease of use) and changes in self-efficacy (ability to use condoms, ability to negotiate use of condoms with partners). Each of these measurable effects of a health promotion programmes is, in itself, an outcome but each is only a 'staging post' on the road to the ultimate outcome of consistent, optimal sexual health, which is consonant with safer sexual practice. They are therefore recognized for their *impact* on the behaviour of the client group and can be measured through research designs such as pre-test/post-test, which can compare the object of intervention before and after delivery of the programme (Cohen et al. 2011).

In contrast, the use of the term 'outcome' is usually seen as a longer-term achievement that is described as summative in nature and can be used to evaluate ultimate goals of a health promotion intervention and/or undertake cost–benefit and cost-effectiveness analyses of specific interventions (Tones and Tilford 2001). Outcome evaluation has been described as 'more likely to be the product of the synergistic effect of many projects' (Springett 1998: 14), which suggests that it is difficult in many cases to attribute an outcome to a single intervention. It is therefore important that when we attempt to evaluate the overall outcome of a programme, we acknowledge that other factors or programmes may also have contributed to the observed change in the clients and/or their environment (Pawson and Tilley 1997). The problem in solving real-life problems in health promotion is that most health promotion interventions are set in highly complex, multi-factorial settings where the ability to attribute change to a simple intervention is complicated by the large number of variables. Thus in the example of the sexual health programme mentioned above, a longer-term outcome would be higher rates of safer sexual practice with concomitant lowered rates of pregnancy and sexually transmitted infections. The difficulty would be in being able to state categorically that this outcome was solely due to the effects of a single health promotion intervention.

Overall, when engaging in evaluation, the decision as to which elements of a programme to evaluate will be crystallized through the formulation of evaluation questions. While the effects on the target group/population will be of primary concern, it is also important to consider studying the effects of both the process and outcomes on other interests. These could include those who commission/fund health promotion initiatives. Commissioners also need to be considered in that they may need to be assured that the methods used are ethically and practically justified, that they are an effective and efficient use of financial and human resource, and that they do not put at risk the client group. In addition, they also need to be supported in managing issues of reputational risk from the implementation of the programme. The wider community within which the initiative is delivered might also be taken into consideration for its facilitating and deleterious effects on the programme. Often issues relating to intellectual disability can cause problems if there is insufficient understanding of this client group and the way in which they will interact with sections of the wider community. Evaluation can have both wide-ranging implications for a range of interests but ultimately it is vital that people with intellectual disabilities are increasingly well served in the health promotion programmes that are designed to enhance their health status.

Summary

- Evaluation is an integral and indispensible element of health promotion programme planning and should be accommodated within the planning process from its beginning.
- Not every element of a health promotion programme can be evaluated and therefore those elements that will yield the greatest learning for key players should be identified and operationalized.
- In the context of intellectual disability, the views of people with such disabilities and their immediate carers should, as far as is possible, always be at the centre of the planning process, which should be participatory, transparent, and open to discussion by all the participants.
- It should be remembered that while short-term outcomes from key objectives can be measured, their contribution to a wider health promotion aim may be difficult to assess, as the lives of any group of clients contain so many variables over which the health promotion practitioner has little to no control.
- Where necessary, those who are inexperienced in planning evaluation strategies should seek assistance from those with well-developed expertise in evaluation.

Web resources

- University of Illinois at Chicago Centre for Health Promotion Research for Persons with Disabilities: http://uic-chp.org/

- Public Health Ontario, Evaluation of Health Promotion Programmes: http://www.thcu.ca/resource_db/pubs/107465116.pdf

- The Development and Evaluation of a Health Promotion Programme for People with Intellectual Disabilities: http://www.specialolympics.ie/Portals/0/public_documents/Health/Health_Promo_Web.pdf

References

Barriball, K.L. and While, A. (1994) Collecting data using a semi-structured interview: a discussion paper. *Journal of Advanced Nursing*, 19: 328–35.

Brolan, C.E., Boyle, F.M., Dean, J.H., Gomez, M., Ware, R.S. and Lennox, N.G. (2012) Health advocacy: a vital step in attaining human rights for adults with intellectual disability. *Journal of Intellectual Disability Research*, 56(11): 1087–97.

Cambridge, P. (1998) Challenges for safer sex education and HIV prevention in services for people with intellectual disabilities in Britain. *Health Promotion International*, 13(1): 67–74.

Cohen, L., Manion, L. and Morrison, K. (2011) *Research Methods in Education*. London: Routledge.

Corby, D., Slevin, E. and Cousins, W. (2013) Improving services through co-operative learning. *Learning Disability Practice*, 16(2): 20–2.

Department of Human Services, Victoria, Australia (2008) *Measuring Health Promotion Impacts: A Guide to Impact Evaluation in Integrated Health Promotion*. Melbourne, VIC: Government of Victoria, Department of Human Services.

Feldman, M.A., Owen, F., Andrews, A., Hamelin, J., Barber, R. and Griffiths, J. (2012) Health self-advocacy training for persons with intellectual disabilities. *Journal of Intellectual Disability Research*, 56(11): 1110–21.

Green, J. and South, J. (2006) *Evaluation*. Maidenhead: Open University Press.

Green, L.W. and Kreuter, M.W (2005) *Health Promotion Program Planning: An Educational and Ecological Approach*, 4th edn. New York: McGraw-Hill.

Harvey, H.D., Fleming, P. and Patterson, M. (2001) A rapid appraisal method for reviewing the effectiveness of workplace smoking policies in large and medium sized organisations. *Journal of the Royal Society of Health*, 121(1): 50–5.

Health Service Executive (HSE) (2012) *New Directions: Personal Support Services for Adults with Disabilities. Review of HSE Day Services and Implementation Plan: 2012–2016*. Monaghan: HSE.

IUHPE (2007) *Global Perspectives on Health Promotion Effectiveness*. Paris: IUPHE.

IUHPE/EC (1997) *The Evidence of Health Promotion Effectiveness – Shaping Public Health in a New Europe*. Brussels-Luxembourg: IUHPE/EC.

Lalonde, M. (1974) *The Health of Canadians*. Ottawa: Ministry of Supply and Services, Government of Canada.

Lane, P., McKenna, H., Ryan, A. and Fleming, P. (2001) Focus group methodology. *Nurse Researcher*, 8(3): 45–59.

Lawson, L., Francis, R., Russell, P. and Veitch, J. (2008) Equality and access to human rights for people with both learning disability and mental illness needs. *Advances in Mental Health and Learning Disabilities*, 2(2): 3–7.

Lyman, G.H. and Kuderer, N.M. (2005) The strengths and limitations of meta-analysis based on aggregate data. *BMC Medical Research Methodology*, 5: 14.

Marmot, M. and Wilkinson, R.G. (eds.) (2006) *Social Determinants of Health*. Oxford: Oxford University Press.

Mitchell, W. (2010) 'I know how I feel': listening to young people with life-limiting conditions who have learning and communication impairments. *Qualitative Social Work*, 9(2): 185–203.

Nutbeam, D. (1998) Evaluating health promotion – progress, problems and solutions. *Health Promotion International*, 13(1): 27–44.

Øvretveit, J. (1998) *Evaluating Health Interventions*. Buckingham: Open University Press.

Parker, R. (2000) Health literacy: a challenge for American patients and their health care providers. *Health Promotion International*, 15(4): 277–83.

Pawson, R. and Tilley, N. (1997) *Realistic Evaluation*. London: Sage.

Rootman, I., Goodstadt, M.S., Hyndman, B., McQueen, D.V., Potvin, L., Springett, J. et al. (eds.) (2001) *Evaluation in Health Promotion: Principles and Perspectives*. Copenhagen: WHO.

Scriven, A. (2010) *Promoting Health: A Practical Guide*, 6th edn. London: Baillière Tindall.

Slevin, E., McConkey, R., Truesdale-Kennedy, M., Laverty, A., Fleming, P. and Livingstone, B. (2010) A health promotion intervention: countering overweight in school children with intellectual disability. *Journal of Applied Research in Intellectual Disabilities*, 23(5): 468.

Slevin, E., Taggart, L., McConkey, R., Cousins, W., Truesdale-Kennedy, M. and Dowling, L. (2011) *A Rapid Review of Literature Relating to Support for People with Intellectual Disabilities and their Family Carers when the Person has Behaviours that Challenge and/or Mental Health Problems; or they are Advancing in Age*. Belfast: University of Ulster.

Springett, J. (1998) *Practical Guidance on Evaluating Health Promotion*. Copenhagen: WHO Europe.

Springett, J. (2001) Appropriate approaches to the evaluation of health promotion. *Critical Public Health*, 11(2): 139–51.

Sweet, M. and Moynihan, R. (2007) *Improving Population Health: The Use of Systematic Reviews*. New York: Millbank Memorial Fund.

Tones, K. (1998) Effectiveness in health promotion: indicators and evidence of success, in D. Scott and R. Weston (eds.) *Evaluating Health Promotion*. Cheltenham: Stanley Thornes.

Tones, K. and Green, J. (2004) *Health Promotion: Planning and Strategies*. London: Sage.

Tones, K. and Tilford, S. (2001) *Health Promotion: Effectiveness, Efficiency and Equity*, 3rd edn. Cheltenham: Stanley Thornes.

United Nations Evaluation Group (UNEG) (2011) *Integrating Human Rights and Gender Equality in Evaluation – Towards UNEG Guidelines*. New York: United Nations

United Nations Evaluation Group (UNEG) (2012) *Ethical Guidelines*. New York: United Nations. Available at: http://www.uneval.org/papersandpubs/documentdetail.jsp?doc_id=102 [accessed 9 July 2012].

Whitehead, M. (1993) The ownership of research, in J. Davies and M. Kelly (eds.) *Healthy Cities: Research and Practice*. London: Routledge.

World Health Organization (WHO) (1986) *Ottawa Charter for Health Promotion*. Geneva: WHO.

World Health Organisation (WHO) (1998a) *Health Promotion Glossary*. Geneva: WHO.

World Health Organisation (WHO) (1998b) *Health Promotion Evaluation: Recommendations to Policy Makers*. Copenhagen: WHO.

World Health Organisation (WHO) (2010) *Better Health, Better Lives: Children and Young People with Intellectual Disabilities and their Families – Empower Children and Young People with Intellectual Disabilities*. Copenhagen: WHO.

World Health Organisation (WHO) (2012) *Global Programme on Health Promotion Effectiveness* (GPHPE). Available at: http://www.who.int/healthpromotion/areas/gphpe/en/index.html

Wright, L. (1999) Evaluation in health promotion: the proof of the pudding?, in E. Perkins, I. Simnett and L. Wright (eds.) *Evidence Based Health Promotion*. Chichester: Wiley.

Index

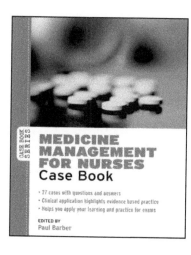

MEDICINE MANAGEMENT FOR NURSES
Case Book

Paul Barber (Ed)

9780335245758 (Paperback)
August 2013

eBook also available

This case book covers the principles and skills involved in a range of medicine management scenarios and will help nursing students integrate their knowledge of physiology, pathophysiology, pharmacology and nursing care. Including 21 case studies, each case gives readers the opportunity to learn about effective medicine management while testing their knowledge and understanding of essential drug groups.

Key features:

- The cases cover a variety of conditions helping students to learn what to do in many types of scenarios
- Includes questions, answers and other self-test features
- Aimed at nurses studying pharmacology/medicine management

www.**openup**.co.uk

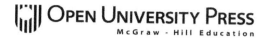

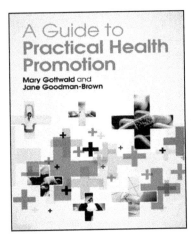

A GUIDE TO PRACTICAL HEALTH PROMOTION

Mary Gottwald and Jane Goodman-Brown

9780335244591 (Paperback)
August 2012

eBook also available

Do you have difficulties deciding which health promotion activities facilitate behavioural change?

This accessible book focuses on the practical activity of health promotion and shows students and practitioners how to actually apply health promotion in practice. The book uses case scenarios to explore how health promotion activities can empower individuals to make decisions that change their health related behaviour

Key features:

- Each chapter uses classic case studies in health promotion
- Includes lists, key points and other succinct tools to give the reader guidance
- Contains activities and specific tasks that can be used in practice

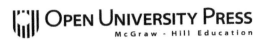

OPEN UNIVERSITY PRESS
McGraw - Hill Education

www.openup.co.uk

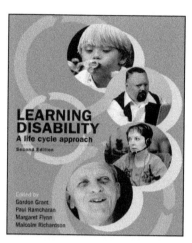

LEARNING DISABILITY

Second Edition

Gordon Grant, Paul Ramcharan, Margaret Flynn and Malcolm Richardson (Eds)

9780335238439 (Paperback)
2010

eBook also available

"It is written with a clearly conveyed in-depth knowledge and in a way that has professional lived experience within the context of the work. The authors have taken into account the emotional, client-centred approach to the modern practitioner's practice ... The book gives a true wealth of good practice scenarios that can only help practitioners be good at what they do and aspire to be."
Lee Marshall, Student Nurse, Sheffield Hallam University, UK

With its spread of chapters covering key issues across the life cycle this text has established itself as the foundational primer for those studying the lived experiences of people with learning disabilities and their families, and outcomes achieved through services and support systems.

Key features:

- Aetiology
- Breaking news (about disability) and early intervention
- Transition to adulthood

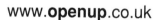
www.**openup**.co.uk

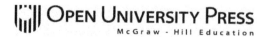
OPEN UNIVERSITY PRESS
McGraw - Hill Education

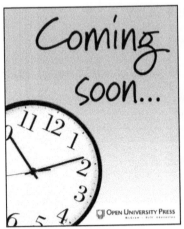

LEARNING DISABILITIES IN HEALTH CARE SETTINGS CASE BOOK

Bob Hallawell

9780335243075 (Paperback)
October 2012

eBook also available

This case book will guide you through the complex and varied ways in which people with Learning Disabilities experience the worlds of health and social care. The practical cases will focus on individuals across the lifespan from children and young people through to older adults to explore shared dimensions of health and social care and support as well as practice specific to each of these arenas.

Key features:

- Links theory to practice
- Each case features questions and guided answers
- Opportunities to assess learning as you go

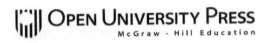

www.**openup**.co.uk

OPEN UNIVERSITY PRESS
McGraw - Hill Education